INTRODUCTORY
NEUROLOGY

INTRODUCTORY NEUROLOGY

James G. McLeod
AO, MB BS, BSc(Med), DPhil(Oxon), FRCP, FRACP, FAA, FTS
*Bushell Professor of Neurology and Bosch Professor of
Medicine, Department of Neurology,
Institute of Clinical Neurosciences, Royal Prince
Alfred Hospital, University of Sydney, Sydney*

James W. Lance
AO, CBE, MD, FRCP, FRACP, FAA
*Professor Emeritus, University of New South Wales;
Consultant Neurologist, Prince of Wales Hospital, Sydney*

Llewelyn Davies
MD, BS, FRACP
*Staff Neurologist and Clinical Senior Lecturer in Neurology,
Institute of Clinical Neurosciences, Royal Prince
Alfred Hospital, University of Sydney, Sydney*

THIRD EDITION

Blackwell
Science

© 1983, 1989, 1995 by
Blackwell Science Pty Ltd
Editorial Offices:
54 University Street, Carlton
  Victoria 3053, Australia
Osney Mead, Oxford OX2 0EL
25 John Street, London WC1N 2BL
23 Ainslie Place, Edinburgh EH3 6AJ
238 Main Street, Cambridge
  Massachusetts 02142, USA

Other Editorial Offices:
Arnette Blackwell SA
  1, rue de Lille, 75007 Paris
  France
Blackwell Wissenschafts-Verlag GmbH
  Kurfurstendamm 57
  10707 Berlin, Germany
Blackwell MZV
  Feldgasse 13, A-1238 Wien
  Austria

First published 1983
Reprinted with corrections 1986
Second edition published 1989
Reprinted 1992, 1993

Typeset by
Page Perfection, Melbourne

Printed in Malaysia

DISTRIBUTORS
Australia
  Blackwell Science Pty Ltd
  54 University Street
  Carlton, Victoria 3053
  (*Orders:* Tel: 03 347-5552)

UK and Europe
  Marston Book Services Ltd
  PO Box 87
  Oxford OX2 0DT
  (*Orders:* Tel: 01865 791155
        Fax: 01865 791927
        Telex: 837515)

North America
  Blackwell Science Inc.
  238 Main Street
  Cambridge, MA 02142
  (*Orders:* Tel: 800 215-1000
        617 876-7000
        Fax: 617 492-5263)

Cataloging in Publication Data

McLeod, James G. (James Graham).
  Introductory neurology.

  3rd ed.
  Includes bibliographies and index.
  ISBN 0 86793 329 1.

  1. Neurology. 2. Nervous system — Diseases.
  3. Nervous system — Diseases — Diagnosis.
  4. Nervous system — Diseases — Treatment.
  I. Lance, James W. (James Waldo), 1926– .
  II. Davies, Llewelyn, 1956– . III. Title.

  616.8

The cover illustration is a stylized version of the spinal cord and roots. (After Shadé, 1966, *The Peripheral Nervous System*. Elsevier Publishing Company, Amsterdam).

Contents

PART 1   NEUROLOGICAL DIAGNOSIS

PART 2   NEUROLOGICAL DISORDERS

PART 3   INVESTIGATION AND TREATMENT OF NEUROLOGICAL DISORDERS

PREFACE TO THE THIRD EDITION

We have been fortunate to recruit the help of Dr Llewelyn Davies as a co-editor of the third edition. The text has been reorganized and every chapter revised to include recent advances in the knowledge of neurology, particularly in the fields of molecular genetics, neuro-imaging and treatment. A number of figures have been re-drawn and new figures added to the text. The book is intended to help undergraduates and residents to take a practical approach to clinical neurology and to relate knowledge of the basic sciences to the mechanisms of diseases of the nervous system.

J. G. McLeod and J. W. Lance

PREFACE TO THE FIRST EDITION

The present book is designed to help the undergraduate medical student relate already acquired knowledge of the basic neurological sciences to the examination of the patient and to diseases of the nervous system. There has been no attempt to discuss in detail all the conditions seen by a neurologist and their treatment since there are many excellent comprehensive textbooks readily available which can and should be consulted. The physiological mechanisms of symptoms and signs are discussed only briefly since the subject has been considered by the authors in another book, *A Physiological Approach to Clinical Neurology* (3rd edn, 1981, Butterworths, London). We are greatly indebted to our colleagues, particularly to Drs R. A. Ouvrier and P. G. Procopis, who have contributed so much by their discussions and in their lectures; to J. Eichorn, L. Hansen and F. Rubiu for the line drawings; and to D. Jones for typing the manuscript.

J. G. McLeod and J. W. Lance

ACKNOWLEDGEMENTS

We are grateful to Drs G. M. Halmagyi, R. Pamphlett and C. MacLeod for their helpful suggestions, to Mr Robert Haynes of the Department of Audio-visual Services, Royal Prince Alfred Hospital and Marcus Cremonese from the Prince of Wales Hospital for drawing some of the figures, and to Ms Margaret Jackson for her patience and skill in typing the manuscript.

Part 1

NEUROLOGICAL DIAGNOSIS

1 | History taking

METHOD OF HISTORY TAKING

Most patients present to their doctors with a problem, with some observations about themselves or symptoms that they consider abnormal or indicative of ill-health. The first and most important measure in helping patients to solve their problems is to take a detailed unhurried history of the development and evolution of their symptoms and then to assess this with a knowledge of the patient's family and personal background. In some neurological disorders, it may be possible to reach a firm diagnosis on the history alone. The acquisition of the clinical skills of history taking and physical examination may eliminate the need for further investigations or at least limit these to the minimum necessary to achieve a final diagnosis. The process of history taking involves a number of steps; the precise sequence in which these steps are taken may vary from one medical school to another, from one doctor to another, or even for the same doctor dealing with different problems. The important point is that the thought process should be logical and should lead to a conclusion. Each aspect of the history should be stated as precisely as possible and not glossed over in general terms.

Before the history is taken, the details of the patient's name, address, date of birth, occupation and other necessary identification data are recorded. After a general enquiry about the presenting symptoms or chief complaints and the purpose of the consultation, notes may be taken about the patient's personal background, family history and past health before going into detail about the problems which chiefly concern him or her. Alternatively, the problem may be analysed carefully as the 'history of the present illness' and then the past, family and personal histories recorded afterwards. The latter approach will be taken to illustrate the case-history of a hypothetical patient, a woman aged 40 years, with a neurological problem.

Presenting symptoms and signs and their duration

Weakness of both legs, 2 years; numbness of both legs, 1 year; urgency of micturition, 6 months.

History of the present illness

This section can be presented in note form or as a narrative, recorded as it unfolds from the patient's own account, sharpened a little here and there by an occasional direct question from the clinician to keep the history within the bounds of relevance and to prevent it from degenerating into a list of doctors consulted, investigations ordered and opinions proffered by neighbours and casual acquaintances.

The nature of the symptoms elicited makes the clinician think in terms of localization of the disorder in the nervous system; whether it originates in cerebral hemispheres, brain-stem, cerebellum, spinal cord, spinal roots, peripheral nerve or muscle, or whether it may be the product of a troubled mind.

The pattern of evolution of symptoms, whether steadily progressive, fluctuating in intensity or remitting for long periods, guides the clinician in assessing the likely pathological cause of the lesion or lesions. In the example given above, the restriction of motor and sensory symptoms to the lower limbs makes one think of a spinal cord lesion and the association with urgency of micturition (disinhibition of bladder reflexes) places the lesion above the conus medullaris, i.e. in the thoracic spinal cord. If the condition is steadily progressive, compression of the spinal cord or a lesion within the spinal cord is likely and warrants immediate investigation. If the condition has fluctuated or remitted one has to entertain the diagnosis of multiple sclerosis. It is important to gauge from the history the *upper limit* of any lesion, if possible. If the patient cited above has also noticed paraesthesiae in the little fingers of both hands, the lesion must be at the level of the eighth cervical segment or above (Fig. 1.1).

Any associated features, precipitating or relieving factors of the symptoms may give a clue as to their nature. This is particularly important in taking a history of any pain, including headache, which should include the following information.

Pain history

- Length of history: when did the pain first start?
- Site: precise part of head, neck, back or other area involved
- Radiation: the distribution of any radicular pain is important for localization (Figs 1.1, 1.2), e.g. low back pain may radiate to the medial malleolus (L4 segment), the outer malleolus (L5 segment), or the back of the heel (S1 segment). Pain is referred to a sclerotome
- Quality of pain: e.g. stabbing (tic douloureux, lightning pains); throbbing, pulsatile (indicating a vascular component); burning (indicating small sensory fibre involvement); constant, tight, colicky, etc.
- Frequency of pain: continuous or intermittent. How many times felt in each day or week?
- Duration of pain: seconds, minutes, hours
- Time of onset: any habitual pattern? Awakening from sleep? At the end of the day?
- Mode of onset: sudden, slowly progressive or preceded by other symptoms e.g. visual disturbance at the onset of migraine headache

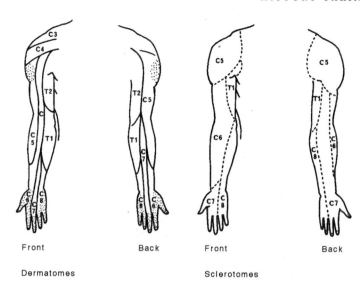

Front   Back   Front   Back

Dermatomes   Sclerotomes

Fig. 1.1   Dermatomes and sclerotomes in the upper limb. If one spinal root only is damaged, sensory loss is usually restricted to the dotted areas shown on the left. Paraesthesiae are generally referred to the dermatome and pain to the sclerotome. (From Lance and McLeod, 1981, with permission of Butterworths, London.)

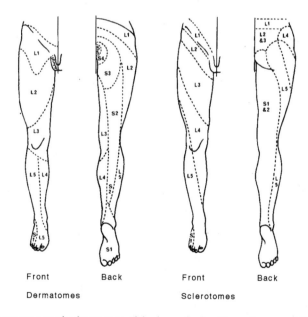

Front   Back   Front   Back

Dermatomes   Sclerotomes

Fig. 1.2   Dermatomes and sclerotomes of the lower limbs. (From Lance and McLeod, 1981, with permission of Butterworths, London.)

- Associated features: nausea, vomiting, dyspnoea, palpitations or other symptoms
- Precipitating factors: movement of head, neck or back. Coughing, sneezing, straining
- Relieving factors: certain postures, pressure over the affected part, bed-rest, heat or cold, various medications and their effects

With any syndrome, the symptoms *first* noticed at the onset and the circumstances in which they appeared are of primary importance in determining the site of origin and possible cause.

Specific interrogation

After the history of the present illness has been clarified as far as possible, the clinician runs through a check list of neurological symptoms to ensure that nothing of relevance has been overlooked, starting at the top of the nervous system and working downwards, asking about the following symptoms:

- Intellectual changes, confusion or loss of memory
- Headaches, fits or faints, drowsiness
- Speech disturbance: dysphasia (is the patient right or left-handed?); dysarthria; dysphonia
- Sense of smell (cranial nerve I)
- Vision (cranial nerve II): impairment or hallucinations of vision; limited to one eye, one half field or bilateral? Details and duration
- Double vision (cranial nerves III, IV, VI)
- Facial paraesthesiae or numbness (cranial nerve V)
- Facial weakness (cranial nerve VII). If facial palsy is apparent from the history, was it accompanied by hyperacusis or impairment of taste on the affected side?
- Hearing, tinnitus and vertigo (cranial nerve VIII)
- Swallowing, coughing and quality of speech (cranial nerves IX, X, XI and central portion of XII)
- Weakness
  unilateral
      hemiparesis: cerebral, brain-stem, or upper cervical cord origin
      monoparesis: cerebral, spinal cord or roots
  bilateral
      quadriparesis: cervical cord or above
      paraparesis: thoracic cord, conus or cauda equina
      proximal: myopathy
      distal: peripheral neuropathy
      fatiguability: myasthenia gravis
- Paraesthesiae or numbness — distribution of the same significance as weakness, with the additional information that: (i) numbness of half of the face and opposite side of the body indicates a brain-stem lesion; (ii) burning sensations down one side of the body with weakness of the other side suggests a

unilateral spinal cord lesion (Brown-Séquard syndrome); (iii) paraesthesiae from a spinal root disturbance are referred to a *dermatome* (Figs 1.1, 1.2)

- Specific symptoms common in multiple sclerosis to be asked about are: (i) tingling down the back on flexing the neck (Lhermitte's sign, electric shock sign) indicating a cervical lesion; (ii) band-like sensations around the trunk or pelvis; (iii) tight wrapping sensations around the legs. The last two symptoms arise from dorsal root entry zones or dorsal columns
- Sphincter disturbance — urgency of, or difficulty in initiating micturition or defaecation; incontinence
- Impotence or failure of ejaculation
- Difficulty with coordination, balance or gait.

Other systems

Since the nervous system does not exist in isolation, the usual questions must be asked about other systems. Those of most relevance to neurological disorders are listed below:

Systemic disturbances such as connective tissue diseases, malignancy or infections — loss of weight; fever, sweating; aches in muscles or joints.

Respiratory disease (such as carcinoma of the lung, tuberculosis, sarcoid, bronchiectasis) which may be related to neurological symptoms — tightness or pain in the chest; dyspnoea; haemoptysis.

Cardiovascular symptoms often associated with cerebral vascular disease — palpitations (cardiac dysrhythmias); angina pectoris; intermittent claudication.

Endocrine disorders drawing attention to the hypothalamus and area around the pituitary fossa — polyuria, polydipsia; symptoms of thyroid or pituitary dysfunction; unexplained weight change; loss of body hair; amenorrhoea, loss of libido, testicular atrophy.

Past history

One of the arts of history taking is to know what of the past history is relevant to the present illness or, indeed, whether it may actually form part of the present illness. If, for example, the patient whose presenting symptoms and signs were given at the beginning of this chapter eventually disclosed that she had suffered loss of vision in the right eye for a period of 3 weeks at the age of 27 years and a tight, band-like sensation around the trunk for 2 months at the age of 35 years, these previous episodes could well be listed at the beginning of the history and would draw attention to the multifocal nature of symptoms experienced by the patient, e.g. transient loss of vision aged 27, band-like sensation around the trunk aged 35, progressive weakness of the legs for the past 2 years, that is, multiple sclerosis.

In the case of epilepsy, mental retardation, or any illness that could have been present at the time of birth or may have been initiated by the birth process, the course of pregnancy and labour and birthweight should be noted. Was the baby given immediately to the mother or was resuscitation, intensive care or a humidicrib required? Milestones of development, the time of sitting, standing, walking and talking, and progress at school, become relevant. Did the child suffer convulsions, with or without a fever? Some 10% of children with febrile convulsions have fits in later life. Head injury, meningitis or encephalitis are obviously of potential relevance to the onset of epilepsy.

A history of headaches, motion sickness, abdominal pain or episodes of vomiting ('bilious attacks') in childhood may augur the development of migraine in adult life.

Recurrent headaches with neck stiffness in the past (perhaps diagnosed as meningo-encephalitis) may suggest repeated bleeding from a cerebral angioma. A history of diabetes, hypertension, tuberculosis, immune disorders or other serious illness should be recorded, as should any operation, even seemingly minor procedures such as the removal of a mole from the skin.

Family history

Many neurological disorders like Huntington's chorea, the heredo-familial ataxias, Charcot-Marie-Tooth disease, muscular dystrophies and some forms of epilepsy are clearly of genetic origin. Other conditions such as migraine and cerebral vascular diseases tend to 'run in families' although no pattern of inheritance has been determined.

Personal and social background

The personality of the patient, his or her relationship with peer groups, spouse, children and attitude to occupation may play an important part in the genesis of symptoms considered to be neurological, because of the constant interaction of mind and body. On the other hand, the development of neurological illness may have a profound impact on the patient's ability to work, to maintain satisfactory relationships with family and friends and to derive benefit and enjoyment from life. One must therefore obtain as accurate a picture as possible of the type of life that a patient is leading and hopes to lead in the future to aid in diagnosis and then to help in counselling once the diagnosis is reached. The financial state of the family must also be assessed to see whether some form of financial assistance through sickness benefits or pensions is required. The emotional state of the patient must be carefully assessed as minor degrees of depression are very common and often relevant.

The nature of the patient's occupation and the details of his or her work must be noted because of the possible relevance to the neurological problem and in case of any workers' compensation or other legal action.

Standard questions about the amount of alcohol consumed, smoking habits, exposure to toxins and consumption of drugs are also of importance. The patient should be asked to list all medications currently being consumed or that have been used in the past since they may be relevant to present symptoms and certainly must be known to the clinician before any pharmaceutical agent is prescribed. Tactful enquiry about sexual preference has become increasingly important as the neurological manifestations of acquired immune-deficiency syndrome (AIDS) are more often encountered.

GUIDE TO DIAGNOSIS FROM THE HISTORY

The concept of taking such a complete medical history may seem daunting to those who are just starting their clinical training. With greater experience the process becomes easier and quicker, and is spiced with interest or even excitement as the clues present themselves to the receptive mind of the clinician. The phlegmatic recording of the history without any attempt being made by the clinician to correlate the facts as they appear, to make deductions and to form a provisional diagnosis during the process, can be a fruitless exercise. The pieces of the puzzle must be fitted into place while the story is evolving so that any missing fragments can be sought later.

The aim of history taking is to establish, as far as possible, whether the illness is likely to be of organic or psychological origin. If it is organic, what part or parts of the nervous system may be implicated? What is the pattern of the illness over a period of time? What are the precipitating and relieving factors? What is the possible pathology? Particular attention should be paid to the following points.

Localization

Do the symptoms arise in one site or multiple sites? Can they be explained on the basis of impairment of a particular system (e.g. posterior columns, spinocerebellar pathways, corticospinal tracts) or a particular vascular territory (internal carotid and its branches, vertebrobasilar system, anterior spinal artery)? Examples of symptoms arising from various sites are:

Cortex   Focal (partial) epileptic seizures. Localizing cerebral symptoms (Chapter 3). Hemianopic or quadrantanopic field defects (Chapter 4).

Thalamus   Contralateral dysaesthesiae (unpleasant burning pain) or sensory loss.

Basal ganglia   Parkinson's disease, involuntary movements (Chapter 15).

Internal capsule   Contralateral hemiplegia (and sometimes limb ataxia) and sensory loss.

Mid-brain   Tectum (superior colliculi): failure of upward deviation of the eyes (Parinaud's syndrome). Tegmentum: third nerve palsy. Contralateral 'wing-beating' (red nucleus) tremor. Contralateral hemiparesis.

Pons and medulla   Ipsilateral facial numbness (and often contralateral numbness of the body). Paresis of VI, VII, IX, X or XII cranial nerves. Dysarthria and dysphagia from involvement of cranial nerves IX–XII is called 'bulbar palsy'. If impairment of speech and swallowing is caused by involvement of corticobulbar pathways rostral to lower cranial nerve nuclei, the condition is called 'pseudobulbar palsy'. Vertigo, tinnitus, deafness (VIII cranial nerve). Ipsilateral Horner's syndrome (sympathetic pathway). Contralateral hemiparesis. Ipsilateral cerebellar signs. Sometimes a lesion in the upper pons may compromise corticopontocerebellar fibres so that limb ataxia is on the same side as the hemiparesis ('ataxic hemiparesis').

Cerebellum   Mid-line: vertigo, ataxia of gait. Hemispheres: ipsilateral inco-ordination (Chapter 8).

Spinal cord   Bilateral: motor and sensory loss below the level of the lesion. Sparing of posterior columns suggests anterior cord compression or anterior spinal artery involvement. Urgency of micturition (Chapter 7). Unilateral: ipsilateral paresis and loss of joint position sense with contralateral loss of pinprick and temperature sensation (Brown-Séquard syndrome). The horizontal level is estimated from any accompanying lower motor neurone lesion, sensory impairment or reflex loss at the segment or segments involved and by the upper limit of the upper motor neurone and sensory tract involvement.

Spinal roots   Weakness, wasting, pain, paraesthesiae, or sensory, motor and reflex loss in the distribution of a particular root or roots as described above.

Peripheral nerves   Sensory and motor symptoms in the distribution of a particular nerve (mononeuritis), several nerves (mononeuritis multiplex) or all peripheral nerves symmetrically (peripheral neuropathy; Chapter 10).

Neuromuscular junction   A purely motor syndrome with fatiguability (myasthenia). Muscles commonly involved are: extra-ocular muscles (ptosis, diplopia, without pupillary changes); bulbar muscles; proximal limb muscles (Chapter 10).

Muscle   A purely motor syndrome with proximal wasting and weakness. Distal muscles may be involved in some myopathies such as dystrophia myotonica (Chapter 10).

Mode of onset

Note the precise sequence of events at the onset of the illness. The initial story given might be one of loss of consciousness. 'I just blacked out, went out like a light'. 'Yes, but what were you doing at the time? Did you notice anything just before you became unconscious?'

Repeating this question in a different form a number of times (because patients often think that minor sensations are of no significance and not worth reporting) often helps to diagnose the cause of the episode. Sample replies might include:

'Well, I just turned my head to one side, then my eyes went dim and I felt giddy' (vertebrobasilar insufficiency).

'My heart started racing and I felt faint' (cardiac dysrhythmia causing syncope).

'I just got out of bed to pass urine and woke up on the floor of the bathroom' (micturition syncope).

'My chest was tight and I couldn't get enough air into my lungs' (anxiety hyperventilation).

'I suddenly felt very frightened, as though it had all happened before' (temporal lobe epilepsy).

The principle is to look for minor symptoms that lead to the major event, for they and they alone may hold the key to the diagnostic doorway.

The evolution (temporal pattern) of the illness

Have the symptoms reached their maximum and then progressively subsided?
For example:

- Headache — viral meningo-encephalitis
- Vertigo, tinnitus — acute labyrinthitis
- Weakness — upper motor neurone: acute stroke
  — lower motor neurone: Guillain-Barré disease (acute polyneuritis)

Have the symptoms relapsed and remitted?
For example:

- Headache — migraine
- Vertigo, tinnitus — Ménière's syndrome
- Weakness — upper motor neurone: multiple sclerosis
  — lower motor neurone: relapsing polyneuritis.

Have the symptoms progressively become worse?
For example:

- Headache — cerebral tumour or other space-occupying lesion
- Vertigo, tinnitus — acoustic neuroma or brain-stem glioma
- Weakness — upper and lower motor neurone: motor neurone disease (amyotrophic lateral sclerosis)

The temporal pattern thus gives some idea of the nature of the pathological process.

CONCLUSION

The history enables an hypothesis to be formed about the site of origin and cause of the patient's symptoms. The physical examination then tests aspects of this hypothesis. After that, further elucidation of the problem may depend on special investigations. Bear in mind that physical examination and diagnostic tests may not help. *Diagnosis often depends entirely on the history.*

2 | Neurological examination

GENERAL

Appearance and behaviour of the patient

During history taking, the emotional state and general intellectual competence of the patient will have become apparent, as well as any abnormal facial appearance, posture or involuntary movements.

Gait and stance

If the patient is able to walk, one observes body posture, swinging of the arms, and movements of the legs and feet, looking for asymmetry or any deviation from normal in the pace, fluidity of movement and maintenance of balance. Balance can be tested more stringently by asking the patient to walk heel-to-toe (*tandem gait*). The patient is then asked to stand with the feet together, then to close the eyes. If the patient is unable to maintain the upright posture with the eyes closed (*Romberg's sign*), proprioceptive information from the lower limbs is deficient.

The patient may be asked to hold the examiner's hands and to stand on the heels, elevating the feet, so that a minor degree of foot-drop can be observed.

MENTAL STATE

Examination of the mental state is often referred to as examination of the higher centres.

Level of consciousness

If the patient is stuporous, the level of consciousness may be assessed by responsiveness to voice, touch or painful stimuli. The examination of the unconscious or uncooperative patient is discussed in Chapter 14.

Orientation in time and place

Does the patient know the day, month and year, his or her name and usual address and the place where he or she is at the moment of examination?

General intellectual function

Note the general appearance, mood, spontaneous speech and response to questions, attitude to others, and whether or not there are disorders of perception.

Delusions   Firmly held incorrect beliefs which may be a feature of confusional states or psychosis.

Illusions   A misinterpretation of sensory stimuli, common in confusional states, delirium and dementia.

Hallucinations   These are sensory perceptions unrelated to external stimuli. Visual hallucinations are common in delirium; auditory hallucinations occur in alcohol and other drug withdrawal states and schizophrenia; and hallucinations of cutaneous sensation, like insects crawling on the skin (*formication*), may also be a feature of drug withdrawal.

Test the interpretation of proverbs (e.g: 'a bird in the hand is worth two in the bush'; 'people in glass houses shouldn't throw stones'). An intellectually impaired person may give a literal rather than a figurative interpretation which is known as 'concrete thought'. Evidence of serious emotional or thought disorder requires psychiatric consultation.

Memory

If patients have recently suffered a head injury they should be asked for their last recollection before impact to assess the duration of *retrograde amnesia*, and their first memory after the accident to assess the duration of *post-traumatic amnesia*. If recent memory is defective, the patient may recite imaginary events to fill in the gaps (*confabulation*, a feature of Korsakoff's psychosis). A commonly used test for registration and short-term retention of memory is to ask the patient to remember a name and address for 5 minutes while the examination continues. Useful tests of attention and immediate recall are the digit span (normally seven numbers forward and five backwards can be repeated), the serial sevens test (subtracting 7 from 100, then from each subsequent remainder) and repetition of the Babcock sentence. The Babcock sentence ('There is one thing a nation must have to be rich and great, and that is a large secure supply of wood') is repeated alternately by examiner and patient until two word-perfect recitations have been obtained, or eight incorrect attempts.

Mini-mental state examination

This is a simple, quick method of scoring the mental state and may be useful for repeated examinations of people with confusional states, or as a screening test for dementia and other disorders of intellectual function. The finding of persistent abnormalities should prompt more detailed neuropyschological assessment (Table 2.1).

Table 2.1   Mini-mental state examination

Test	Max. score	Patient's score
Orientation		
What is the (year, season, date, day, month)?	5	( )
Where are you (country, state, town, hospital, ward)?	5	( )
Retention		
Name 3 objects, then ask patient to repeat these	3	( )
Give 1 point for each correct answer		
Repeat them until patient has learnt them all		
Count the number of trials and record		
Calculation and attention		
Serial 7s. 1 point for each correct answer	5	( )
Stop after 5 answers. If patient cannot, or will not, do this, ask him to spell 'world' backwards (0–5 points)		
Recall		
Ask patient to name the 3 objects learned earlier	3	( )
Give 1 point for each correct answer		
Language		
Name a pencil and a watch (2 points)	9	( )
Repetition: ask patient to repeat a short sentence (0 or 1 point)		
3-stage command. 'Take a piece of paper in your right hand, fold it in half and put it on the floor' (3 points)		
Read and obey the following:		
'Close your eyes' (0 or 1 point)		
Ask patient to write a sentence of his own choice. It must contain a subject and verb and make sense (0 or 1 point)		
Copying: ask patient to copy 2 intersecting pentagons (0 or 1 point)		
Total score	30	( )

SPEECH AND HANDEDNESS

If speech is entirely normal, this should be stated and preference for using the right or left hand noted, since language is a function of the dominant hemisphere (the left hemisphere in over 50% of left-handers as well as in 96% of right-handers).

Speech defects should be described as: (i) aphasia, or dysphasia — a disturbance of language, causing difficulty in understanding the spoken word or expressing thoughts in words, discussed further in Chapter 3; (ii) dysarthria — faulty articulation despite normal word comprehension and selection. (iii) dysphonia — impaired timbre of the voice from disorders of the vocal cords.

Localization of cortical dysfunction

If there is no perceptual or communication disorder this section may be omitted.

Disordered perception

- Spoken word (sensory dysphasia: Wernicke area)
- Written word (dyslexia: dominant parieto-occipital area)
- Tactile recognition (agnosia: parietal lobe)
- Visual or tactile inattention (unilateral neglect of bilaterally presented stimuli: parietal lobe)
- Spatial relation to environment (losing way in familiar surroundings: non-dominant parietal lobe)

Disordered expression

Inability to select words and name objects (aphasia: Broca and Wernicke areas); inability to write (agraphia: dominant parietal lobe); inability to calculate (acalculia: dominant parietal lobe); inability to distinguish right from left (right–left disorientation: dominant parietal lobe); inability to perform routine tasks (apraxia: dominant parietal or frontal lobes); inability to draw, construct diagrams (constructional apraxia: either parietal lobe); inability to dress oneself (non-dominant parietal lobe).

SKULL

The size and shape of the skull are observed and the circumference measured if microcephaly or hydrocephalus are suspected (Figs 2.1 and 2.2 for normal values). The skull may be palpated, with attention to the fontanelles in young children. When relevant (suspected angioma or vascular tumour), the examiner listens for a bruit over the orbits, temples and mastoid processes. For auscultation over the orbits, the patient is asked to close both eyes while the bell of the stethoscope is placed over one eye. The patient is then asked to open the other eye. This minimizes artefactual sounds from eyelid tremor.

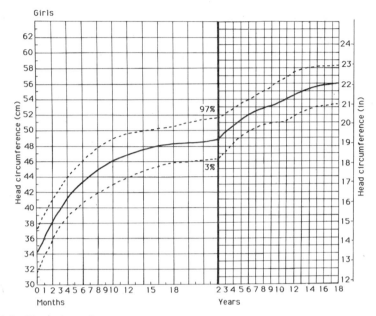

Fig. 2.1 Head circumference in girls. (From Nellhaus, 1968, *Pediatrics*, **41**, 106, with permission of the author and publisher, copyright American Academy of Pediatrics 1968.)

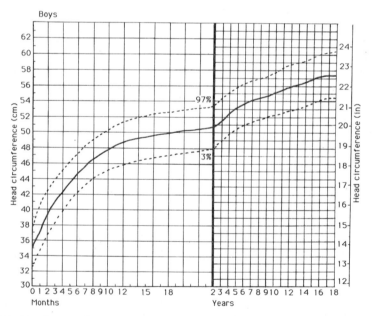

Fig. 2.2 Head circumference in boys. (From Nellhaus, 1968, *Pediatrics*, **41**, 106, with permission of the author and publisher, copyright American Academy of Pediatrics 1968.)

SPINE

The spine is examined for evidence of deformities, such as kyphosis, scoliosis or lordosis. The area of the spine appropriate to the symptoms is particularly inspected for any abnormality such as a tuft of hair in the lumbosacral region which may indicate an underlying spina bifida or other congenital anomaly. The cervical, thoracic or lumbar spine is then moved actively and passively through the full range to determine limitation of movement. Tenderness may be sought by pressure between the spinous processes and lateral to them (over the zygapophyseal joints). Sometimes a smart blow over the suspected area of the spine may reproduce spinal root pain but this test must be employed with discretion.

Resistance to flexing the neck (neck rigidity) is found with meningeal irritation (subarachnoid haemorrhage, meningitis) as well as with local lesions. Another sign of meningeal irritation is inability to extend the leg at the knee joint when the lower limb is flexed at the hip (Kernig's sign).

In lumbosacral root irritation, *straight leg raising* (the extended lower limb being passively flexed at the hip joint by the examiner) is limited by pain on the affected side.

The examiner listens for a bruit over the carotid artery in patients with cerebral vascular insufficiency, and over the spine if·a spinal angioma is suspected.

CRANIAL NERVES

Cranial nerves are discussed in detail in Chapter 4.

Cranial nerve I (olfactory nerve)

It is important to test the sense of smell in patients with dementia (olfactory groove meningioma), ocular palsies (sphenoid wing meningioma) and after head injury (the olfactory filaments are often damaged by shearing strain at the moment of impact).

Cranial nerve II (optic nerve)

Visual acuity

Visual acuity, right and left, should be recorded at 6 m from a Snellen's chart, with the patient wearing glasses if necessary (e.g. VAR 6/6 VAL 6/9 [corrected]). In the USA, normal vision is recorded (in feet) as 20/20.

Ophthalmoscopic examination of the fundi

The key point in the examination of the fundi is for the patient to be able to fix on an external object with one eye while the other eye is being examined. This means that the examiner's head must remain vertical so as not to obscure the vision of the patient's fixating eye.

Note especially the optic disc: what is its colour? (pallor of the temporal half, or the whole of the disc), the optic cup (enlarged in glaucoma, diminished in papilloedema), pulsation of the veins where they pass over the rim of the optic cup (absent in papilloedema) and the circumference of the disc (which is swollen and the margins blurred in papilloedema).

The state of the vessels in the periphery (arteriovenous nipping, haemorrhages, micro-aneurysms) is also noted and the surface of the retina scanned for abnormalities (exudates, choroiditis or retinitis pigmentosa).

Visual fields

The patient is first confronted by the examiner, meeting his or her gaze, while the binocular fields are tested with the examiner's arms outstretched, moving the index finger on the right then the left hand, then both together in the outer quadrants of the fields of vision. In this way a complete homonymous hemianopia or visual inattention to one side can be detected.

Each eye is then tested individually with the other eye covered, the examiner bringing a finger, or preferably a white- or red-headed pin, from the periphery toward the centre of each quadrant. The blind spot should be defined and compared in size with that of the examiner. If a field defect is suspected, it is advisable to advance the pin at right angles to the presumed junction between abnormal and normal parts of the visual field so that a scotoma, hemianopia or quadrantanopia can be clearly defined. Colour vision should also be tested with Ishihara test charts, particularly if optic neuritis, past or present, is suspected.

Pupillary response to light

This is described later in further detail.

Cranial nerves III (oculomotor), IV (trochlear) and VI (abducens) and the ocular sympathetic nerve

Orbit

Prominence of the eye (proptosis, exophthalmos) is noted.

Ptosis

A partial ptosis may be congenital, myopathic, myasthenic or part of a Horner's syndrome (in which case the ipsilateral pupil will be small and sweating may be impaired over the same side of the forehead). A complete ptosis is usually part of a third nerve palsy, in which case the pupil is usually dilated. Ptosis must be distinguished from blepharospasm in which the orbicularis oculi is actively contracting.

Pupils

The size, shape and symmetry of the pupils are noted.

Pupillary responses   Accommodation: normal pupils constrict as the eyes converge (*near response*). Light reflex: the normal pupil contracts briskly in the eye to which the light is directed (direct response) and also in the opposite eye (consensual response).

- Afferent limb — optic nerve
- Efferent limb — Edinger-Westphal nucleus and third cranial nerve

Assuming the third nerve is intact bilaterally, the optic nerve contribution to the reflex may be assessed by swinging a torch from one eye to the other at a rate of about once every 2 seconds. If there is impaired conduction in one optic nerve, the direct response to light in that eye will be insufficient to prevent dilatation of the pupil on that side as it recovers from the consensual constriction induced by shining the light in the sound eye. The effect will thus be pupillary constriction while the light is shone in the sound eye and pupillary dilatation when the light is swung to the eye on the affected side (*swinging torch* or *Marcus Gunn* sign). The effect may not be observed initially, but after one of two swings of the torch, the pupillary response of the affected eye rapidly fatigues.

Ocular movements

Ocular movements are tested in the horizontal plane by asking the patient to look laterally to right and left (saccadic movements) and then to follow the examiner's finger to right and left (pursuit movements), maintaining the lateral position long enough to observe whether nystagmus develops. Vertical eye movements are tested with eyes looking to right and left as well as straight ahead in order to test the actions of the individual muscles. The patient should be asked if he sees a double image in any of the positions of gaze, and if so the paretic muscle should be identified (p. 51). If nystagmus is present it should be further analysed (pp. 59–61).

Cranial nerve V (trigeminal nerve)

Motor

The patient is asked to open the jaw to ensure that it opens in the mid-line and does not deviate to one side (the jaw deviates to the side of a lower motor neurone lesion because of unequal action of the pterygoid muscles). The power of jaw closure is then tested and the masseter and temporalis muscles palpated. The pterygoid muscles may be tested together by assessing the strength of jaw-opening or separately by asking the patient to thrust the jaw sideways.

Sensory

Each of the three divisions of the trigeminal nerve is then tested by touch and pinprick with particular attention being paid to the anatomical distribution of sensory loss and to whether or not there is dissociation of painful and tactile sensation. Sensation on both sides of the face should be compared. Bear in mind that the territory of the second division extends only halfway between the nose and the angle of the mandible (Fig. 4.22). If a subtle lesion is suspected an added refinement is to test for two-point discrimination (the points being separated by 2 mm) on the lip of one side then the other.

Reflexes

Corneal reflex   The corneal reflex is tested by applying a wisp of cotton wool to the lateral aspect of the cornea (not the conjunctiva); the stimulus induces a blink response. The examiner's hand rests on the patient's cheek so that the stimulus can be applied gently to the cornea, using the fingers with delicacy, and not by a frontal assault which induces a startle response.

- Afferent pathway — trigeminal nerve, first division (part of the cornea is sometimes supplied by the second division)
- Efferent pathway — facial nerve

Jaw jerk   A tap on the relaxed, partly open jaw with a percussion hammer evokes a barely perceptible contraction of the jaw-closing muscles in most normal subjects. An exaggerated jaw jerk is an important sign of a bilateral upper motor neurone lesion involving corticobulbar pathways.

- Afferent pathway — third division of trigeminal nerve
- Efferent pathway — third division of trigeminal nerve

Glabella tap sign   Repeatedly tapping the mid-forehead at a rate of about 1/second induces a bilateral blink response, which is rapidly suppressed in most normal subjects. A continued blink response to each tap is often observed in Parkinson's disease. The mechanism is obscure.

Cranial nerve VII (facial nerve)

Motor

The face should be inspected for evidence of asymmetry (e.g. palpebral fissures, drooping of the angle of the mouth, loss of nasolabial fold) or abnormal movements (e.g. tics, dyskinesia, myokymia, fasciculations). Power of the facial muscles is tested by asking the patient: (i) to elevate the eyebrows by looking upwards, and observing the corrugation of the forehead; (ii) to close the eyes firmly, and observing whether the eyelashes are buried equally on both sides after which the examiner should attempt to open the eyelids against resistance; (iii) to smile broadly, observing the depth of the nasolabial folds.

All three sections of the facial nerve should be tested in this manner since the upper face is relatively spared by an upper motor neurone lesion. An upper motor neurone source of lower facial weakness can usually be confirmed by inducing the patient to laugh or smile spontaneously (if a feeble joke does not produce this effect, the examiner may have to resort to tickling) in which case the smile becomes symmetrical.

Sensory

The nervus intermedius can be tested by applying a bent pin to the posterior aspect of the external auditory canal. Sensation in this area may be diminished

(Hitzelberger's sign) in early compression of the seventh nerve, by acoustic neuroma for example, but this sign has not proved reliable in our hands.

Taste

Taste can be tested by applying a salty or sweet solution to the anterior two-thirds of each side of the protruded tongue in turn. Taste fibres travel with the lingual nerve but cross to the facial nerve in the chorda tympani so that taste is impaired if the facial nerve is compromised proximal to the junction with the chorda tympani (as it often is in Bell's palsy; Fig. 4.24).

Reflexes

Corneal reflex and glabella tap sign as described under cranial nerve V. In frontal lobe lesions, contraction of the orbicularis oris may follow percussion of the closed lips (pouting response).

Cranial nerve VIII (acoustic and vestibular nerves)

Acoustic (auditory) nerve

Hearing is tested grossly by blocking one ear with a finger while the threshold of the other ear is determined by whispered or spoken voice at varying intensities. Normally the whispered word can be heard at a distance of about 60 cm. If one ear is deaf, the nature of the deafness is determined by two clinical tests after ensuring that the external auditory meatus is not obstructed.

Rinné test   The base of a vibrating tuning fork (128, 256, or 512 Hz) is placed on one mastoid process until it can no longer be heard. The vibrating prongs are then held next to the ear. If the tone is then audible, 'air conduction' (AC) is said to be better heard than 'bone conduction' (BC), which is normally so and is also the case in mild perceptive (nerve) deafness. Bone conduction is better than AC in conduction deafness (due to external or middle ear disease). In severe nerve deafness the sound may be conducted through bone to the normal ear, thus giving a spurious result.

Weber's test   The base of a vibrating tuning fork is placed on the middle of the forehead. The sound is heard better on the normal side in the case of nerve deafness but is referred to the deaf ear in the case of conduction deafness (because of the lack of competing auditory stimuli through the normal channels).

It must be borne in mind that tuning fork tests use frequencies lower than those of the normal conversational range and that they are highly fallible. Audiometry is recommended in any case of deafness (Chapter 4).

Vestibular nerve

Positional vertigo and nystagmus may be sought by lowering the patient's head backwards over the end of the examination couch, first to one side, then to the other (Hallpike's test). Other tests include Romberg's test and the stepping test (Chapter 4). Electronystagmography and caloric testing are necessary if a lesion is suspected.

Cranial nerves IX (glossopharyngeal nerve) and X (vagus nerve)

Observe quality of speech and coughing for dysphonia, from weakness of closure of the vocal cords (paralysis of vagus or its recurrent laryngeal branch), or for a nasal intonation from palatal weakness. Look at the posterior pharynx for unswallowed saliva and check swallowing while the patient drinks a glass of water. Movement of the palate is observed: (i) during voluntary activity with the patient saying 'ah'; (ii) during reflex activity after touching the posterior pharyngeal wall with a wooden probe or tongue depressor ('gag reflex').

If both voluntary and reflex movement are impaired bilaterally (bulbar palsy), or the palate fails to elevate on one side, the lesion is of the lower motor neurone. If the palate cannot be elevated voluntarily but moves normally in the gag reflex, the lesion involves the upper motor neurone ('pseudobulbar palsy').

Sensory

The posterior pharyngeal wall is innervated by the glossopharyngeal nerve and sensation is tested by means of a wooden probe (a pin is too unkind) first on one side then the other.

Reflex

The gag reflex is described above. The cough reflex is usually not tested.

Cranial nerve XI (spinal part of the accessory nerve, arising from cervical cord segments 1–5)

This is solely motor, supplying the upper trapezius and the sternomastoid muscles. Its integrity is tested by instructing the patient to shrug the shoulders upwards against the pressure of the examiner's hand and to turn the head firmly against pressure while the sternomastoid muscles are palpated. Wasting and weakness of the affected muscles are noted.

Cranial nerve XII (hypoglossal nerve)

The patient protrudes the tongue and then pushes it into one cheek and then the other against pressure from the examiner's hand. With a unilateral lesion of the lower motor neurone, the tongue deviates to the side of the lesion (since the action of the hyoglossus muscle is to push the tongue forwards), and pressure exerted against the cheek is diminished on the affected side. Slight deviation of the tongue may be seen with an upper motor neurone lesion, but in this case the deviation is to the side of the hemiparesis; i.e. opposite to the side of the lesion. Wasting and fasciculation of the tongue may be noted on the side of the lesion, or bilaterally, in the case of bulbar palsy. Since a tremor may develop in a protruded tongue and obscure fasciculations, these are best sought with the tongue at rest on the floor of the mouth. Coarse undulations of the tongue musculature (myokymia) may be observed with central lesions such as brain-stem gliomas.

MOTOR SYSTEM

More detail on the motor system can be found in Chapter 5.

Inspection

The patient, wearing the minimum of clothing compatible with age and sex, lies comfortably on an examination couch in the supine position. The following are closely observed:

- Posture and development of the trunk and limbs: symmetry of the upper limbs is checked. Shortening of one forearm by more than 1 cm suggests some disturbance of the opposite hemisphere (parietal region) at birth or in early childhood. Asymmetry of the hands, fingernails and of the lower limbs may provide supporting evidence. The patient then holds both arms in front of the body and closes the eyes while the examiner observes whether either arm drifts downwards from the horizontal level. This is a quick check of pyramidal, proprioceptive and cerebellar function since all are required to maintain posture. The lower limbs are similarly inspected. Pes cavus may suggest a congenital anomaly, such as spina bifida, or an hereditary disorder such as a spinocerebellar degeneration or peroneal muscular atrophy (Charcot-Marie-Tooth disease)
- Involuntary movements
- Muscle wasting — degree, distribution
- Muscle fasciculations

Muscle tone

'Muscle tone' does not refer to the firmness or flabbiness of the muscle bellies but to the activity of the stretch reflexes, usually assessed by the resistance encountered on stretching the muscle at increasing velocities.

Diminished muscle tone may be inferred from posture. If the patient's elbows are resting on a firm base with the forearms held vertically, the wrist usually assumes a resting posture at an angle of about 30° above the horizontal line. If muscle tone is diminished (hypotonia) the wrist is held at or below the horizontal level. One foot may be seen to rest on a lower level than the other if that limb is hypotonic.

Muscle tone in the upper limbs is examined by passively flexing and extending the elbows and the wrists, and by pronating and supinating the wrists. If the patient has been noticed not to swing one arm on walking (as in Parkinson's disease), the tone of the shoulder muscles should be examined by rotary movements at the shoulder joint. The cogwheel rigidity of Parkinson's disease may be enhanced by asking the patient to make a mental calculation, clench the jaw, turn the head from side to side or to clench the fist on the opposite side. Muscle tone in the lower limbs is assessed by passively flexing and extending the hip, knee and ankle joints at varying velocities. Changes in muscle tone (hypotonia in disorders of the lower motor neurone and cerebellum; hypertonia in upper motor neurone lesions or Parkinson's disease) are discussed in Chapter 5.

Power

The examination of muscle power is best conducted in an orderly sequence, proceeding from proximal to distal muscles, testing abductors before adductors and flexor groups before extensors, so that any pattern of weakness becomes apparent while the examination is in progress. This is of particular importance in detecting an upper motor neurone ('pyramidal') pattern of weakness in which the flexors of the lower limbs (including the dorsiflexors of the ankles as part of the flexor synergy) are preferentially impaired. The exact manner in which each muscle group is most easily tested is best learned at the bedside and requires considerable practice so that the examination is carried out rapidly and accurately. When testing the power of the hip flexors it is helpful to keep one hand under the heel of the opposite foot. If the patient is not trying hard to flex the hip (because of pain, malingering or hysteria), normal counter pressure is not felt on the opposite side (Hoover's sign).

Muscle power may be graded on the Medical Research Council (MRC; United Kingdom) scale:

0   no movement
1   a flicker is perceptible in the muscle
2   the muscle can move the limb if the force of gravity is eliminated by supporting the limb
3   the muscle can elevate the limb against the force of gravity
4   the muscle can move the limb against resistance supplied by the examiner
5   normal power

The problem with the MRC scale is that most muscular weakness falls between 4 and 5 so that one has to resort to the cumbersome intermediate gradings of 4.25, 4.5 and 4.75.

If weakness of the lower limbs extends upwards to the trunk, the upper limit of motor deficit can sometimes be ascertained by asking the patient to try to sit up without using the arms. If the umbilicus deviates upwards, it indicates that the lower abdominal muscles are weaker than the upper (lesion around the T10 level). If expansion of the thoracic cage on deep inspiration is less in the lower part of the chest than the upper, it suggests that the lesion lies at the T5/6 level.

REFLEXES

Tendon jerks

A brisk reflex contraction of most muscles can be obtained by tapping their tendons (or a bony attachment) with a percussion hammer so that the muscle is vibrated or transiently stretched, thus stimulating the primary endings of the muscle spindle. An afferent volley set up by percussion then traverses the mono-synaptic arc, causing a reflex contraction (Fig. 5.6). This is a means of testing the integrity and excitability of various segmental levels in the spinal cord.

The patient lies supine with the upper limbs flexed, the elbows being sup-ported on the examination couch and the forearms and hands resting lightly across the abdomen. The percussion hammer is lightly flicked from one radial styloid process to the other so that the amplitude of the supinator reflex on each side may be compared. The bicep jerk is tested by tapping each biceps tendon separately. Each arm is then gently drawn across the abdomen to make the triceps tendon taut so that the triceps jerk may be tested. To elicit the finger jerk, the patient lightly clenches his or her fingers against the examiner's fingers so that tapping the examiner's fingers with the percussion hammer will transmit a vibration wave or brief stretch to the patient's finger flexors, which thus evokes the finger jerk. If the thumb is noted to flex with the fingers, this thumb reflex is known as *Hoffman's sign*. Hoffman's sign is traditionally elicited by flipping the terminal phalanx of the index or middle finger which transmits a vibratory stimulus to the tendons of finger and thumb flexors which is similar to that evoked by percussion of the fingers. Hoffman's sign is found whenever reflexes are brisk and is not specific for an upper motor neurone lesion.

To test knee jerks it is easiest to place one hand under both knees, lifting so that the lower limbs are partly flexed at the knees and the percussion hammer can be flicked from one ligamentum patellae to the other, to detect any asymmetry of knee jerks. The ankle jerks are most simply tested with the lower limbs abducted at the hips and the knees flexed, a position similar to the frog-kick used in swimming breast-stroke. The foot is then grasped by the examiner, moved rapidly up and down to ensure that the muscle is relaxed, then placed in the mid-position before the tendo Achillis is tapped. These minor points of technique are important because the reflex will not be detected if the patient is voluntarily holding the ankle rigidly in position, or if the tendon is so slack that the vibration from percussion is not transmitted, or if the ankle is sharply dorsiflexed so that the calf muscle is stretched so much that the ankle jerk is reflexly inhibited.

If reflexes are brisk, repetitive discharge of the stretch reflex arc (*clonus*) may be demonstrated by maintaining the appropriate muscle on stretch.

Superficial reflexes

These are best considered as protective reflexes by which stimulation of the skin induces a contraction of the underlying or surrounding muscles (comparable with the corneal reflex).

Abdominal reflexes

A pin is drawn briskly but lightly across the four quadrants of the abdomen in sequence, from outside inwards, running down along the line of the derma-tomes. The stroke should not be so firm as to scratch the skin of the abdomen. The abdominal muscles are seen to contract in response to the stimulus.

Cremasteric reflexes

A brisk stroke on the inner side of the thigh produces contraction of the cremasteric muscle, causing the testis to retract.

Bulbocavernosus reflex

A sharp squeeze or gentle pinprick applied to the glans penis induces a contraction in the bulbocavernosus muscle which can be felt in the perineum at the base of the penis.

Anal reflex

A stroke or pinprick in the circumanal region induces contraction of the external sphincter which can be seen (or felt by a finger per rectum). The bulbocavernosus and anal reflexes are important to test in patients with sphincter disturbance, impotence or other symptoms suggesting a cauda equina or conus lesion.

Plantar responses

The lateral aspect of the sole (S1 dermatome) is stimulated by a firm stroke with a blunt object and the movement of the great toe is observed. The normal response of adults and children over the age of 12 months is flexion of the great toe (flexor plantar response). If flexor reflexes are released by damage to cortico-reticulospinal pathways, as happens in most upper motor neurone lesions, the great toe extends as it does normally in infancy. Extension of the great toe (extensor plantar response, upgoing toe or positive Babinski response) is often accompanied by abduction of the other toes. Although the movement of the great toe is extension in anatomical terms, it is part of a flexor protective reflex in physiological terms. This can be clearly seen in patients with an upper motor neurone lesion of the spinal cord (which releases flexor reflexes from brain-stem control), in which case repeated stroking of the sole causes first a Babinski response, then dorsiflexion of the ankle as well, then flexion of the entire lower limb which becomes more marked with each stroke of the sole (flexor spasms).

The presence and the briskness of reflexes is indicated by the following symbols:

0 or −   absent
+   diminished
++   normal
+++   increased
++++   clonus present

Normal reflexes, the segments that mediate them and the way in which they are recorded, are listed in Table 5.1. The jaw jerk is included here because it is of relevance to the level of an upper motor neurone lesion, but other cranial nerve reflexes have been omitted.

An extensor plantar response is indicated by a reversed arrow (↑). Primitive reflexes released in frontal lobe disorders include pouting and sucking responses, grasp reflexes and the palmar-mental response (contraction of the chin muscles ipsilateral to a firm stroke across the thenar eminence).

COORDINATION

If position sense and motor pathways are intact, coordination tests assess cerebellar function (see also Chapter 8).

Upper limbs

The following tests of coordination are commonly used:

Rhythmic repetitive movement

Tapping the fingers rapidly on a table or other surface for instance. Dysrhythmia may be heard as well as seen.

Alternating movements

Tapping the opposite hand or thigh with pronation-supination of the wrist for example. If speed decreases and amplitude of hand movement increases as the alternating movement continues, this is known as *dysdiadochokinesia.*

Rebound phenomenon

The patient is asked to elevate the extended arms briskly in front of the body and halt them in a given position. In cerebellar disorders, the movement is slow to start and slow to stop so that the affected limb shoots past the intended endpoint (*rebound phenomenon*).

Finger–nose test

The patient is asked to touch the tip of his nose, then touch the examiner's finger which is held in front of the patient, then to touch his own nose again. The movement should be performed slowly, then rapidly, to bring out any possible defect. Abnormalities that may be noted are: (i) dysmetria — the finger falls short of the target or exceeds it (past-pointing) or deviates to one side or the other (usually to the side of a cerebellar lesion); (ii) action tremor — a tremor accompanies the movement throughout its duration. Action tremor is not of cerebellar origin and must not be confused with intention tremor; (iii) intention tremor — the amplitude of tremor increases as the target is approached.

Lower limbs

Rapid tapping movement of the feet

The patient makes rapid voluntary movements with the foot against the examiner's hand.

Heel–knee–shin test

The patient lifts one leg, then places it on the knee and runs it down the shin of the other leg.

Toe–finger test

The patient lifts his leg so as to touch the examiner's finger, which is moved from point to point. Intention tremor may be seen.

In cases of cerebellar disturbance, certain features may have been noted earlier in the examination:

- Posture. The head may be held on one side with the occiput to the side of the lesion
- Gait. The patient may walk with a wide base and turn in a series of steps ('by numbers'), a form of decomposition of movement, or may deviate to the side of the lesion. When asked to walk on the spot with the eyes closed, the patient may rotate to one side
- Hypotonia of the affected side. If the knee jerk is tested when the patient is sitting on the examination couch with the legs suspended, the leg may swing to and fro after the reflex contraction, an undamped or pendular knee jerk
- Nystagmus
- Dysarthria

SENSORY SYSTEM

See also Chapter 6. Various forms of sensibility may be tested.

Light touch

A wisp of cotton wool is used as the testing stimulus.

Pain sensation

Superficial pain sensation is tested by pricking the skin with a pin. The patient may be asked to distinguish the sensation elicited by the sharp and blunt ends of the pin.

Temperature sensation

A cold object is applied to the skin and the sensation of coldness experienced from different areas is compared by the patient. An elaboration of this test is to use test tubes filled with water at 7° C above and below the skin temperature, so that the patient can detect the difference between heat and cold in various areas.

Proprioception

This is often called 'joint position sense' but also depends on muscle afferent fibres. It is tested by asking patients (with eyes closed) to state the direction of movement taking place at a joint when it is passively moved by the examiner. Movements at distal joints of toes and fingers are commonly tested but, if proprioceptive loss is gross, movement at wrist or elbow, ankle or knee may have to be tested. If the upper limbs can be maintained in a constant outstretched posture without drifting away and without unintended movements of the fingers, it is unlikely that formal examination will discern any proprioceptive loss in the upper limbs.

Vibration sense

This is examined by placing the base of the vibrating tuning fork (128 Hz) on bony prominences such as the terminal interphalangeal joints of fingers and toes. Normally, vibration sense is preserved at these distal joints but if not it should be tested at more proximal joints such as ankles, knees, wrists and elbows.

Two-point discrimination

The pulps of the finger should be able to distinguish two points separated by 3 mm and the sole or dorsum of the foot if the separation of the points is increased to 3 cm.

Stereognosis

The ability to distinguish the size or texture of small objects is tested by placing coins or various materials in each hand while the patient's eyes are closed.

Figure writing (graphaesthesia)

A test of fine sensibility similar to stereognosis is to trace on the patient's skin a figure between 1 and 9, which should be identified by the patient with eyes closed.

In practice, these tests are not necessarily all employed in examination of every patient. Sensory testing is guided by the history. If the patient has experienced paraesthesiae or numbness in a certain area, that area is tested first and compared with the nearest adjacent normal area. The pin or other testing object is then advanced from the area of sensory impairment toward the normal area until a line of demarcation is reached where sensation becomes normal. In this way, the distribution of sensory loss can be mapped rapidly and determined to be of peripheral, spinal root, spinal cord or cerebral origin.

GENERAL EXAMINATION

Other systems should also be examined in the normal way with particular emphasis on examination of the pulse, heart, abdomen and lymph glands. The blood pressure must always be recorded, in both lying and standing positions if there have been symptoms of postural hypotension. The radial pulses are asymmetrical in subclavian stenosis and a bruit may be heard above the clavicle. The blood pressure should be recorded in each arm separately in patients with suspected cerebral vascular insufficiency. The texture of the skin, distribution of body hair, testicular size and breast development are indicators of pituitary function which may be impaired by tumours in or near the pituitary gland or by a longstanding increase in intracranial pressure. Testicular atrophy is found in dystrophia myotonica.

REFERENCE

Aids to the Examination of the Peripheral Nervous System (1986). Baillière-Tindall, London.

3 | Focal cerebral lesions and speech

Lesions in different anatomical sites of the cerebral hemispheres have specific clinical features.

FRONTAL LOBES

The frontal lobes are usually divided into the precentral region or motor cortex, and the prefrontal region.

Prefrontal lobes (areas 9, 10, 11, 12, 13)

Information concerning the function of the prefrontal lobes comes largely from studies on patients with gunshot wounds and other injuries, and from patients subjected to prefrontal leucotomies. Clinical features of prefrontal changes are:

Personality change
Loss of insight; carelessness about appearance, dress and habits; shallowness of emotion; jocularity, facetiousness and making simple jokes and puns; lowering of intelligence, difficulty in concentrating, impairment of judgement and of grasping situations as a whole; difficulty in changing from one mental activity to another, repetition of phrases (*palilalia*) or words (*echolalia*).

Grasp reflex
This is a primitive reflex, normally found only in infants, that consists of flexion of thumb and fingers on stroking the skin of the palm between thumb and index fingers. It becomes disinhibited in frontal lobe lesions.

Sucking and pouting reflexes
These are other primitive reflexes that become disinhibited. Lightly stroking the lips produces a sucking movement, and tapping the closed lips causes contraction of the circumoral muscles ('pouting').

Tonic innervation or perseveration
This is a persistence of muscular contraction which may be seen, for example, in a failure to relax the grip or in the repetition of an action after it has become inappropriate.

Incontinence

The patient may be unconcerned by this and urinate in inappropriate places.

Epileptic seizures

These may be a symptom of frontal lobe tumours, infarcts and other lesions.

Unilateral anosmia

This may result from meningiomas of the olfactory groove (p. 42).

Unilateral optic atrophy with papilloedema in the other eye

This is also known as Foster-Kennedy syndrome and may result from frontal lobe tumours (p. 48).

Incoordination and ataxia (Brun's frontal ataxia)

This may occur and is probably caused by interruption of the cortico-ponto-cerebellar pathways (Chapter 8).

Frontal apraxia of gait

This may result from bilateral parasagittal frontal lesions. The patient can make walking movements while lying down but is unable to walk spontaneously while standing.

Precentral region (areas 4 and 6)

Lesions in the precentral region of the frontal lobe involving the motor areas characteristically cause:

Weakness in the form of a hemiparesis or monoparesis

This will depend on the site of the lesion.

Expressive aphasia

If the posterior part of the third frontal gyrus in the dominant lobe is involved, expressive or Broca's aphasia results (Fig. 3.1).

Jacksonian (focal motor) fits with an irritative lesion

If the frontal adversive fields (area 8) are involved, the head and eyes will deviate, usually to the opposite side.

Complex partial seizures

These may occur with irritative lesions in the supplementary motor area.

TEMPORAL LOBES

Temporal lobe lesions cause the following:

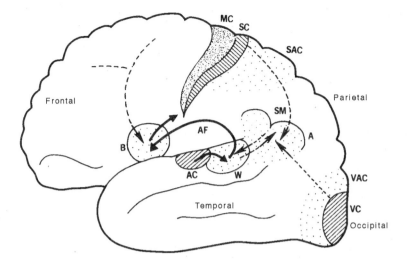

Fig. 3.1   The neurological basis for language skills.

Speech: The basic speech circuit comprises: primary auditory cortex (AC), association cortex (Wernicke's area, W), arcuate fasciculus (AF), Broca's area (B), motor cortex (MC) and corticobulbar pathways. This circuit is responsible for repetition of the spoken word and is influenced by input from dominant frontal and parietal lobes.

Language: The supramarginal (SM) and angular (A) gyri form a language integrating centre with afferent inflow from the visual cortex (VC) and visual association cortex (VAC) for the interpretation of the written word, from Wernicke's area for the spoken word and from the sensory cortex (SC) and sensory association cortex (SAC) for kinaesthetic information. Connections between the language integrating centre and the motor cortex are also responsible for writing and other motor skills.

Visual field defects

Disease of either temporal lobe may result in a superior quadrantanopia on the opposite side due to involvement of Meyer's loop (Figs 4.4, 4.6).

Aphasia

Disease involving the posterior part of the superior gyrus of the dominant temporal lobe will result in a *Wernicke's* or *receptive aphasia* i.e. difficulty in understanding spoken or written words, and jargon aphasia (Fig. 3.1).

Epilepsy

The patient may suffer from complex partial seizures (p. 187).

Hearing defects

Hearing is bilaterally represented in the transverse convolutions of Heschl in the superior temporal gyrus (Fig. 3.1). Hearing defects due to cortical lesions are very rare and are encountered only with bilateral temporal lobe lesions.

Memory disturbances

The hippocampal region of the temporal lobes is essential in laying down new memories. Bilateral hippocampal lesions result in severe memory defects, characterized by an inability to consolidate information. Unilateral lesions do not usually cause disturbance of memory.

Emotion

Emotional disturbance, such as sudden outbursts of anger, may be features of temporal lobe lesions.

PARIETAL LOBES

Lesions of the parietal lobes cause the following:

Disorders of tactile sensation

Since the parietal lobes are the main receiving area in the cerebral cortex for the somatic sensory pathways, lesions involving this area (3, 1, 2) of the brain may result in sensory impairment. Irritative lesions may result in 'sensory fits' of a Jacksonian type. Destructive lesions result in impairment of spatial and discriminative aspects of sensation, so called 'cortical sensory loss', in which there may be impairment of two-point discrimination, astereognosis (inability to recognize shape and texture of an object), impairment of position sense and tactile inattention or extinction (failure to recognize a stimulus on one side of the body when both sides are touched simultaneously). Other modalities of sensation may be intact.

Disorders of motility

Hypotonia and wasting of the contralateral limbs is occasionally seen and is referred to as 'parietal lobe wasting'.

Visual defects

Homonymous hemianopia or visual inattention to the opposite half-fields may be detected. Optokinetic nystagmus is impaired to the side of the lesion (p. 60).

Gerstmann's syndrome

In dominant parietal lobe lesions there may be agraphia (impairment of ability to write), acalculia (inability to calculate), finger agnosia (inability to recognize and identify fingers correctly), and left-right disorientation. These four clinical features are together known as Gerstmann's syndrome. This is rarely seen in its fully developed form but isolated components of the syndrome are common in parietal lobe lesions. There may also be dyslexia (difficulty in reading) and an ideomotor apraxia.

Apraxias

Apraxia is the inability to carry out a purposive movement, the nature of which the patient understands, when there is no accompanying motor impairment, sensory loss or ataxia. The following types of apraxia are recognized:

Ideomotor apraxia   The patient has no difficulty in formulating the idea of a simple act that he is instructed to carry out, but he finds himself unable to execute it. Thus he may not protrude his tongue to command, but will spontaneously lick his lips; he cannot make a fist, but he can grasp an object spontaneously.

Ideational apraxia   This is a disturbance of more complicated tasks, e.g. putting on a hat, pouring out a glass of water.

Ideomotor and ideational apraxia are caused by lesions of the parietal or medial frontal lobes, particularly in the dominant hemisphere. Lesions of the corpus callosum may also produce an ideational apraxia.

Dressing apraxia   This is difficulty in putting on garments correctly and is usually due to a lesion of the non-dominant parietal lobe. It is closely related to constructional apraxia.

Constructional apraxia   This is a disorder of visuo-spatial function. The patient has difficulty in drawing common objects (e.g. a bicycle), or copying designs with matchsticks or blocks. This is caused most commonly by a non-dominant parietal lobe lesion, but may also be seen in dominant lobe lesions. Patients with dressing and constructional apraxias frequently have difficulty with navigation. This may range from difficulty with reversing a car to an inability in finding the way out of a room.

Disorders of the body image

These are usually associated with lesions of the non-dominant parietal lobe. There may be unilateral neglect of the opposite side which may be motor, sensory or visual. Hemiplegic patients may ignore the paralysed limb (*auto-topagnosia*) or even deny their hemiplegia (*anosagnosia*). The non-dominant parietal lobe appears to serve the same function for visuo-spatial integration as the dominant parietal area does for speech.

OCCIPITAL LOBES

Lesions of the occipital lobes characteristically result in visual field defects (Fig. 4.6). A destructive lesion involving the whole of one occipital lobe will result in a congruous contralateral homonymous hemianopia. Bilateral occipital lesions will result in cortical blindness with preservation of pupillary reflexes, a clinical state that may be difficult to distinguish from hysteria. Some patients with bilateral lesions may be unaware of, or deny, their blindness (*Anton's syndrome*). Lesions involving visual association areas 18 and 19 will result in the inability to recognize faces or objects even though they can be seen (visual agnosia). Irritative lesions of the primary visual cortex may cause epileptic fits with an unformed visual aura (coloured or flashing lights), while formed hallucinations may be evoked from the visual association cortex.

SPEECH DISORDERS

ANATOMY AND PHYSIOLOGY

In 1861 Paul Broca pointed out that disturbed language output results from damage to a specific area of the brain; the posterior part of the third frontal gyrus of the dominant hemisphere (*Broca's area*). This area lies immediately in front of the cortical region supplying the muscles of the face, jaw, tongue, palate and larynx, in other words, the muscles of speech production.

In 1874 Carl Wernicke described an area at a site in the left hemisphere in the posterior aspect of the superior temporal gyrus adjacent to the auditory area. Damage to Wernicke's area results in loss of comprehension of speech.

Wernicke's and Broca's areas are connected by a bundle of nerve fibres, the arcuate fasciculus. When a word is heard, the output from the primary auditory area is received by Wernicke's area. If the word is spoken, the pattern is transmitted from Wernicke's area to Broca's area and then on to the motor area that controls the speech muscles. Interconnections with other areas in the parietal lobe of the dominant hemisphere are necessary for reading and spelling (Fig. 3.1).

The left hemisphere is dominant (i.e. concerned with language function) in over 90% of right-handed people. In left-handed people the left hemisphere is dominant in more than 50%, so that only a small number of people have a dominant right hemisphere.

Motor pathways for speech

The descending motor pathways for articulation are: (i) the corticobulbar tracts which arise from the precentral gyrus and travel to the fifth, seventh and twelfth cranial nerve nuclei and to the nucleus ambiguus: (ii) the corticospinal tracts to the diaphragm and intercostal muscles. The cerebellum and basal ganglia also play a role in the coordination of articulation.

DEVELOPMENT OF SPEECH

The understanding of language begins in infancy well before speech emerges. The successful development of speech requires normal hearing.

Vocalization develops during the first year. The first words normally appear at about 12 months of age. By 2 years of age the average child will understand several hundred words and regularly use some 200. However very wide individual variations occur and a few normal children may use only a dozen or so words by their second birthday.

The average age of first using two-word phrases is 18 months and by 2 years of age nearly 90% are using simple word sequences. Girls are usually slightly more advanced than boys in language development.

Delayed speech

There may be a delay in learning to speak up to the age of 3–3½ years (developmental delay) that is not explicable by any demonstrable anatomical, auditory, intellectual, metabolic or psychiatric disturbance. This condition is compatible with a high order of intelligence, and motor and social development proceeds normally. Comprehension of speech is frequently normal. A positive family history is often obtained. Boys are affected about three times as frequently as girls, and a proportion of them have difficulty later in learning to read, write and spell. A speech therapist should be consulted for children who are not putting two words together by 2 years of age. Defective hearing is another important cause of delayed speech that should be identified early in life to enable therapeutic intervention.

Mental retardation is a common cause of delayed speech; brain damage and psychiatric disturbances are other important causes of delayed speech.

Developmental dyslexia

Developmental dyslexia is a difficulty in learning to read, displayed by normally intelligent children who have intact sensory mechanisms and are not emotionally disturbed, and has been estimated to affect 10–20% of primary school children. There is no underlying structural lesion of the brain. In addition to the reading disability the child often has difficulty in writing. Intensive intervention may alter the course of this disorder.

APHASIA

Aphasia is a disorder of the higher language functions of speech. Several different types are recognized.

Expressive (Broca's) aphasia

Lesions of Broca's area in the posterior part of the third frontal gyrus of the dominant hemisphere produce a *non-fluent aphasia*. There is a sparse output of words and the speech that is produced is uttered slowly, with great effort and poor articulation. It lacks small grammatical words and endings and most of the words used are nouns or verbs, so that it takes on a telegraphic quality. Asked about the weather, such a patient may say 'sunny', and if urged to produce a full sentence he may say 'weather... sunny'. Broca's aphasia is usually associated with hemiparesis. The speech lacks normal rhythm and melody (*dysprosody*).

Receptive (Wernicke's) aphasia

Wernicke's aphasia is caused by lesions in Wernicke's area in the posterior part of the superior temporal gyrus in the dominant hemisphere. It is a *fluent aphasia*: the patient produces well articulated, long phrases or sentences with a normal grammatical skeleton, having normal rhythm and melody. Speech may be faster than normal. However, the speech is abnormal in that its content is defective. Circumlocution, non-specific words (e.g. 'thing') and incorrect words are all used. The term *paraphasia* is used to describe the substitution of syllables (phonemic substitution), or words which are often nonsense words. Patients with Wernicke's aphasia have a failure of understanding and an inability to repeat simple phrases. Comprehension of written language, as well as spoken language, may be affected. Wernicke's aphasia, if produced by a stroke, has a good prognosis and substantial spontaneous recovery often occurs.

Nominal aphasia

This is an inability to name objects. It occurs in the recovery phase of most aphasias, but also in a pure form with lesions in the parieto-temporal region of the dominant hemisphere.

Transcortical aphasia

In this disorder the ability to repeat test phrases is intact because the basic speech circuit of Wernicke's area → arcuate fasciculus → Broca's area is spared. There is impairment of spontaneous speech because the input from frontal and parietal areas of the cortex to the basic speech circuit is prevented by a transcortical lesion. This disturbance is most often encountered with a 'watershed infarction' at the junction of middle cerebral and anterior cerebral arterial territories.

Conduction aphasia

This is a result of a lesion localized to the arcuate fasciculus. Spontaneous speech is impaired by substitutions, but comprehension is good in contrast to transcortical aphasia. Repetition is impaired.

DYSARTHRIA

Dysarthria is a disorder of articulation. The motor pathways for the production of sound are disordered but the patient has no difficulty in comprehending or expressing himself in writing or by gesture. He has no difficulty in the mental formation of words or sentences, nor any difficulty in the handling of verbal symbols.

Dysarthria must be distinguished from aphasia. A simple rule of thumb is that when speech is transcribed, correct English sentences are produced in dysarthria but not in dysphasia.

Cortical lesions

On occasion, small areas of damage in the area of the motor strip in the dominant hemisphere that subserves the muscles of articulation can produce distorted speech without aphasia.

Upper motor neurone lesions

Since the muscles of articulation are bilaterally innervated, it is usually necessary to damage both corticobulbar tracts in order to cause spastic dysarthria. Bilateral capsular lesions, brain-stem vascular lesions, motor neurone disease and multiple sclerosis are some of the possible aetiological factors in this type of speech disorder.

On examination, the jaw jerk and facial reflexes are found to be brisk; the tongue may appear small and contracted and cannot be fully protruded; swallowing may be affected, and there may be emotional lability.

The complete syndrome is sometimes called *pseudobulbar palsy*. The speech is slow and forced and the patient has particular difficulty in enunciating labial and dental sounds.

Extrapyramidal lesions

In Parkinson's disease, articulation is slow and slurred and the speech is monotonous, lacking inflection and low in volume.

In both spastic dysarthria and extrapyramidal disorders, but especially the former, there is usually poor coordination of the respiratory muscles and diaphragm, so that speech is often in short, breathless sentences.

In athetosis (e.g. in cerebral palsy from birth hypoxia) the voice is slow, consonants are pronounced poorly if at all and speech is accompanied by inappropriate involuntary movements.

Cerebellar lesions — ataxic dysarthria

Coordination of articulation becomes impaired. The speech is slow and slurred and there may be an unnatural separation of syllables ('scanning speech'). This is seen in multiple sclerosis, Friedreich's ataxia and cerebellar degenerations.

Lower motor neurone lesions

The tongue becomes wasted, the palate weak, and the facial muscles incapable of adequate movements. This condition is known as *bulbar palsy* and can occur in poliomyelitis, motor neurone disease, medullary tumours and syringobulbia. Phonation may also be impaired and the speech becomes slurred and indistinct. Labial sounds usually suffer first. In palatal palsy, speech has a nasal quality and there is difficulty with sounds such as 'ing' and 'egg'.

Myopathies

Myopathies and myasthenia result in similar disturbances to bulbar palsy. In myasthenia the speech disturbance becomes apparent after the patient speaks for some time.

DYSPHONIA

This is an inability to approximate the vocal cords normally for speech or coughing, giving a husky or gravelly quality to the voice. It occurs in bulbar palsy, recurrent laryngeal nerve paralysis and rarely as a focal dystonia which may be mistaken for an hysterical manifestation.

EXAMINATION OF THE PATIENT WITH A SPEECH DISORDER

Disorders of speech are distressing to the patient since they severely impair the ability to communicate and to play a useful role in life. It requires patience on the part of the physician to make contact with such patients and to elucidate the nature of their condition.

The first thing to determine is the nature of the speech disorder. If it is aphasia, the following outline of examination is useful:

- Ensure that the patient is alert, mentally clear and intellectually unimpaired. Examination periods should be limited to 15–20 minutes because fatigue interferes with responses to tests.
- Determine whether the patient is right- or left-handed when writing or playing games
- Estimate the probable level of education for reading and writing
- Note spontaneous speech. Is it slow or fast, fluent or non-fluent? Is it grammatical?
- Can the patient understand spoken language? Test the response to simple verbal commands, e.g. put out your tongue, close your eyes, put your right hand on your head, touch your right ear with your left hand
- Can the patient repeat words and sentences?

- Can the patient read? Make sure there are no organic visual defects. Test the understanding of simple written commands. Give the patient sentences from newspapers and books to read
- Can the patient write? Test spontaneous writing, e.g. name and address, letter to a relative. See if the patient can write to dictation and copy
- Can he name common objects?

REFERENCES

Adams R. D. and Victor M. (1993) *Principles of Neurology*, 5th edn. McGraw-Hill, New York.

Damasio A. R. (1992) Aphasia. *New England Journal of Medicine*, **326**, 531–539.

Geschwind N. (1965) Disconnection syndromes in animals and man. *Brain*, **88**, 237–294, 585–644.

Mesulam M-M. (1985) *Principles of Behavioural Neurology*. F. A. Davis, Philadelphia.

4 | Cranial nerves

CRANIAL NERVE I: THE OLFACTORY NERVE

The olfactory portion of the nasal mucous membrane contains bipolar cells, the central processes of which form the olfactory filaments that pass through the cribriform plate to the olfactory bulb. The olfactory tract runs back and divides into medial and lateral olfactory striae; central connections are made in the prepyriform area, amygdala and other structures.

The sense of smell is tested separately at each nostril with test odours, e.g. tobacco, coffee, peppermint and cloves. Pungent and irritating test substances such as ammonia should be avoided, since they stimulate the trigeminal nerve endings.

Loss of sense of smell (anosmia) may result from: (i) local causes, e.g. colds, sinusitis, deviated nasal septum; (ii) head injury, with or without fracture of bone, causing damage to the olfactory filaments as they pass through the cribriform plate; (iii) meningiomas, gliomas and other tumours in the anterior cranial fossa which directly involve the olfactory bulb and central pathways; (iv) meningitis, acute or chronic, which damages the olfactory filaments.

CRANIAL NERVE II: THE OPTIC NERVE

Light falls on the rods and cones of the retina, which lie on its outermost layer. Impulses are transmitted from these end-organs through a relay of bipolar cells to the ganglion cell fibres which enter the optic nerve.

The macula, on the temporal side of the optic disc, is the area of the retina specialized for central vision and the perception of detailed images; it has a high concentration of cones and contains no rods.

An object in the left temporal field of vision will cast an image on the right temporal and left nasal retinae. An object in the upper field of vision will cast an image on the inferior retinal quadrants.

Fibres from the temporal region of the retina course through the temporal half of the optic nerve, the upper temporal fibres lying in its upper temporal quadrant. The nasal half of the retina is represented in the nasal half of the optic nerve. The macular fibres occupy a central position (Fig. 4.1).

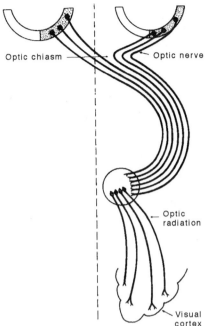

Fig. 4.1   Visual pathways.

In the *optic chiasm* the nasal fibres from each retina cross while those from the temporal halves remain uncrossed. The crossed and uncrossed fibres unite to form the optic tracts (Fig. 4.1).

The anatomical relations of the optic chiasm are important (Figs 4.2, 4.3). Above it lies the cavity of the third ventricle and on its lateral aspects are the internal carotid arteries before they divide into the anterior and middle cerebral vessels. Anterior to the chiasm lie the anterior cerebral vessels and the anterior communicating artery. Posteriorly lies the interpeduncular fossa area, and below lies the pituitary gland in the sella turcica.

In the optic tracts, the fibres from the lower retinal quadrants are laterally placed and those from the upper retinal quadrants are medial.

The fibres from the optic tracts pass back to the *lateral geniculate body*, from where they relay to the *visual cortex* in the occipital lobes by way of the *optic radiation* (geniculo-calcarine tract; Fig. 4.1). This tract is situated posteriorly in the internal capsule. The lowermost fibres of the optic radiation pass over the antero-superior aspect of the temporal horn of the lateral ventricle (Meyer's loop). These fibres are derived from the inferior quadrants of the corresponding hemiretinae (Fig. 4.4).

The remainder of the optic radiation passes through the parietal lobes close to the temporal and occipital horns of the lateral ventricle to terminate in the visual or striate cortex (area 17) which lies on either side of the calcarine fissure. The uppermost fibres of the optic radiation terminate in the upper lip (cuneus); the

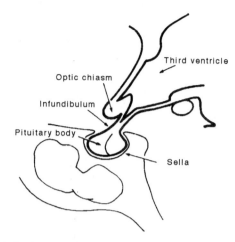

Fig. 4.2   Anatomical relations of the optic chiasm in the sagittal plane.

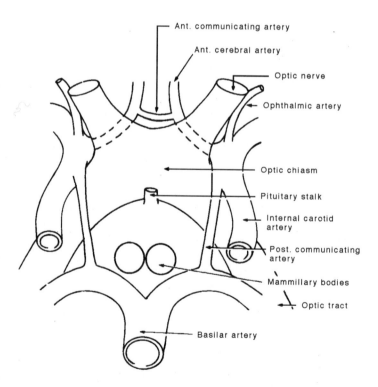

Fig. 4.3   Anatomical relations of the optic chiasm viewed from below.

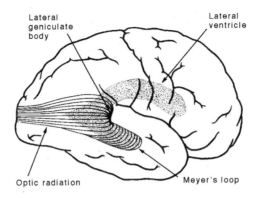

Fig. 4.4   Optic radiation. (Modified from Ranson and Clark 1959, *The Anatomy of the Nervous System*, 10th edn. W. B. Saunders, Philadelphia.)

lowermost fibres terminate in the lower lip (lingual gyrus). The macular area is represented posteriorly, and the most peripheral parts of the retina are represented anteriorly in the visual cortex (Fig. 4.5).

The blood supply of the visual cortex is derived chiefly from the posterior cerebral artery, but the middle cerebral vessels may supply the tip of the occipital pole thus accounting for macular sparing in some cases of posterior cerebral artery occlusion.

The examination of the second cranial nerve includes testing of visual acuity, ophthalmoscopic examination and charting of the visual fields. It is described in detail in Chapter 2.

Anatomical classification of visual field defects

Some of the more common types of visual field defect are shown in Fig. 4.6.

Retina
Detachment of the retina, retinitis pigmentosa and glaucoma give rise to characteristic field defects. An island in the visual field where vision is absent or defective is known as a 'scotoma'.

Optic nerve
In papilloedema (pp. 47–48), the blind spot is increased in size and later the peripheral field becomes uniformly diminished. In optic neuritis (p. 49), central or paracentral scotomata may develop. Complete lesions of the optic nerve result in total blindness of the affected eye.

Chiasmal lesions
The most common lesions of the chiasm are those caused by pressure from tumours arising either in the pituitary fossa or above the sella, such as, suprasellar cysts, craniopharyngiomas and meningiomas (Figs 4.2, 4.3). The chiasm may also

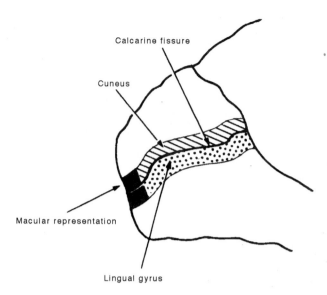

Calcarine fissure

Cuneus

Macular representation

Lingual gyrus

Fig. 4.5 Visual cortex. (Modified from Ranson and Clark 1959, *The Anatomy of the Nervous System*, 10th edn. W. B. Saunders, Philadelphia.)

be invaded by gliomas, it may be compressed by the third ventricle in obstructive hydrocephalus (Fig. 4.2), or it may be compressed by an enlarging aneurysm on one of the nearby arteries (Fig. 4.3).

Pressure in the mid-line, initially involving crossing fibres, gives rise to a bitemporal hemianopia (Fig. 4.6). If pressure is from below, inferior nasal fibres will be involved first, giving a bitemporal superior quadrantanopia. If pressure is from above, an inferior quadrantanopia will result.

Pressure effects from tumours however are rarely symmetrical. Some tumours compress one optic nerve together with crossing fibres from the other eye, thus giving rise to a scotoma in one eye and a superior temporal quadrantanopia in the other. Asymmetry of the visual field defects is the rule in chiasmal lesions.

Optic tracts

The optic tracts may be compressed by pituitary tumours, temporal lobe tumours, aneurysms and other expanding lesions. Homonymous hemianopia results, but it is usually incongruous (i.e. it is not bilaterally symmetrical) and incomplete.

Optic radiation

Lesions of the optic radiation result in homonymous field defects. Lesions in the temporal lobe may involve Meyer's loop, causing a superior homonymous quadrantanopia on the contralateral side (Fig. 4.6). Lesions in the parietal lobe may cause an inferior homonymous quadrantanopia or inattention to the opposite half-field. Complete homonymous hemianopia may result from a more extensive lesion.

When there is a lesion of the striate cortex of one occipital lobe, such as infarction following occlusion of one posterior cerebral artery, a contralateral symmetrical (congruous) homonymous hemianopia will be present (Fig 4.6). When the striate cortex of both occipital lobes is affected, usually by an infarct resulting from occlusion of the basilar artery (of which both posterior cerebral arteries are terminal branches), *cortical blindness* results. A characteristic feature of this condition is that patients may deny or be unaware of their loss of vision (Anton's syndrome). Since the reflex pathways for the pupillary reflexes are not involved, and therefore the pupils react normally to light, the condition can be misdiagnosed as hysterical blindness. Cortical blindness may be a transient phenomenon in migraine and may follow a relatively minor head injury in children and adolescents.

Papilloedema

Papilloedema refers to oedema of the optic papilla or disc, without reference to its underlying cause. It is commonly caused by raised intracranial pressure.

The optic nerve is a direct extension of the central nervous system. The dura mater fuses with the periosteum of the orbit, and the pia mater and arachnoid

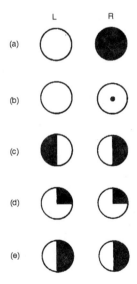

Fig. 4.6 Field defects: (a) right optic nerve lesion; (b) right central scotoma e.g. retrobulbar neuritis; (c) bitemporal hemianopia caused by a chiasmal lesion; (d) right superior quandrantanopia resulting from a left temporal lobe lesion; (e) right homonymous hemianopia from a deep left hemisphere or left occipital lobe lesion.

mater fuse with the sclera. The optic nerve is therefore surrounded by the sub-arachnoid space, and a rise in central cerebrospinal fluid pressure is freely conducted to the optic subarachnoid space (Fig. 4.7).

Early signs of papilloedema are distension of the veins, loss of venous pulsation and blurring of the upper and lower disc margins; the temporal margin is last to become blurred. The next stage is filling in of the physiological cup and elevation of the disc above the retinal levels. Oedema may spread out like a fan across the retina and haemorrhages may appear around the disc. Eventually secondary optic atrophy follows. Causes of papilloedema include:

- Intracranial neoplasms, especially of the posterior fossa or temporal lobe. Papilloedema occurs less commonly in slow growing tumours when pressure readjustments occur. A tumour near one optic foramen compressing the optic nerve may protect that nerve from raised intracranial pressure resulting in unilateral optic atrophy with papilloedema in the opposite eye (Foster--Kennedy syndrome)
- Abscesses, subdural haematomas and other space-occupying lesions
- Hydrocephalus from any cause including meningitis and subarachnoid haemorrhage
- Intracranial venous thrombosis
- Benign intracranial hypertension (pp. 262–263)
- Metabolic disorders, e.g. hypoparathyroidism, emphysema
- Malignant hypertension
- Ischaemic optic neuropathy from disease of the posterior ciliary artery which supplies the area around the optic disc (Fig. 4.7)

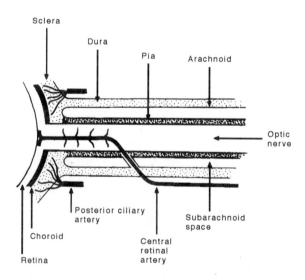

Fig. 4.7   Pial membranes and subarachnoid space surrounding optic nerve. (Modified from Hayreh, S.S., *Transactions of the American Academy of Ophthalmology and Otolaryngology* 1974, **78**, OP241–54.)

Optic neuritis

Optic neuritis is an inflammation of the optic nerve. If the inflammation is sufficiently anterior to cause swelling of the optic disc, the appearance is described as *papillitis*. If it is situated more posteriorly so that the direct effects of inflammation are not visible ophthalmoscopically it is called *retrobulbar neuritis*. The symptoms of optic neuritis are usually blurring or dimness of vision, pain in and behind the eye and pain on eye movement. Examination reveals impaired visual acuity and colour vision, a central or paracentral scotoma, and a relative afferent pupillary defect (Marcus Gunn pupil; p. 19).

The most important and common cause of optic neuritis is multiple sclerosis (Chapter 20); about 50–60% of patients with optic neuritis will eventually develop multiple sclerosis. Other causes include neuromyelitis optica, herpes zoster and other viral infections, meningitis and encephalitis, but in many cases no cause is determined.

Optic atrophy

Optic atrophy is the result of degeneration of optic nerve fibres. Clinically, there is impaired visual acuity, poor colour vision, a central or paracentral scotoma in the visual field and pallor of the optic disc on ophthalmoscopic examination.

Causes include: (i) compression of optic nerves by tumours, aneurysms; (i) optic neuritis, most commonly in multiple sclerosis; (iii) papilloedema, with secondary optic atrophy; (iv) toxic causes (e.g. tobacco, lead, alcohol); (v) vitamin deficiencies (e.g. pernicious anaemia); (vi) hereditary causes (e.g. Leber's optic atrophy and some hereditary ataxias); (vii) other causes such as trauma, syphilis, retinal artery occlusion (with secondary optic atrophy) and retinal degeneration.

CRANIAL NERVES III, IV AND VI

The third, fourth and sixth cranial nerves innervate the extra-ocular muscles. Their chief function is to control ocular movement.

Ocular movements

The ocular movements are carried out by three pairs of muscles: superior and inferior recti; medial and lateral recti; superior and inferior oblique muscles. In order to understand the function of individual muscles it is necessary to know their planes of action.

The medial and lateral recti move the eye in a horizontal plane, parallel to the floor of the orbit. The superior and inferior recti move the eye in a vertical plane when the eye is turned outwards. If the eye is turned inwards the superior and inferior recti act as rotators of the eye (Fig. 4.8).

The superior and inferior oblique muscles act in a vertical plane when the eye is turned inwards; the superior oblique then acts as a pure depressor and

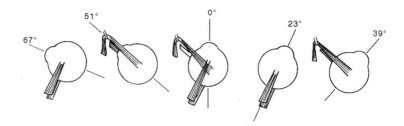

Fig. 4.8 The positions and actions of the superior and inferior rectus muscles, and superior and inferior oblique muscles, in different positions of gaze of the right eye. (Modified from Cogan, 1956.)

the inferior oblique as an elevator. If the eye is turned outwards the superior and inferior oblique muscles act as rotators of the eye (Fig. 4.8).

From a practical point of view, when testing the actions of the eye muscles, the superior oblique depresses the eye and the inferior oblique elevates it when the eye is turned inwards; the superior rectus elevates and the inferior rectus depresses the eye when it is turned outwards. The actions of the medial and lateral recti are to adduct and abduct the eye in the horizontal plane, respectively, (Fig. 4.9).

The oculomotor (III) nerve innervates the superior rectus, medial rectus, inferior rectus and inferior oblique; the trochlear (IV) nerve supplies the superior oblique and the abducens (VI) nerve innervates the lateral rectus muscle.

Squint or strabismus

This is the term applied to lack of parallelism of the visual axes of the two eyes. It is important to distinguish between a *paralytic squint*, which is caused by weakness or paralysis of an ocular muscle, and a *non-paralytic* or *concomitant* squint which is often congenital and is caused by ocular muscle imbalance.

Paralytic squint   A paralytic squint may become apparent only on horizontal or vertical eye movements. It is accompanied by double vision (diplopia) in the direction of the gaze of the weakened muscle.

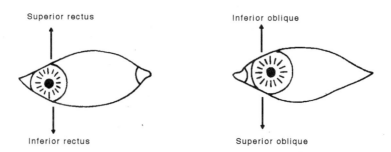

Fig. 4.9 Direction of action of the ocular muscles. (From Lance and McLeod, 1981, with permission of Butterworths, London.)

Non-paralytic squint   This is present when both eyes are at rest and is equal for all positions of the eye. The term *esotropia* refers to one eye being adducted at rest while *exotropia* refers to the eye being in the abducted position at rest. If the fixing eye is covered, the movements of the affected eye are full. A non-paralytic squint is usually not associated with diplopia.

Diplopia

Diplopia, or double vision, occurs when there is paresis of one or more ocular muscles. Because the image is projected into the macula of one eye and into some other part of the retina of the other eye, the patient will see two objects since the images are not falling on the corresponding part of both retinae as they normally do. If a horizontally acting muscle is weak, the patient will report that the images are side-by-side; if a vertical muscle is weak, then one image will be above the other.

Clinically, the paretic muscle is most easily determined by asking the patient to follow the examiner's finger with the eyes as it is moved in different directions. Find the position of gaze in which the two images are maximally separated. Then: (i) the direction in which separation is greatest is the direction of action of the paralysed muscle; (ii) the more peripheral of the two images is the false image and is seen by the affected eye. If, for instance, the right lateral rectus muscle is paralysed, the two images will be separated maximally when the eyes are deviated to the right and the false image will be the one on the extreme right. If the patient has difficulty in distinguishing the real image from the false image, covering one eye with a red glass enables the source of the images to be identified.

III Oculomotor nerve

The nucleus of the third nerve lies in the mid-brain at the level of the superior colliculus (Figs 4.10, 4.11). It consists of: (i) the main oculomotor nucleus, which is the motor nucleus for the medial rectus, superior rectus, inferior rectus, inferior oblique and levator palpebrae superioris muscles; (ii) Edinger-Westphal nucleus which controls pupillary constriction.

The oculomotor nerve passes through the red nucleus to emerge from the mid-brain in the angle between the cerebral peduncles and the pons (Fig. 4.11). It then passes forwards between the posterior cerebral and the superior cerebellar arteries, close to the posterior communicating artery (Fig. 13.2) to enter the cavernous sinus through the dura mater near the posterior clinoid process (Figs 4.10, 4.12, 13.2). It then passes through the cavernous sinus and superior orbital fissure to supply the appropriate extra-ocular muscles. The nerve to the inferior oblique muscles has a parasympathetic branch which goes to the ciliary ganglion. Sympathetic fibres from the plexus around the internal carotid artery join the first division of the trigeminal nerve in the cavernous sinus.

Lesions of the third nerve

These result in varying degrees of paralysis of the muscles that it supplies. A complete lesion of the third nerve results in ptosis and paralysis of all extra-

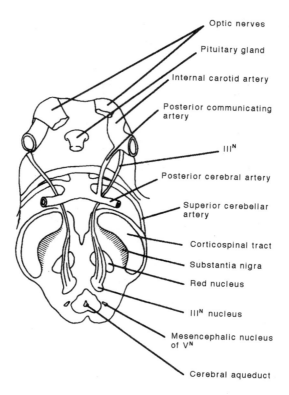

Optic nerves

Pituitary gland

Internal carotid artery

Posterior communicating
artery

III^N

Posterior cerebral artery

Superior cerebellar
artery

Corticospinal tract

Substantia nigra

Red nucleus

III^N nucleus

Mesencephalic nucleus
of V^N

Cerebral aqueduct

Fig. 4.10 Origin and course of oculomotor (III) nerve. (Modified from *Grant's Atlas of Anatomy*, 1978, 7th edn. Williams & Wilkins, Baltimore.)

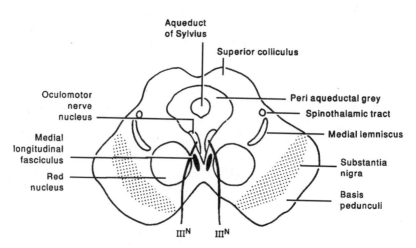

Aqueduct
of Sylvius

Superior colliculus

Oculomotor
nerve
nucleus

Peri aqueductal grey

Spinothalamic tract

Medial lemniscus

Medial
longitudinal
fasciculus

Red
nucleus

Substantia
nigra

Basis
pedunculi

III^N III^N

Fig. 4.11 Section of mid-brain at the level of superior colliculi.

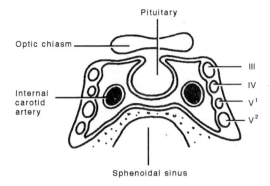

Fig. 4.12 Coronal section of the cavernous sinuses showing the position of cranial nerves in the walls.

ocular muscles except the superior oblique and the lateral rectus. The eye is deviated outwards. The pupil is widely dilated and unreactive.

The third nerve may be affected: (i) in the mid-brain, e.g. vascular lesions, glioma. Long tracts are commonly affected as well, causing a contralateral hemiplegia. The brachium conjunctivum may be involved as it passes through the red nucleus leading to cerebellar ataxia and 'red nucleus tremor'; (ii) in its intracranial course, e.g. aneurysms (usually on the posterior communicating artery), meningitis, vascular lesions (diabetes), cavernous sinus thrombosis, tumours; (iii) in the superior orbital fissure (together with the fourth nerve and first division of the fifth nerve) or within the orbit, e.g. inflammatory lesions, tumours, granulomas.

Extrinsic compressive lesions usually affect the pupilloconstrictor fibres resulting in a dilated unreactive pupil, but in an intrinsic lesion of the third nerve of vascular origin, such as occurs in diabetes or migraine, the pupil is often spared.

IV Trochlear nerve

The trochlear nerve arises from its nucleus at the level of the inferior colliculus in the mid-brain. The fibres from the nucleus course dorsally and decussate completely in the roof of the mid-brain to emerge behind the inferior colliculi (Fig. 4.13). The nerve then passes anteriorly and ventrally around the cerebral peduncles and enters the cavernous sinus through the dura below the posterior clinoid processes (Fig. 4.12). It enters the orbit through the superior orbital fissure.

Lesions of the fourth nerve

These cause paralysis of the superior oblique muscle with extorsion of the eye and weakness of downward gaze, resulting in vertical and torsional diplopia (one image is rotated with respect to the other). Patients adopt a posture with the head tilted towards the opposite shoulder. The nerve may be involved by conditions similar to those that affect the oculomotor nerve.

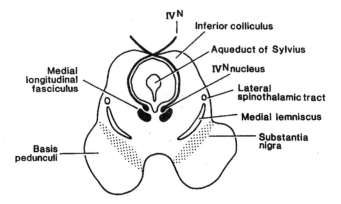

Fig. 4.13 Transverse section of mid-brain at level of the inferior colliculi showing the course of the trochlear nerve.

VI Abducens nerve

The sixth nerve nucleus is situated in the pons beneath the fourth ventricle at the level of the facial colliculus (Fig. 4.14). Fibres leave the nucleus and course anteriorly through the tegmentum of the pons to emerge from the brain-stem at the lower border of the pons (Fig. 4.14). The nerve then passes forwards and laterally over the tip of the petrous temporal bone, pierces the dura mater alongside the dorsum sellae and enters the cavernous sinus (Fig. 4.12). It subsequently enters the orbit through the superior orbital fissure.

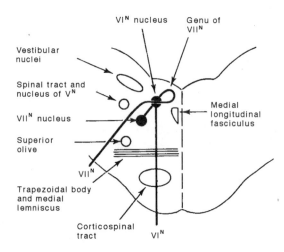

Fig. 4.14 Section of pons showing course of abducens (VI) and facial (VII) nerves.

Lesions of the sixth nerve

These result in paralysis of abduction of the eye and may be due to causes similar to those which produce lesions of the third and fourth nerves. Because of its long intracranial course, the sixth nerve is often involved secondarily to raised intracranial pressure; the pressure results in the nerve being stretched as it passes over the tip of the petrous temporal bone. This is an example of a 'false localizing sign', since the sixth nerve palsy is not the result of a primary lesion of the nerve. Infection of the petrous temporal bone, resulting from chronic middle ear infection, or invasion by carcinoma, may involve the sixth nerve causing double vision and the first division of the fifth nerve, causing pain above the eye (Gradenigo's syndrome; p. 169).

Conjugate movements of the eyes

Saccadic movements of the eyes rapidly fixate the image of a new object on the macula; *pursuit* movements are slower and enable the image of a moving target to remain on the macula. Saccadic movements are generated through the pathway from the frontal eye fields to the pontine paramedian reticular formation (PPRF) for horizontal conjugate gaze, and to the rostral interstitial nucleus of the medial longitudinal fasciculus (RiMLF) in the mid-brain for vertical gaze. Pursuit movements are controlled by pathways from the occipital areas to the dorsolateral pontine nuclei (Figs 4.15, 4.16).

The *medial longitudinal fasciculus* is a fibre tract that runs in the brain-stem in close relationship to the third, fourth and sixth nerve nuclei (Fig. 4.15). It co-ordinates the actions of the nerves to the extra-ocular muscles with each other and with the vestibular apparatus thus maintaining visual fixation during rapid head movements (vestibulo-ocular reflexes), and it relays impulses for the horizontal conjugate gaze from the abducens (VI) nucleus in the pons to the medial rectus subnucleus in the mid-brain.

Control of horizontal conjugate eye movements

Figure 4.15 relates to this section.The following regions of the brain are involved in the control of horizontal conjugate gaze:

Frontal   Voluntary saccadic eye movements are initiated from the frontal eye fields (area 8) at the posterior end of the second frontal convolution. Cortico-fugal fibres pass through the internal capsule and course downwards to the mid-brain where they supply the RiMLF. The fibres then decussate at the rostral end of the mid-brain and terminate in the PPRF near the sixth nerve nucleus.

Posterior parietal region   A centre for conjugate eye movements also exists in the posterior parietal region. This is concerned with tracking (pursuit) movements of the eyes in response to visual stimuli.

Pontine centre   There is a pontine centre for ipsilateral horizontal saccades situated in the region of the sixth nucleus (PPRF).

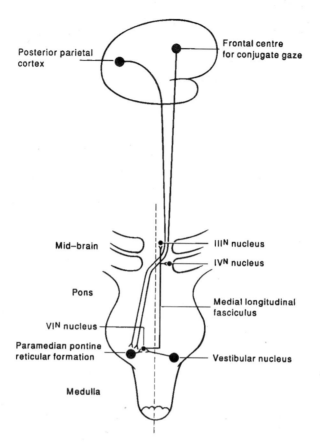

Fig. 4.15 Pathways for horizontal eye movements. Voluntary saccadic eye movements are initiated in the frontal centre for conjugate gaze (area 8). Descending pathways cross at the rostral end of the mid-brain and terminate in the pontine paramedian reticular formation (PPRF) near the sixth nerve nucleus. The PPRF is the brain-stem saccadic pulse generator and activates one group of neurones in the sixth nerve nucleus to abduct the ipsilateral eye, and other neurones of the nucleus to adduct the contralateral eye via the medial longitudinal fasciculus. Smooth pursuit movements are controlled through a pathway arising from the posterior parietal and other posterior cortical areas.

Control of vertical conjugate eye movements

Refer to Fig 4.16 for this section. The following regions of the brain are involved in vertical conjugate gaze:

Cortical centre in the frontal lobes   This is the same as that for horizontal gaze. Descending pathways decussate above the level of the superior colliculi.

The RiMLF in the mid-brain   The RiMLF causes upward and downward eye movements and projects predominantly ipsilaterally to the oculomotor and trochlear nuclei.

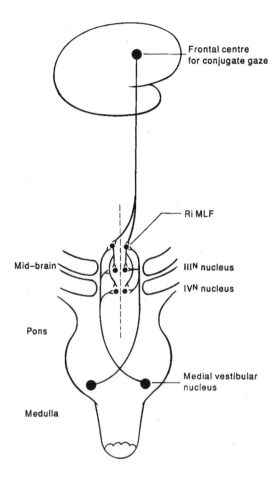

Frontal centre
for conjugate gaze

Ri MLF

Mid-brain

III^N nucleus

IV^N nucleus

Pons

Medial vestibular
nucleus

Medulla

Fig. 4.16 Pathways for vertical eye movements. Vertical saccadic eye movements are generated from the frontal centre for conjugate gaze (area 8). Descending pathways cross to terminate in the rostral interstitial nucleus of the medial longitudinal fasciculus (RiMLF), which innervates the third and fourth nerve nuclei.

Lesions resulting in gaze palsies

Horizontal gaze palsies   In considering disorders of ocular movements it is of great clinical importance to distinguish supranuclear lesions (which do not cause diplopia because both eyes continue to move along parallel axes) from nuclear and infranuclear lesions which can cause diplopia.

Cerebral lesions may be *irritative or paralytic*. Irritative lesions of the frontal region, and sometimes of the parietal region, may result in turning of the head and eyes to the side opposite the lesion, e.g. in focal epilepsy (versive seizures). Paralytic lesions, such as occur after strokes and injuries, cause a deviation of the eyes to the side of the lesion because of the unopposed stimulus arising from the opposite cortex.

Pontine lesions (e.g. vascular and demyelinating disorders, encephalitis, gliomas, Wernicke's encephalopathy) may cause impairment of conjugate eye movements to the side of the lesion. Usually this is accompanied by nystagmus and involvement of neighbouring cranial nerves, nuclei and long tracts.

Vertical gaze palsies   Cerebral lesions, especially if irritative, may cause impairment of vertical as well as horizontal conjugate gaze, but the vertical component is relatively insignificant.

Irritative lesions of the tectum and perhaps basal ganglia may cause the oculogyric crises that are seen in postencephalitic Parkinsonism. Paralytic lesions usually are in the region of the superior colliculus (e.g. pinealoma) and cause various types of vertical gaze palsies, which may be seen in *Parinaud's syndrome*. This consists of paralysis of vertical eye movements, impaired vergence, retractory nystagmus and pupils that do not react to light but may continue to react to accommodation. Unlike Argyll Robertson pupils, they are not constricted or irregular. Loss of vertical saccadic eye movements, particularly down gaze, with retention of reflex movement is characteristic of progressive supranuclear palsy (Steele-Richardson syndrome).

Paralysis of vergence

Impairment of vergence is seen with lesions of the mid-brain in the region of the superior colliculus. However, many normal people have difficulty converging the eyes.

Internuclear ophthalmoplegia

An important disorder of eye movement is caused by a lesion of the medial longitudinal fasciculus. It is characterized by weakness of adduction of one eye on conjugate lateral deviation, associated with nystagmus in the opposite (abducting) eye (Fig. 4.17). It may be bilateral or unilateral. If lesions are caudally placed, near the sixth nerve nucleus, vergence is intact. With more rostrally placed lesions, near the third nerve nucleus, vergence may be affected. Bilateral internuclear ophthalmoplegia is often caused by multiple sclerosis, but the unilateral condition more often results from vascular lesions. Mild forms may be detected by observing the visual axes during saccadic movements as the examiner asks the patient to glance rapidly from one of the examiner's fingers to the other.

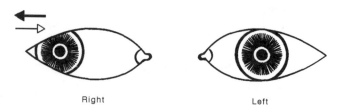

Right   Left

Fig. 4.17 Internuclear ophthalmoplegia. The left eye does not adduct (lesion of the left medial longitudinal fasciculus) and there is nystagmus in the abducting right eye.

Nystagmus

Nystagmus is a disorder of eye movements characterized by involuntary rhythmic oscillations. The eyes normally remain stationary if the tonic innervation of the muscles is equal and opposite in all directions. The tonic innervation of the ocular muscles is derived from various sources, e.g. cerebral, brain-stem, labyrinthine, ocular and cervical cord (neck muscles). Any interruption of these pathways may cause alteration in tone giving rise to nystagmus. Nystagmus may be *pendular* (oscillating) or *jerk* (rhythmic). See Figs 4.18, 4.19.

Pendular nystagmus

This is characterized by sinusoidal oscillations that are approximately equal in rate for the two directions of movement (Fig. 4.18). It can be due to loss of vision and of the normal reflex tonic innervation from the retina. It can also occur in acquired lesions of the brain-stem or cerebellum.

Jerk nystagmus

The oscillations are composed of involuntary rapid eye movements (saccades) in one direction and slower drifts in the other, producing a sawtooth waveform on electronystagmography (Fig. 4.19). The direction of the nystagmus is designated by the direction of the fast component. Nystagmus may be horizontal, vertical or rotatory.

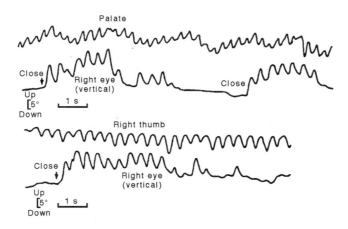

Fig. 4.18 Pendular nystagmus. Oculographic recordings from the right eye show a regular 3–4 Hz vertical pendular oscillation of the eyes, which was present only when the eyes were closed. (It was absent even in the dark.) There was a synchronous pendular oscillation (i.e. tremor) of the palate and of the right thumb. The lesion was in the central tegmental tract in the mid-brain; amplitude calibrations apply only to the eye movements. (From Halmagyi 1994, Central eye movement disorders. In: *Principles and Practice of Ophthalmology*. Eds D. M. Albert and F. A. Jakobiec. W. B. Saunders, Baltimore. 2411–2444).

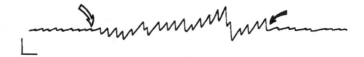

Fig. 4.19 Peripheral vestibular nystagmus. Oculographic recording shows a left beating nystagmus that was obvious only when visual fixation was removed (open arrow) and was quickly suppressed again when visual fixation was permitted (filled arrow). Peripheral vestibular nystagmus can be detected clinically by viewing the fundus of one eye while occluding the other. This patient had acute vestibular neuritis. Upward defections indicate rightward eye movements; downward deflections indicate leftward eye movements. Bars represent 10 degrees and 1 second (From Halmagyi 1994, Central eye movement disorders. In: *Principles and Practice of Ophthalmology.* Eds D. M. Albert and F. A. Jakobiec. W. B. Saunders, Baltimore. 2411–2444).

Opsoclonus is the term applied to rapid multidirectional eye movements usually associated with severe brain disease.

Oscillopsia is the visual sensation of movement of the environment experienced by subjects with nystagmus.

Nystagmus retractorius (retractory nystagmus) is a quick rhythmic retraction of the eyes, seen in Parinaud's syndrome on attempted convergence.

Causes of jerk nystagmus

Optokinetic nystagmus   This is a normal phenomenon when the eyes are following a series of objects moving across the field of vision, e.g. looking out of a train window. The slow phase represents the normal pursuit movement of the eyes and the fast phase represents the corrective movement which brings the eyes back to the central position (saccadic movement). Optokinetic responses can be elicited clinically with a rotating drum marked with vertical stripes and may be helpful in determining the site of a lesion causing hemianopia. The optokinetic responses remain normal in lesions of the optic tract; impairment of optokinetic responses occurs with a cerebral lesion. With unilateral cerebral lesions (with or without hemianopia), particularly those in the parieto-occipital region, the opticokinetic responses will be disturbed when the stimulus moves towards the site of the lesion.

Vestibular nystagmus   Each vestibular system exerts a tonic effect causing drift of the eyes to the opposite side. Normally vestibular effects are balanced so that the eyes are stable. Damage to the vestibular system causes an imbalance so that the eyes drift towards the damaged canal until a fast corrective movement restores them to mid-point (jerk nystagmus). This type of nystagmus is seen normally during rotation (the slow component is opposite to the direction of rotation). Clinically, vestibular nystagmus is seen in disease of the labyrinth or vestibular nerve (e.g. labyrinthitis, Ménière's disease, vestibular neuronitis) or their connections in the brain-stem (e.g. multiple sclerosis, vascular lesions, encephalitis). The slow component is directed towards the side of the lesion and the jerk component to the opposite side.

Vertical nystagmus is nearly always the result of a lesion of the central nervous system, usually in the brain-stem. It almost never occurs in lesions of the labyrinth or vestibular nerve. Down-beating nystagmus (fast-phase downwards) suggests a lesion at the level of the foramen magnum.

Nystagmus in cerebellar lesions   Nystagmus is common in disorders affecting the cerebellum, particularly if its connections with the vestibular nuclei are involved. The fast component of cerebellar nystagmus is directed towards the side of the lesion.

Nystagmus from weakness of ocular movements   Nystagmus may occur where there is weakness of conjugate lateral gaze. This can occur in normal individuals at extremes of ocular deviation, in fatigue, myasthenia, sedative drug intoxication and in cerebral lesions which affect conjugate gaze (frontal, occipital, brain-stem). The fast phase is in the direction of gaze.

Congenital nystagmus   Congenital nystagmus may be either pendular or jerk and may be inherited. Some people are able to induce nystagmus voluntarily.

The pupils

In examining the pupils one should note their size, equality, regularity and reaction to light and accommodation. The size of the pupil depends upon the reciprocal actions of the sphincter muscle, which is innervated by the parasympathetic nerves, and the dilator muscle, which is innervated by the sympathetic nerves (Fig. 4.20).

The *sympathetic pupillodilator fibres* arise in the hypothalamus, descend in the lateral tegmentum of the mid-brain, pons and medulla to synapse on cells of the intermediolateral column at C8 and T1.

Preganglionic sympathetic fibres leave the cord at the first thoracic segment and course through the ventral roots and white rami to the superior cervical ganglion where they synapse.

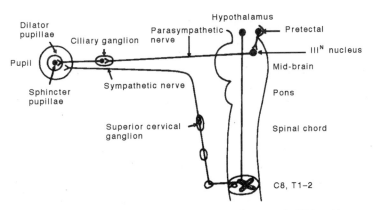

Fig. 4.20   Innervation of the pupil. (From Lance and McLeod, 1981, with permission of Butterworths, London.)

Postganglionic fibres travel from the superior cervical ganglion along the common carotid artery to its bifurcation. Most fibres responsible for sweating and vasomotor function of the face travel with the external carotid artery, but those responsible for sweating on the medial aspect of the forehead, and the pupillodilator fibres, travel with the internal carotid artery to the carotid siphon. At the petrous temporal bone, and at the cavernous sinus, the sympathetic pupillodilator fibres join and course with the first division of the trigeminal nerve.

The *parasympathetic pupilloconstrictor fibres* arise in the Edinger-Westphal nucleus and course in the third nerve to the ciliary ganglion where they synapse. The postganglionic fibres emerge as the ciliary nerves.

The light reflex

The afferent pathway of the light reflex is from the retina, along the optic nerve to the optic tract where the fibres part from those that are destined for the lateral geniculate body and instead go to the pretectal region. There is a pathway from the pretectal region to part of the third cranial nerve nucleus (Edinger-Westphal nucleus) of both sides, thus accounting for direct and consensual light reflexes. The efferent pathway is in the third nerve (Fig. 4.21).

In a lesion of the third nerve, the pupil will be dilated. The direct light reaction, and the consensual response elicited by shining a light in the other eye, will be absent. However, the consensual reaction of the unaffected eye will be present when a light is shone in the affected eye.

In bilateral blindness due to cortical lesions (but not optic nerve or tract lesions), direct and consensual reflexes of both eyes will be present.

Accommodation reflex

The accommodation reflex is pupillary constriction associated with convergence of the eyes ('near response'). The descending pathways project from the parieto-occipital cortex to the mid-brain (Edinger-Westphal nucleus). Any lesion involving the pupilloconstrictor fibres will impair the reaction of accommodation. Selective impairment of accommodation may occur in some mid-brain lesions.

Relative afferent pupillary defect

This is also known as the Marcus Gunn pupil or swinging torch sign (p. 19).

Adie's pupil (tonic pupil of Adie; Holmes-Adie syndrome)

This condition occurs mainly in females and the onset is usually sudden with the complaint of blurred vision. One pupil becomes larger than the other, but the pupillary abnormality is bilateral in 20% of cases. The pupil reacts very sluggishly to light and accommodation, but will pass slowly through the full range of constriction on prolonged exposure to light. On relaxation, dilatation proceeds slowly. Knee and ankle jerks may be absent and the syndrome must therefore be distinguished from tabes dorsalis which it superficially resembles (p. 118). Because of denervation supersensitivity of receptors, the instillation of 2.5% methacholine eyedrops causes Adie's pupil, but not the normal pupil, to constrict. On slit-lamp examination, the margin of the iris may be seen to undulate.

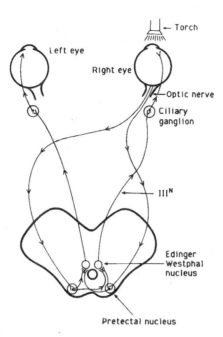

Fig. 4.21   Pathways of the pupillary light reflex for direct and consensual responses. (Modified from Duke-Elder & Scott, 1971, *System of Ophthalmology*, XII. Kimpton, London.)

Pathological changes have been demonstrated in the ciliary ganglion. Synaptic transmission is impaired in the spinal monosynaptic reflex arc, accounting for the absent reflexes.

Horner's syndrome

Horner's syndrome results from a lesion of oculosympathetic fibres anywhere along their pathway, e.g. brain-stem, cervical cord, first thoracic root, cervical sympathetic trunk or intracranial course (Fig. 4.20). The characteristic features are:
- Ptosis (sympathetic fibres supply the smooth muscle of upper eyelids) although it should be noted that the ptosis in Horner's syndrome is only partial and never complete as it is in a third nerve palsy
- Pupillary constriction
- Enophthalmos
- Anhidrosis of one side of the face if the lesion is proximal to the carotid bifurc-ation (since sympathetic fibres to the face course with the external carotid artery). Anhidrosis of the medial side of the forehead occurs if the lesion is distal to the bifurcation

Argyll Robertson pupil

Douglas Argyll Robertson, an Edinburgh physician, described pupils that are small, irregular, unequal, dilate poorly with mydriatics and react to accommodation but not to light. They are observed most commonly in syphilis, but are also occasionally seen in some other disorders, e.g. diabetes. The site of the lesion is uncertain but is probably in the pretectal region. Pseudo-Argyll Robertson pupils may occur in mid-brain lesions. They also do not react to light, but they are neither small nor irregular.

CRANIAL NERVE V: THE TRIGEMINAL NERVE

The fifth nerve contains motor and sensory fibres. It arises from the lateral aspect of the inferior surface of the pons by two roots; a large sensory and a small motor root (Fig. 13.2). The roots pierce the dura mater to join the trigeminal or Gasserian ganglion which lies between two layers of dura mater on the apex of the petrous temporal bone.

Sensory root

The sensory root, the ganglion cells of which lie in the Gasserian ganglion, has three main divisions which are summarized below.

Ophthalmic division   This passes through the lateral wall of the cavernous sinus to enter the orbit through the superior orbital fissure (Fig. 4.12). It supplies sensation to the nose, forehead, scalp and upper lid as well as to the cornea and the mucous membrane of the frontal sinuses (Fig. 4.22). Dura mater of the falx and superior surface of the tentorium is supplied by the tentorial nerve arising from the ophthalmic division.

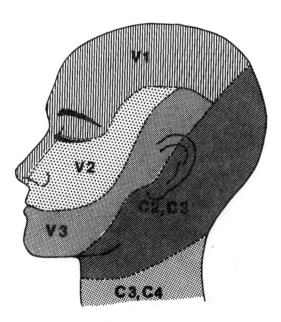

Fig. 4.22   Cutaneous innervation of the face. (Modified from Brodal, 1969, *Neurological Anatomy in Relation to Clinical Medicine*, 2nd edn. Oxford University Press, Oxford.)

Maxillary division The maxillary division courses through the foramen rotundum into the pterygopalatine fossa and then enters the orbit through the inferior orbital fissure. It leaves the orbit as the infra-orbital nerve. It supplies the skin of the lower lid, alae nasae, the upper lip and a 2–3 cm strip on the face, anterior to a line which extends from the outer angle of the mouth through a point midway between the outer canthus of the eye and the ear (Fig. 4.22).

Mandibular division This division leaves with the motor root through the foramen ovale. It supplies the skin of the lower jaw, part of the face, tragus and anterior part of the pinna (Fig. 4.22); it also innervates the mucous membrane of the cheek, the anterior two-thirds of the tongue and the floor of the mouth. Meningeal branches supply the dura mater above the tentorium.

Motor root

The motor root innervates the temporalis muscle, the masseter, pterygoids, anterior belly of the digastric, mylohyoid, tensor tympani and tensor palati muscles.

Central connections of the fifth nerve

Sensory nucleus

The sensory nucleus is in three parts (Fig. 4.23):

Main sensory nucleus The main sensory nucleus, which is in the lateral part of the pons, receives the sensory fibres concerned with tactile and sensibility; second order neurones cross to the quintothalamic tracts, near the medial lemniscus.

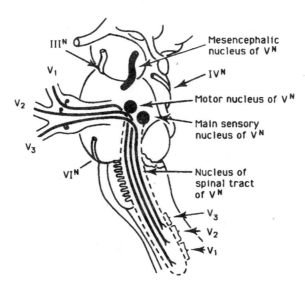

Fig. 4.23 Nuclei and fibre tracts in the brain-stem of the trigeminal nerve. (Modified from Brodal, 1965, *The Cranial Nerves. Anatomy and anatomico-clinical correlations*, 2nd edn. Blackwell Scientific Publications, Oxford.)

Nucleus of the spinal tract   This extends downwards in the lateral part of the medulla to about the level of C2 where it is continuous with the substantia gelatinosa. It receives the pain and temperature fibres from the fifth nerve. The ophthalmic division terminates in the more caudal part, and the mandibular division terminates in the most cephalic part of the nucleus. Second order neurones cross to the quintothalamic tracts.

Mesencephalic nucleus   This nucleus lies cephalad to the main sensory nucleus and receives the muscle afferent fibres which run in the motor root.

Motor nucleus

The motor nucleus is situated in the mid-pons, medially to the main sensory nucleus.

Lesions of the fifth nerve

Central lesions of the fifth nerve in the brain-stem are usually associated with palsies of other cranial nerves and involvement of long tracts. A lesion in the pons may cause loss of tactile sensation over the trigeminal nerve distribution with preservation of painful sensation which is relayed in the spinal tract. A lesion in the medulla, e.g. syringobulbia, posterior inferior cerebellar artery thrombosis (PICA syndrome), may cause loss of pain and temperature sensation (spinal tract of V), but preservation of light touch (main sensory nucleus in pons). Peripheral lesions may give rise to pain, paraesthesiae and sensory loss over the distribution of the trigeminal nerve. Such lesions may result from a neuroma of the fifth nerve, herpes zoster (pp. 246–247), or compression by adjacent tumours (e.g. meningioma, acoustic neuroma).

Trigeminal neuralgia

Refer also to pp. 178–180. This is a distressing disorder, characterized by *paroxysmal brief* attacks of severe unilateral facial pain in the distribution of the fifth nerve, usually in its second and third divisions. The condition affects usually, but not exclusively, middle-aged people. The pain is burning and jabbing and tends to be precipitated by chewing, cold, talking, swallowing, or touching 'trigger zones'. There are no sensory abnormalities detectable on neurological examination. The probable causes include spontaneous repetitive discharges from the Gasserian ganglion or spinal nucleus of the fifth nerve, or pressure on roots by tumours or small arteries.

The pain of trigeminal neuralgia, or *tic douloureux* has to be differentiated from constant, dull facial pain due to: pressure on the fifth nerve; pain arising in sinuses, teeth, eyes (glaucoma) and temporomandibular joints; or atypical facial neuralgia.

CRANIAL NERVE VII: THE FACIAL NERVE

The seventh cranial nerve consists of two parts:

The facial nerve   This innervates the muscles of facial expression, together with the stapedius, stylohyoid and posterior belly of the digastric muscles.

The nervus intermedius   This carries taste fibres from the anterior two-thirds of the tongue and parasympathetic secretory fibres to the lacrimal, submandibular and sublingual glands.

Facial nerve

The nucleus of the facial nerve is situated caudally in the lateral part of the pons. The emerging fibres pass backwards to form a loop around the sixth nerve nucleus beneath the facial colliculus, before passing ventrolaterally to emerge from the lateral aspect of the caudal part of the pons (Fig. 4.14). Together with the eighth nerve and nervus intermedius the facial nerve enters the internal auditory meatus and courses laterally in the facial canal of the petrous temporal bone. It turns sharply backwards on the medial aspect of the middle ear to form the genu, where the geniculate ganglion is situated, and then downwards to emerge from the skull at the stylomastoid foramen (Fig. 4.24). It pierces the parotid gland and divides into branches which supply the muscles of the face as well as the stylohyoid and posterior belly of digastric muscles.

Supranuclear fibres are derived from: (i) corticobulbar tracts, that arise mainly from area 4, and which are crossed; however, the upper part of the facial musculature receives a bilateral upper motor neurone innervation; (ii) extrapyramidal fibres that are concerned with emotional expression.

Nervus intermedius

Efferent fibres originate from the cells of the superior salivary nucleus close to the facial nucleus. Those destined for the lacrimal gland leave the nervus intermedius near the geniculate ganglion in the greater superficial petrosal nerve (Fig. 4.24). Those destined for the sublingual and submaxillary glands travel in the chorda tympani.

Afferent fibres, which convey taste from the anterior two-thirds of the tongue and travel in the lingual and chorda tympani nerves, have their cell nuclei in the geniculate ganglion. They terminate centrally in the nucleus of the tractus solitarius.

Lesions of the facial nerve

It is important clinically to distinguish between upper and lower motor neurone lesions.

Upper motor neurone lesions

Upper motor neurone lesions of the face are commonly seen in strokes in which there is a capsular haemorrhage or infarction. As well as a hemiplegia there is weakness of the facial musculature. This is usually noted as asymmetry, with

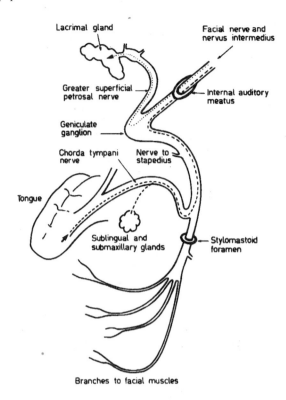

Fig. 4.24   The facial nerve. (Modified from Walton, 1977, *Brain's Diseases of the Nervous System*, 8th edn. Oxford University Press, Oxford.)

drooping of the angle of the mouth and loss of the nasolabial fold. The upper part of the face, i.e. frontalis and the orbicularis oculi muscles, is nearly always involved to a lesser extent than the lower part of the face because of the bilateral corticobulbar innervation of the relevant part of the facial nucleus. Facial movements in response to emotional reactions are often normal, even though voluntary movements are impaired, since emotional expression is mediated through fronto-pontine pathways. Sometimes, the upper and lower face are equally affected and then the facial palsy can be distinguished clinically from a lower motor neurone paralysis by the retention of emotional expression.

Lower motor neurone lesions

These facial lesions are exemplified by *Bell's palsy*. This is a relatively common condition of uncertain aetiology, characterized by sudden onset of facial weakness or paralysis. The upper and lower facial muscles are equally affected and are paralysed for both voluntary and involuntary movements. The patient cannot close the eye, pout, or whistle, and the angle of the mouth droops.

If the lesion is proximal to the level of separation of the chorda tympani, taste over the anterior two-thirds of the tongue will be lost. If the lesion lies proximal to the greater superficial petrosal nerve, lacrimation will also be impaired (Fig. 4.24). If the nerve to stapedius is involved, there will be hyper-acusis, i.e. an intensification of loud noises.

Facial palsies may also occur in: (i) pontine lesions, when they are usually accompanied by lateral rectus palsy and long tract signs; (ii) peripheral neuropathies; (iii) fractures of the petrous temporal bone; (iv) middle ear infections; (v) geniculate herpes (Ramsay-Hunt syndrome; p. 246); (vi) acoustic neuromas (pp. 81, 253) or other tumours.

CRANIAL NERVE VIII: THE VESTIBULO-COCHLEAR NERVE

The eighth nerve contains two groups of fibres: those in the cochlear branch, which are concerned with hearing and those in the vestibular branch which are concerned with posture and equilibrium.

The cochlear nerve

The peripheral processes of the cochlear nerve are in contact with the cells of the spiral organ of Corti in the inner ear. The cell bodies lie in the spiral ganglion, and the central processes pass with the eighth nerve through the internal auditory meatus to enter the brain-stem at the lower border of the pons, where they synapse in the cochlear nucleus. Fibres cross in the trapezoid body, synapse in the superior olivary complex of nuclei, pass rostrally in the lateral lemniscus to the medial geniculate body and inferior colliculus and thence to the auditory cortex in the superior temporal gyrus. Hearing is bilaterally represented in the cerebral cortex.

The major symptoms of disease of the cochlear nerve are tinnitus (a sensation of noise or ringing in the ears, usually a whistling or hissing sound) and deafness. The clinical examination of hearing is described in Chapter 2.

Audiometric testing (measuring of hearing threshold at various frequencies) enables more accurate assessment of auditory function to be made and should always be performed when hearing loss is suspected from clinical examination. Specialized audiometric tests, such as loudness recruitment and tone decay, help to localize the lesion causing deafness to cochlea, nerve or brain-stem.

Causes of nerve deafness
* *Cochlea:* Noise; old age; drugs, e.g. aminoglycosides, diuretics; congenital and hereditary causes; trauma; Ménière's disease
* *Nerve:* Cerebellopontine angle tumour; vascular lesions; trauma; hereditary causes

Cortical deafness is very rare and requires the presence of bilateral lesions in the superior temporal gyrus.

Vestibular nerve

The vestibular branch of the eighth nerve is concerned with the maintenance of posture and balance. It receives afferent impulses from the utricle, saccule and semicircular canals in the labyrinth (Fig. 4.25). There are three semicircular canals on each side; an anterior–vertical, a posterior–vertical and a horizontal canal, which are arranged in planes at right angles to one another. The posterior–vertical canal is in a vertical plane parallel to that of the anterior vertical canal of the other side.

When the head is inclined 30° forwards from the horizontal, the lateral semicircular canals are vertical. This is the position adopted when caloric tests are performed. The semicircular canals respond to angular acceleration. In contrast, the otolith organs in the utricle and saccule signal the static position of the head in space and respond to linear acceleration (Fig. 4.25).

The vestibular nerve has its cell bodies in the vestibular ganglion of Scarpa in the internal auditory meatus. The central processes pass in the vestibular nerve to the lower border of the pons. There the cochlear and vestibular nerves part company, the vestibular nerve passing more medially to terminate in the vestibular nuclei. The vestibular nuclei have four main parts and are connected to: (i) the anterior horn cells of the spinal cord by the vestibulospinal tract; (ii) the ocular

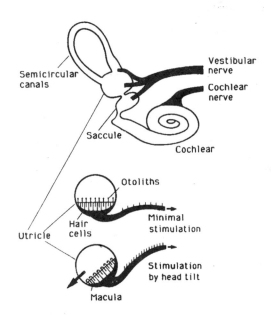

Fig. 4.25 Schema of the internal ear showing a stylized version of the otolith organ in the utricle. When the head is in such a position that otoliths hang from hair cells, labyrinthine stimulation is maximal, as indicated by the vertical strokes (representing nerve impulses) superimposed on the branch of the vestibular nerve. (From Lance and McLeod, 1981, with permission of Butterworths, London.)

motor neurones by the medial longitudinal fasciculus; (iii) the floccolonodular lobe of the cerebellum; (iv) the reticular formation (Fig. 4.26).

Examination of the vestibular function of the eighth nerve

Disorders of the vestibular branch of the eighth nerve may be manifested by clinical signs of nystagmus, disturbance of gait, balance and muscular control. Neurological examination should include tests for nystagmus, past-pointing, ataxia, Romberg's sign and stepping tests. There are two special tests of vestibular function that are of particular importance.

Caloric tests   The patient lies on a couch, face up, with the neck flexed 30° to the horizontal plane and eyes looking straight ahead. In this position the horizontal canals are vertical. Cool water at 30° C is run into one ear for 40 seconds and the slow phase velocity of the evoked nystagmus (fast component is directed to the opposite side with cold water) is measured. The opposite ear is then similarly irrigated and the same measurements made. The procedure is then repeated with warm water (44° C) which, in normal subjects induces a nystagmus that beats to the same side as the irrigation. Nystagmus is usually recorded electrically by electronystagmography (ENG) which allows nystagmus to be recorded in darkness. The nystagmus is exaggerated in darkness, by eliminating visual function. Two major types of abnormality may be observed:

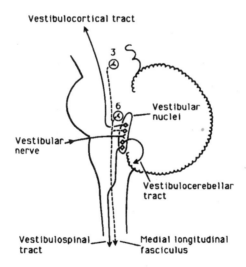

Fig. 4.26 Some anatomical connections of the vestibular nuclei. Fibres ascending to the nuclei responsible for eye movement in the median longitudinal fasciculus take origin from all four of the large vestibular nuclei, and descending fibres from the medial nucleus only. The vestibulospinal tract arises from the lateral vestibular nucleus in which cells are arranged somatotopically, thus permitting the effects of cerebellovestibular connections (not shown) to be distributed to localized areas of the spinal cord. (From Lance and McLeod, 1981, with permission of Butterworths, London.)

(1) *Canal paresis*   This term indicates a diminished or absent response to caloric irrigation of one ear and occurs with destructive peripheral lesions, e.g. labyrinthitis, vestibular neuronitis, Ménière's disease, acoustic neuroma.

(2) *Directional preponderance*   This is a term used to describe the unmasking of latent imbalance of tonic vestibular mechanisms. Cold water in the left ear and warm water in the right ear both cause nystagmus to the right. If these reactions are more pronounced than corresponding reactions producing nystagmus to the left there is said to be a right directional preponderance. It occurs mainly with brain-stem lesions but can also be present in peripheral lesions. The directional preponderance can be interpreted as a latent nystagmus to that side and is therefore toward the side of a cerebellar lesion but away from the side of a vestibular lesion.

Combined responses, i.e. canal paresis with directional preponderance, may also occur.

Positional tests   Disease or damage to the otolith organ (e.g. trauma, vascular disease, infection) may result in giddiness and nystagmus on sudden head movements. The condition is known as positional vertigo.

In order to test for positional nystagmus, the Hallpike test is used. The patient sits on a couch and the head is held while the patient is rapidly moved into the supine position with the neck extended 30–40° below horizontal and rotated to one side. In normal people, there is no nystagmus. In positional vertigo, rotatory nystagmus towards the lowermost ear (if this is the affected one) will develop after a latent interval and will fatigue in less than a minute. On sitting up again, nystagmus may recur. In brain-stem and cerebellar lesions, there is no latent interval and the nystagmus continues without fatiguing.

Stepping test (Unterberger test)   The patient closes the eyes or is blindfolded and holds the arm extended horizontally in front while marking time on the same spot for one minute. Rotation occurs to the side of the vestibular lesion.

Vertigo

Vertigo may be defined as an illusory perception of movement of the body in relation to the environment, or of apparent movement of the surroundings in relation to the body. There is usually a sense of turning either of the person, or of the outside world. However, the patient may complain of a rocking movement, or of a tendency to veer to one side when walking, or that the outside world tends to move towards or away from him or her. Vertigo is the commonest symptom of labyrinthine disorders, but does not occur exclusively in these conditions.

The maintenance of equilibrium and posture and the awareness of the position of the body in space depend upon visual impulses from the retina, labyrinthine impulses, and proprioceptive impulses from joints and muscles of the neck, trunk and limbs. Disturbances of equilibrium may therefore have origins other than disease of labyrinthine pathways.

It is very important to obtain a careful history from patients who complain of disorders of equilibrium. Patients may say they suffer from 'dizziness' or 'giddiness', but this should not be described as vertigo unless there is some sense of rotation or movement of the person or the environment. True vertigo is often accompanied by nausea or vomiting. Dizziness or giddiness in many cases may really be a feeling of light-headedness or faintness or weakness, and not a true disturbance of equilibrium. It is essential to find out what sensation the patients actually experience during their attacks and to realize that their definitions of dizziness and giddiness may be different from those used in medical practice.

Causes of vertigo

Lesions of the vestibular nerve and labyrinth
These can be divided into six main lesions or disturbances:

(1) *Labyrinthine (aural) vertigo* This tends to occur in acute attacks, lasting for only 1–2 hours. Often there is associated tinnitus and deafness. Causes include Ménière's disease, acute labyrinthitis and vascular lesions of the labyrinth.

Ménière's disease is a condition in which recurrent attacks of severe vertigo are associated with tinnitus and deafness. It is commonly unilateral and runs a protracted course. It occurs mainly in middle age and the pathology is degeneration of the organ of Corti due to increased endolymphatic pressure. There is an end-organ (cochlear) deafness and a canal paresis on caloric testing.

(2) *Lesions of the eighth nerve:* (i) Cerebellopontine angle tumours or meningeal inflammation involving the eighth nerve directly are rare causes of vertigo. Deafness and tinnitus are associated; (ii) vestibular neuronitis (epidemic vertigo). A severe, prostrating vertigo which usually starts suddenly and is not associated with deafness or tinnitus. It lasts for days and is accompanied by nausea and vomiting. There may be a preceding viral infection. Caloric testing usually demonstrates a canal paresis, but there may be a directional preponderance; (iii) drugs. Ototoxic drugs (e.g. aminoglycosides and salicylates) do not cause vertigo, but ataxia. Disequilibrium due to bilateral loss of vestibular function can be caused by many drugs including alcohol, anticonvulsants and sedatives.

(3) *Brain-stem lesions* Lesions of the brain-stem (e.g. vascular lesions) and multiple sclerosis can cause a severe and prolonged vertigo associated with nystagmus. Short duration vertigo (minutes, hours) may be a symptom of a transient ischaemic attack. Brain-stem lesions should be suspected if vertigo is prolonged for several weeks. There is no associated deafness or tinnitus but there is vertical nystagmus. Brain-stem nuclei or tracts are involved. There is directional preponderance without canal paresis on caloric testing and electronystagmography shows that nystagmus does not become more pronounced when the eyes are closed, in contrast to vestibular nystagmus.

(4) *Cerebellar disturbances*   Vertigo occurs particularly if the vestibular connections with the flocculonodular lobe are involved (Fig. 8.3).

(5) *Cortical disturbances*   Vertigo may occur as an aura of migraine. Benign recurrent vertigo is a condition often confused with Ménière's disease. The cause is uncertain but it is thought to be a periodic syndrome allied to migraine.

(6) *Ocular disturbances*   Dizziness that is not true vertigo may be experienced by some people on looking down from heights, or when ocular palsies result in double vision; or it may accompany optokinetic nystagmus when a subject looks at fast-moving objects.

CRANIAL NERVE IX: THE GLOSSOPHARYNGEAL NERVE

The glossopharyngeal nerve arises from a series of rootlets on the lateral surface of the medulla and courses with nerves X and XI through the jugular foramen (Fig. 4.27). It lies in the neck in association with the carotid vessels and jugular

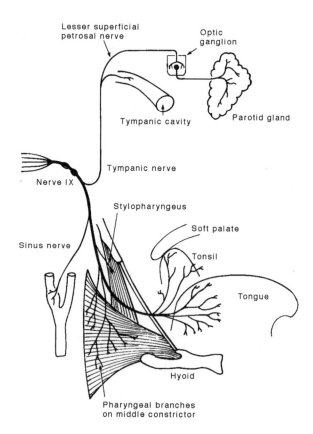

Fig. 4.27   The glossopharyngeal nerve. (Modified from *Grant's Atlas of Anatomy*, 1978, 7th edn. Williams and Wilkins, Baltimore.)

vein. It contains motor fibres which arise from the nucleus ambiguus and innervates the stylopharyngeus muscle. Afferent fibres which run in the glossopharyngeal nerve have their cell bodies in the petrosal ganglion of the nerve. Peripheral
branches carry sensory impulses from the posterior third of the tongue, tonsils, soft
palate and posterior wall of the pharynx; centrally directed fibres terminate in the
nucleus of the tractus solitarius. A tympanic branch transmits sensation from the
tympanic cavity. Secretory fibres arise in the inferior salivatory nucleus and travel
to the parotid gland (Fig. 4.27).

Together with the vagus nerve and central part of the accessory nerve, the
glossopharyngeal nerve is examined clinically by means of the gag reflex, and
by testing palatal and pharyngeal sensation.

The glossopharyngeal nerve is very rarely involved in isolation. In association
with the vagus and accessory nerves it may be compressed by tumours of the
posterior fossa in the jugular foramen or in the upper part of the neck.

Glossopharyngeal neuralgia

The characteristics of glossopharyngeal neuralgia are similar to those of trigeminal
neuralgia. Intense paroxysmal pain of brief duration is experienced in the side of
the throat and may radiate to the ear because the sensory part of the vagus nerve
is usually implicated in the discharge. Attacks may be precipitated by swallowing.

CRANIAL NERVE X: THE VAGUS NERVE

The vagus nerve contains both motor and sensory fibres (Fig. 4.28). It leaves the
medulla and passes through the jugular foramen to enter the carotid sheath with
nerves IX and XI.

Motor fibres   These are derived from the nucleus ambiguus in the medulla,
whence fibres travel in the vagus to supply the muscles of the palate, pharynx and
larynx. General visceral efferents also run in the vagus to the parasympathetic
ganglia of the vagal plexuses that innervate the thoracic and abdominal viscera.
They have their cell bodies in the dorsal nucleus of the vagus beneath the floor of
the fourth ventricle.

Sensory fibres   These supply the dura mater of the posterior fossa and part of
the ear and external auditory meatus and terminate centrally in the sensory nucleus
of the fifth nerve. Fibres supplying sensation to larynx, trachea, oesophagus,
thoracic and abdominal viscera terminate centrally in the nucleus of the tractus
solitarius.

Lesions of the vagus nerve

Paralysis of the palate   This will result from lesions involving the nucleus
ambiguus or the vagus above its pharyngeal branch. A unilateral paralysis causes
few symptoms, but on examination the palate does not fully elevate on the
affected side and the uvula is drawn to the unaffected side. With bilateral palatal

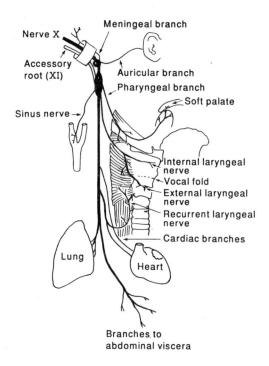

Fig. 4.28   The vagus nerve. (Modified from *Grant's Atlas of Anatomy*, 1978, 7th edn. Williams and Wilkins, Baltimore.)

palsies, fluids and food regurgitate into the back of the nose on swallowing and speech takes on a nasal quality; words are characteristically mispronounced, e.g. 'eng' instead of 'egg'.

Paralysis of the pharynx   There may be no symptoms from a unilateral lesion, but with a bilateral lesion swallowing becomes difficult and the pharyngeal reflex is lost.

Paralysis of the larynx   Unilateral paralysis will result from a lesion of the recurrent laryngeal nerve. There may be no symptoms, but usually the voice is hoarse. The affected cord will be seen to lie near the mid-line. Unilateral paralysis will also result from lesions above the nodose ganglion, but there will be an associated paralysis of the palate and pharynx. Bilateral paralysis of the larynx results in hoarse voice, difficulty in coughing and respiratory stridor.

Visceral effects of vagal injury   These are rarely conspicuous clinically. A tachycardia may follow bilateral vagal injury, e.g. Guillain-Barré syndrome.

Causes of vagus nerve lesions

Nuclear lesions in the medulla   These may result from poliomyelitis, motor neurone disease, diphtheria, syringobulbia, or vascular occlusions.

Posterior fossa tumours   These usually involve nerves IX, XI and XII also.
Damage to the main trunk of the vagus in the neck by tumours or trauma
If the lesion lies above the superior laryngeal nerve there will be anaesthesia of
one side of the larynx, with total ipsilateral vocal cord paralysis.
Involvement of the recurrent laryngeal nerve   This could be due to lymph-
adenopathies or carcinoma in the neck or thorax, or on the left side by an aortic
aneurysm. It may also be affected by a mononeuritis of viral or immune origin.
There will be unilateral cord paralysis, but no sensory loss.

CRANIAL NERVE XI: THE ACCESSORY NERVE

The central accessory nerve is functionally part of the vagus nerve and supplies
motor fibres to the palate and pharynx.

The spinal accessory nerve is purely motor and supplies the sternomastoid and
trapezius muscles through its spinal branch, which arises from C1–5 segments,
ascends through the foramen magnum and leaves the skull through the jugular
foramen. It may be damaged by tumours in the posterior fossa or at its exit from
the skull, or in its peripheral course behind the sternomastoid muscle and across
the floor of the posterior triangle of the neck. It is also vulnerable to surgical trauma
during lymph node biopsy and other procedures. Lesions may result in weakness
and wasting of the sternomastoid and upper part of the trapezius muscle.

CRANIAL NERVE XII: THE HYPOGLOSSAL NERVE

The hypoglossal nerve is the motor nerve to the tongue and its fibres originate
from the hypoglossal nucleus in the medulla. The nerve fibres emerge on the
ventral aspect of the medulla between the olives and pyramids and leave the
skull through the hypoglossal canal to supply the muscles of the tongue (Fig. 4.29).

A unilateral lesion results in wasting of one side of the tongue. On protrusion,
the tip of the tongue deviates to the paralysed side. Fasciculations may be observed
when the tongue lies at rest on the floor of the mouth. In bilateral lesions, the
tongue may be shrunken and wasted, and protrusion may be impossible. Dysarthria
and dysphagia result.

Nuclear lesions in the medulla may occur in poliomyelitis, motor neurone
disease, vascular occlusions and syringobulbia. Basal meningitis, or infections or
injuries of the occipital bone may affect the nerve in its infranuclear course. It
may sometimes be injured by operations on the neck.

BULBAR PALSY

Bulbar palsy is the result of weakness or paralysis of muscles supplied by the
medulla oblongata (the 'spinal bulb') which are mainly those of pharynx, larynx

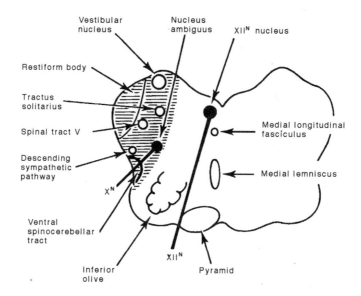

Fig. 4.29 Section of medulla, at the level of the inferior olives. Shaded area is that supplied by the posterior inferior cerebellar artery.

and tongue, producing difficulty with speech and swallowing. Causes include acute disorders such as diphtheria, Guillain-Barré syndrome, brain-stem infarction, poliomyelitis and chronic progressive disorders such as motor neurone disease, tumours or aneurysms in the posterior fossa. Myasthenia gravis may also cause bulbar weakness.

PSEUDOBULBAR PALSY

Pseudobulbar palsy is an upper motor neurone disorder affecting the muscle of pharynx, larynx and tongue resulting from bilateral corticobulbar tract lesions. The palate cannot be elevated fully voluntarily, but responds briskly in the gag reflex. Speech and swallowing become slow and difficult, and the tongue appears small and cannot be protruded fully. The jaw jerk and facial reflexes are exaggerated. The patients frequently have marked emotional lability. Pseudo-bulbar palsy is seen particularly in hypertensive cerebrovascular disease, motor neurone disease and multiple sclerosis, although a parasagittal tumour must always be excluded.

BRAIN-STEM DISORDERS

The cranial nerve nuclei and their connections, the ascending and descending long tracts, and the cerebellar peduncles are all closely related to one another anatomically in the brain-stem so that lesions in this area usually involve more than one structure.

The brain-stem may be damaged by vascular lesions, demyelination, tumours, infections and degenerative diseases. The clinical features of brain-stem disorders depend upon the anatomical site of the lesion. Common neurological manifestations of brain-stem involvement are unilateral or bilateral pyramidal tract signs or sensory disturbances, associated with cranial nerve palsies.

Mid-brain lesions

Lesions involving the *superior colliculi* and *tectal* region result in *Parinaud's syndrome* (p. 58). This is most commonly seen in pineal tumours but also occurs with multiple sclerosis and vascular lesions.

More anteriorly placed lesions of the tegmentum of the mid-brain at this level may cause third nerve palsy and contralateral hemiplegia as a result of destruction of the corticospinal tracts in the cerebral peduncles (*Weber's syndrome*); or contralateral cerebellar ataxia and a gross wing-beating tremor of the arms (*rubral tremor*) from involvement of the brachium conjunctivum near the red nucleus, together with corticospinal tract signs (*Benedikt's syndrome*); or contralateral cerebellar ataxia and tremor alone (*Claude's syndrome*; see Fig. 4.11).

Decerebrate rigidity results from a mid-brain lesion and is manifested by opisthotonus and extension of the arms and legs. It may be caused by mid-brain tumours, vascular, traumatic and other lesions, or by herniation of the mid-brain through the tentorial notch as a result of raised intracranial pressure.

Lesions of the pons

There may be hemiplegia and sensory disturbances on the side opposite the lesion; ataxia on the same side as the lesion as a result of damage to cerebellar peduncles; palsies of nerves VI, VII, VIII; internuclear ophthalmoplegia when the medial longitudinal fasciculus is involved; nystagmus; or Horner's syndrome. Both pupils may be small in a bilateral lesion, when consciousness is usually impaired. Spontaneous vertical eye movements ('ocular bobbing') may be observed.

The *Millard-Gubler* syndrome is a unilateral VI and/or VII nerve palsy with a crossed hemiplegia resulting from a lesion at the base of the pons.

Lesions of the medulla

The lateral part of the medulla is classically affected by infarction in the distribution of the posterior inferior cerebellar artery (*lateral medullary syndrome*; *Wallenberg's syndrome*; Fig. 4.29). The most common cause of this is occlusion of one vertebral artery. Clinical features include: nausea, vomiting, giddiness (vestibular nucleus); hiccoughs; pain and numbness over the ipsilateral side of face (fifth nerve nucleus, descending tract of fifth nerve); dissociated sensory loss of the contralateral side of the body (spinothalamic tract); ipsilateral cerebellar ataxia (cerebellum, inferior cerebellar peduncle); dysphagia, palatal weakness, hoarseness and vocal cord paralysis (nucleus ambiguus); ipsilateral loss of taste (tractus solitarius); and ipsilateral Horner's syndrome (descending sympathetic tract). Ipsilateral facial palsy may sometimes be seen, depending on the anatomical variations of the blood supply. The pyramidal tracts are spared.

Cerebellopontine angle tumours

Acoustic neuromas are the most common tumours in this region but meningiomas, cholesteatomas, trigeminal neuromas and, rarely, aneurysms can also cause a cerebellopontine angle syndrome.

Acoustic neuromas

Such neuromas arise from nerve VIII and unilateral nerve deafness is the chief symptom. The tumours may enlarge to involve the neighbouring nerves V and VII, causing loss of sensation over the ipsilateral side of the face and a depressed corneal reflex and facial paralysis. Ipsilateral cerebellar ataxia may result from compression of the cerebellar hemisphere, and hemiplegia and hemi-anaesthesia from pressure on the long tracts in the brain-stem. The diagnosis should be made when the tumour is small by investigating patients with nerve deafness thoroughly.

REFERENCES

Brodal A. (1965) *The Cranial Nerves. Anatomy and Anatomico-clinical Correlations*, 2nd edn. Blackwell Scientific Publications, Oxford.

Leigh R. J. and Zee D. S. (1991) *The Neurology of Eye Movements*, 2nd edn. F. A. Davis, Philadelphia.

Dyck P. J., Thomas P. K., Griffin J. W., Low P. A. and Poduslo J. F. (1993) *Peripheral Neuropathy*, 3rd edn. W. B. Saunders, Philadelphia.

5 | Motor system

FUNCTIONAL DIVISION OF MOTOR PATHWAYS

The motor system may be considered in terms of five main functional divisions: the lower motor neurone (final common pathway), the corticospinal (pyramidal) tract, extrapyramidal tracts, cerebellum and cerebral cortex (Fig. 5.1).

Lower motor neurone

The lower motor neurone innervates a motor unit which comprises an anterior horn cell (motoneurone) with an axon that divides to supply 2–1500 muscle fibres (Fig. 5.2) that all contract when the motor unit is active. The force of contraction in a muscle depends on the number of active motoneurones, their size and their rate of firing (up to about 100 Hz). Motor units are recruited in an orderly fashion, from the smallest to the largest, in a given muscle. Disorders of the lower motor neurone involve the motor unit, e.g. poliomyelitis and motor neurone disease (affecting anterior horn cells), intervertebral disc protrusions (which may compress motor roots), plexus lesions and peripheral neuropathies. The motor unit may also be affected by failure of neuromuscular transmission (myasthenic syndromes) or disorders of muscle fibres (myopathies).

The corticospinal (pyramidal) tract

This major motor pathway arises chiefly, but not exclusively, from the precentral gyrus of the cerebral cortex, and decussates in the pyramids at the lower end of the medulla. The descending fibres terminate directly, or via an interconnecting neurone, on the anterior horn cells (Fig. 5.3). A pure lesion of the lateral corticospinal tract is rarely seen because the tract is accompanied throughout its course by an extrapyramidal pathway, the reticulospinal tract. Disorders involving the corticospinal tract (and accompanying corticoreticulospinal fibres) are spoken of clinically as *upper motor neurone lesions*. Such disorders are very common and are seen, for example, after strokes or injuries involving the spinal cord.

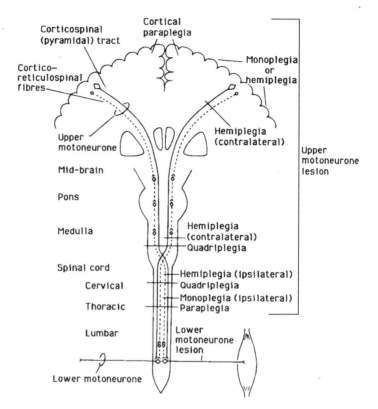

Fig. 5.1 Diagram of upper and lower motor neurones showing the levels of the nervous system, where they may be affected and the distribution of weakness that results. The pyramidal tract is accompanied by corticoreticulospinal fibres (interrupted lines), damage to which causes spasticity. (From Lance and McLeod, 1981, with permission of Butterworths, London.)

Extrapyramidal tracts

Descending pathways other than the pyramidal tract are connected with the spinal motoneurone pool mainly through interneurones and play a role in voluntary movement (Fig. 15.1). These arise from the frontoparietal cortex, basal ganglia, cerebellum and other nuclei in the brain-stem and, after interconnections, finally project downstream as rubrospinal, reticulospinal and vestibulospinal pathways. *Extrapyramidal disorders* are manifested chiefly as abnormalities of muscle tone, posture and movement. The commonest extrapyramidal disorder is Parkinson's disease (Chapter 15).

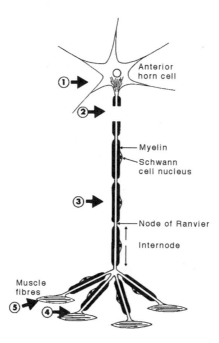

Fig. 5.2   Lower motor neurone. Lower motor neurone disorders may result from diseases of (1) the anterior horn cell, (2) motor roots or (3) peripheral nerve. Disorders of the neuromuscular junction (4) and muscle fibres (5) may simulate lower motor neurone lesions by affecting the distal parts of the motor unit.

Cerebellum

The cerebellum has reciprocal connections with sensorimotor cortex, reticular formation, vestibular nuclei and spinal cord (Figs 8.3–8.5). It participates in the programming of ballistic (rapid) movement and feedback control of ramp (slow) movements. Cerebellar disorders are characterized by hypotonia, incoordination and ataxia (Chapter 8).

Cerebral cortex

At the highest level, damage to association and frontal areas of the cerebral cortex, which are involved in transforming thought into action, may impair or prevent willed movement. These disorders are known as *apraxias* (p. 35). For example, in an ideational apraxia which follows damage to the dominant parietal lobe, a movement cannot be performed as instructed although the appropriate motor pathways are intact (Chapter 3).

REFLEXES

There is a hierarchy of human motor control that proceeds from the most simple reflex movement, the monosynaptic tendon jerk, to complex voluntary motor actions such as fine finger movements. Reflex activity plays a prominent part in the maintenance of posture and the execution of movement.

The simplest reflex is the stretch reflex (Fig. 5.4). The *muscle spindle*, the stretch receptor in muscle, consists of specialized muscle fibres supplied with nuclear bag and nuclear chain nerve endings whose afferents are Group Ia and II nerve fibres. The muscle spindle (with its intrafusal fibres) lies parallel to the extrafusal muscle fibres. When the muscle spindle is stretched, impulses pass along Group Ia afferent fibres which synapse monosynaptically with *alpha motoneurones*. These in turn discharge, causing the muscle to contract. The smaller diameter Group II muscle afferents from muscle spindles exert mainly inhibitory effects on extensor motoneurones and facilitatory effects on flexor motoneurones, i.e. they act as flexor reflex afferents (FRA) and this reflex action becomes apparent

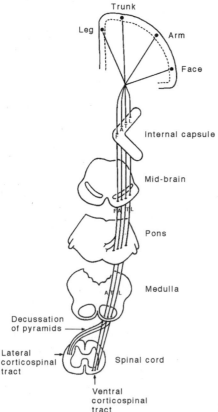

Fig. 5.3 Pathways of corticospinal tracts.

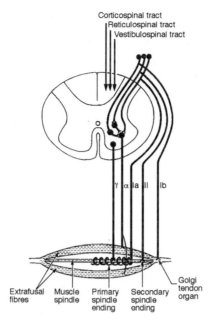

Fig. 5.4   Stretch reflex arc. Group Ia afferent fibres, connected to the primary spindle endings, synapse directly with alpha motoneurones in the anterior horn whose axons innervate the extrafusal muscle fibres. Group Ib afferent fibres are connected to Golgi tendon organs. Group II afferent fibres connected to secondary spindle endings are mainly inhibitory on extensor motoneurones and facilitatory on flexor motoneurones. The gamma motoneurones innervate the muscle spindle. Descending motor pathways (corticospinal, reticulospinal, vestibulospinal) regulate alpha and gamma motoneurone excitability.

in spasticity. *Golgi tendon organs* lie near tendons and are connected to Ib afferents; these are highly sensitive to active contraction and also to sudden increases in tension. *Gamma motoneurones* which innervate the muscle spindle and regulate its tension and thereby its sensitivity to stretch, also lie in the anterior horn of the spinal cord. Their action during movement is to cause contraction of the muscle spindle fibres so that afferents can continue to act as sensors during contraction when the extrafusal fibres shorten. *Supraspinal control* of alpha and gamma motoneurones is derived from corticospinal, vestibulospinal, reticulospinal and rubrospinal pathways (Fig. 5.4).

Tendon reflexes

Clinically the reflex arc is tested by way of the tendon or stretch reflexes. A brisk tap over the tendon or a vibration wave induced by percussion of bone to which the tendon attaches, stretches the muscle spindle and excites the monosynaptic reflex causing the extrafusal muscle fibres to contract (Fig. 5.5). This is an example of a *phasic stretch reflex* in which there is excitation from a more or less synchronous afferent volley of action potentials. Reflexes that are commonly tested clinically and the segments through which they operate are shown in Table 5.1.

Table 5.1 Commonly tested tendon reflexes

Reflex	Segment
Jaw jerk	Fifth cranial nerve (motor nerve)
Biceps jerk	C5, 6
Brachioradialis (supinator) jerk	C5, 6
Triceps jerk	C7
Finger-flexion jerk	C8
Knee jerk	L3, 4
Ankle jerk	S1

Alteration in tendon reflexes

Tendon jerks vary in amplitude from person to person but are normally symmetrical.

Depression of reflex activity Reflexes may be depressed because of impairment of function of parts of the reflex arc in: (i) the gamma motoneurone; fusimotor activity may be depressed in spinal shock and probably in acute cerebellar

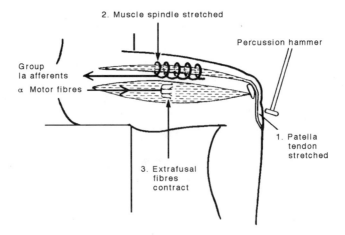

Fig. 5.5 Mechanism of a tendon reflex. A brisk tap with a percussion hammer stretches the tendon (1) and the muscle spindle (2), initiating a volley of impulses in the Group Ia afferent fibres that excites the alpha motoneurone thus causing the extrafusal fibres to contract (3).

lesions. As a result, the muscle spindle becomes less sensitive to stretch; (ii) afferent fibres, e.g. peripheral neuropathy and dorsal root lesions; (iii) anterior horn cells, e.g. poliomyelitis or motor neurone disease; (iv) efferent fibres, e.g. peripheral neuropathy and ventral root lesions; (v) muscles, e.g. myopathy; (vi) the contraction of antagonists, e.g. poor relaxation and extrapyramidal rigidity.

Selective damage to the muscle spindles is not known clinically; they do not share in the muscular atrophy of motor neurone disease.

In general, reflexes are much more sensitive to damage to the afferent pathways than to the efferent pathways.

Exaggeration of reflex activity   The most common pathological cause of increased tendon reflexes is an upper motor neurone lesion, but they may also be exaggerated as a result of anxiety, after exercise and in thyrotoxicosis.

Reinforcement of reflexes

Reflex activity may be heightened by *reinforcement*, e.g. a depressed biceps jerk may become brisker if the patient is asked to squeeze an object hard with the opposite hand at the time the reflex is being elicited, or lower limb reflexes may be enhanced by the patient pulling with one hand against the other (*Jendrassik manoeuvre*).

Reflexes should not be considered absent unless reinforcement has been attempted. The effort increases alpha motoneurone activity in the spinal cord and thus increases the sensitivity of the stretch reflex.

Spread of reflexes

Sometimes in normal people, and frequently in patients with upper motor neurone disease, what is known as a *spread of reflexes* is seen. For example, if a supinator jerk is elicited, the biceps and triceps as well as the brachioradialis may contract briskly in response to the tap over the radius. This is due to both alpha motoneurone hyperexcitability in the spinal cord and local mechanical spread of a wave of vibration that excites muscle spindles in distant muscles causing them to contract reflexly (Fig. 5.6). Primary endings in muscle spindles are very sensitive to vibration.

Tonic reflexes

Tonic reflexes (as distinct from phasic reflexes) are those that are excited by a sustained asynchronous afferent stimulus. In cats, there is some evidence that different alpha motoneurones subserve the phasic and tonic reflexes but there is no evidence that this is so in man. Tonic stretch reflexes may become apparent in normal people during anxiety and postural adjustment or voluntary muscle contraction. They cannot usually be detected in relaxed normal human subjects. They are increased in upper motor neurone lesions (spasticity) and some extrapyramidal disorders (rigidity). Application of a vibrator to the muscle belly or tendon elicits a tonic reflex contraction in man (tonic vibration reflex or TVR), that has some application in physiotherapy.

Superficial cutaneous reflexes

These are polysynaptic reflexes that are often relayed through several spinal segments. (Table 5.2).

Table 5.2   Polysynaptic reflexes that are often relayed through more than one segment

Reflex	Segment
Corneal	Cranial nerve V and VII
Abdominal	
Upper	T9, 10
Lower	T11, 12
Cremasteric	L1, 2
Plantar	S1
Bulbocavernosus	S2, 3, 4
Anal	S3, 4, 5

MUSCLE TONE

Muscle tone is a clinical term used to describe the resistance of muscles to passive movement. The resistance is determined partly by mechanical factors (joints, ligaments and viscoelastic properties of muscle), and partly by background and reflex contraction of the muscle (the tonic stretch reflex).

Normal subjects are capable of learning to relax to the point where no muscular activity is present at rest and no muscular activity is provoked by limb movements of slow or moderate velocity. In subjects who are standing or seated however, there will be tonic muscular activity in the postural muscles at least and often a small degree of activity in the non-postural muscles (co-contraction). Increases in this muscle activity may occur (but with a longer latency than seen with phasic tendon jerks) in response to perturbations of posture. It is this muscle activity which comprises the variable element of tone.

Tone will be decreased when there is an interruption of the stretch reflex arc, such as may occur in peripheral neuropathies and other lower motor neurone disorders. Tone is also decreased in cerebellar disorders and immediately after spinal cord injuries (spinal shock), probably as a result of decreased responsiveness of the muscle spindle to stretch, consequent upon a depression of fusimotor activity.

Tone is increased in upper motor neurone disorders, when it increases in proportion to the velocity at which the muscle is stretched (*spasticity*). It is also increased in certain extrapyramidal disorders such as Parkinson's disease, when it is

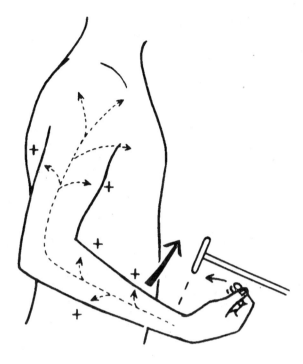

Fig. 5.6   The radial ('supinator') jerk. Percussion of the radius initiates a vibration wave that stimulates primary spindle endings as it traverses muscle bellies, causing a reflex contraction (+) of biceps, triceps, brachioradialis, finger flexors and extensors. The limb moves in the direction of the stronger muscles so that the elbow and fingers flex, the reaction of a normal 'supinator' or radial jerk. Multiple muscle contractions are observed more clearly in upper motor neurone lesions, a finding termed 'reflex irradiation'. (From Lance and McLeod, 1981, with permission of Butterworths, London.)

relatively insensitive to the velocity of stretch and is often interrupted by tremor (*cog-wheel rigidity*). *Dystonia* is a term used to describe a transient or persistent increase in tone that is associated with co-contraction of antagonistic muscles and assumption of an abnormal posture.

LOWER MOTOR NEURONE DISORDERS

Lower motor neurone disorders may result from disease or damage to the anterior horn cell (e.g. poliomyelitis, motor neurone disease, syringomyelia), motor root (e.g. cervical or lumbar disc protrusions, malignancy) or peripheral nerve (e.g. Bell's palsy, nerve injuries, peripheral neuropathy). See Figs 5.1 and 5.2.

Clinical features of lower motor neurone disorders

Muscle weakness

This may range from slight weakness (paresis) to total paralysis.

Muscle wasting

Peripheral nerve lesions result in muscle wasting and weakness in the distribution of the damaged nerve. Root injuries result in wasting that follows a segmental distribution. Anterior horn cell disease may give rise to diffuse weakness and wasting.

Fasciculation

Coarse fascicular twitches, caused by spontaneous contraction of one or more motor units, are seen in lower motor neurone disorders, especially in chronic degenerative diseases of the anterior horn cell, such as motor neurone disease. *Benign fasciculations* occur frequently in normal people, especially if the muscle is in a state of tension. Benign fasciculations are coarse, and usually affect the same motor unit repeatedly. Fasciculations in the calves due to S1 root irritation are a common finding in middle-aged and elderly subjects. Pathological fasciculations due to degeneration of nerves or nerve cells are an irregular twitching seen in various parts of a relaxed muscle; minutes may elapse before the same motor unit contracts for a second time. As a general rule, fasciculation has pathological significance only when the muscle concerned is atrophied or weak.

Myokymia is a related phenomenon to fasciculation. It is an irregular undulation of superficial muscle fibres. It commonly occurs around the eye and is usually benign but persistent facial or limb myokymia may be a sign of involvement of the appropriate efferent pathway. Widespread facial myokymia is seen in structural lesions of the pons (e.g. brain-stem glioma, multiple sclerosis).

Fibrillation

This is an electromyographic term and refers to spontaneous electrical activity in individual muscle fibres after denervation (Fig. 5.7).

Hypotonia

Tonic stretch reflexes are diminished in proportion to the degree of muscular weakness.

Tendon reflexes

These are depressed in proportion to the degree of damage to the efferent limb of the reflex arc. They may, however, be increased if there is an associated upper motor neurone lesion (e.g. motor neurone disease).

Contractures

Progressive shortening of muscle bellies in paralysed muscles or in their antagonists may result in deformities of the limb (contractures).

Trophic changes

These are partly a result of disuse, and partly a result of vasomotor (autonomic) involvement. The skin is cold, cyanosed, smooth and dry. Toe-nails, finger-nails and bones become osteoporotic and brittle.

Electromyogram (EMG)

The features of denervation are: spontaneous fibrillation, positive sharp waves, a reduced pattern of motor unit activity on maximum voluntary effort and polyphasic, large amplitude motor units of long duration (Figs 5.7, 5.8).

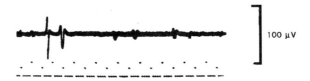

100 μV

Fig. 5.7 Spontaneous fibrillation, recorded through a concentric needle electrode from a denervated muscle. Time marker: 5 ms intervals.

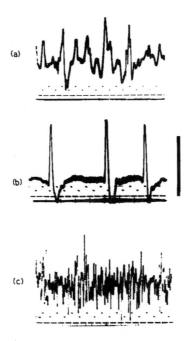

(a)

(b)

(c)

Fig. 5.8 Electromyogram recorded on maximum voluntary effort from (a) normal muscle, (b) denervated muscle, (c) muscular dystrophy. Time marker: 5 ms intervals. Calibration 2 mV (a+c), 5 mV (b).

DISORDERS OF THE NEUROMUSCULAR JUNCTION AND MUSCLES

Failure of neuromuscular transmission causes fatiguability and weakness of muscles and is seen most commonly in myasthenia gravis. Diseases of muscle fibres (myopathy) cause wasting and weakness of muscles. Muscular dystrophies are genetically determined myopathies.

Clinical features

Muscle weakness

In myopathies, muscle weakness is usually proximal and may be restricted to particular muscle groups. In myasthenia gravis, the characteristic feature is weakness after sustained or repeated effort (muscle fatiguability); extra-ocular, bulbar and proximal limb muscles are most commonly affected. It is not unusual for myasthenia to be confined to the ocular muscles (ocular myasthenia).

Muscle wasting

Muscle wasting may be severe in myopathies but is not a feature of myasthenia gravis. In myopathies, muscle wasting and weakness may be restricted to particular muscle groups, especially proximal muscles.

Fasciculation

This is absent.

Hypotonia

Tone is reduced in proportion to the degree of muscle weakness.

Reflexes

Reflexes are depressed when muscle wasting is advanced, but may not be affected in the early stages since muscle spindles are spared.

Contractures

Contractures occur in wasted muscles.

Trophic changes

Trophic changes may be seen in paralysed limbs.

Electromyogram

The electromyographic features of myopathies are a full pattern of activity on maximum voluntary effort but the individual motor unit potentials are of short duration, polyphasic and of reduced amplitude (Fig. 5.8).

UPPER MOTOR NEURONE DISORDERS

The descriptive terms *upper motor neurone disorder, pyramidal tract disorder* and *corticospinal tract disorder* are all used synonymously in clinical medicine. This is not an accurate use of terms in an anatomical or physiological sense, but it is hallowed by tradition. Pure pyramidal tract lesions are rarely seen clinically; accompanying corticoreticulospinal fibres are usually involved as well.

The major contributions to the pyramidal tract in man arise from the precentral and postcentral gyri, and from the paracentral lobule (Fig. 5.9), with significant contributions from Brodman's areas 5, 6 and 7. Only 2–3% of the fibres arise from Betz cells.

The corticospinal and corticobulbar fibres have a definite topographical distribution on the cortex (Fig. 5.10). This mapping is referred to as the motor *humunculus* (little man). At the lowermost part of the precentral gyrus are the areas for larynx and pharynx, above which are the areas for palate, mandible and tongue, and then the centres for lower and upper face. The upper face has a bilateral representation like the pharynx and larynx and sternomastoid muscles. Lower limb areas lie in the upper part of the motor strip and paracentral lobule so that lesions in the parasagittal region (e.g. meningiomas), or sagittal sinus thrombosis, may cause lower limb paralysis with sparing of the upper limbs (Fig. 5.1). Conversely tumours and vascular lesions in the lower part of the motor strip may involve the opposite side of the face and upper limb exclusively.

The corticospinal and corticobulbar tracts descend in the corona radiata to the internal capsule, where they occupy mainly its posterior limb; the fibres from the face and shoulder lie anteriorly, and those for the lower limb, posteriorly

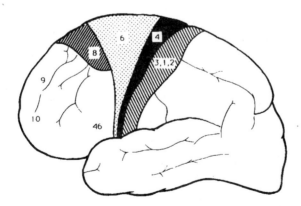

Fig. 5.9 Origin of corticospinal tracts from cerebral cortex. Most of the fibres in the corticospinal tracts arise from the motor cortex (area 4), premotor cortex (area 6) and somatosensory cortex (areas 3, 1, 2). The supplementary motor cortex (area 8) plays an important part in programming movements. (Modified from D. Cogan, 1966, *Neurology of the Ocular Muscles*, 2nd edn. Courtesy of Charles C. Thomas, Springfield, Illinois.)

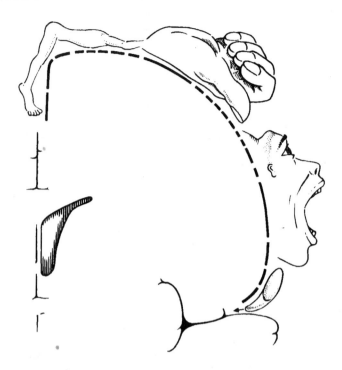

Fig. 5.10 Topographical distribution of origin of corticospinal tracts from cerebral cortex (after Penfield).

(Fig. 5.3). The face and upper limb may be selectively paralysed by thrombosis of the recurrent branch of the anterior cerebral artery (Heubner's artery) which supplies the relevant area of the internal capsule.

In the mid-brain, the corticospinal tract runs in the middle three-fifths of the cerebral peduncles; in the pons it becomes broken into scattered bundles amidst transverse fibres and islands of pontine grey matter; in the medulla the fibres come together again to form the pyramids (Fig. 5.3). About 70–90% of the fibres cross to the other side of the medulla in the decussation of the pyramids. Most of the uncrossed fibres run in the ventral corticospinal tract, and cross before terminating on the anterior horn cells chiefly of the neck and trunk muscles. Corticospinal tract fibres terminate on anterior horn cells either directly or through internuncial cells.

The pyramidal tract is not essential for most voluntary movements which can be carried out by primates after the pyramids have been sectioned. However, in contrast to the extrapyramidal motor system, it is responsible for fine and skilled movements, particularly of the hands and fingers. It also has an inhibitory effect on antigravity muscles and promotes abduction of upper limbs and flexion of lower limbs, i.e. it breaks up the pattern of reflex standing in man (flexed upper limbs and extended lower limbs) which is determined mainly by extrapyramidal pathways.

Clinical features of upper motor neurone disorders

The commonest cause of an upper motor neurone disorder is a vascular lesion involving the internal capsule. This is the most common type of stroke and since the corticospinal and corticobulbar fibres are close together in this region, they are all affected. This gives rise to a paralysis (*hemiplegia*) or weakness (*hemiparesis*) of the opposite side of the body (Fig. 5.1). The main features of hemiplegia from any cerebral lesion, which should be contrasted with those of lower motor neurone disorders, are described below.

Muscle weakness

This always affects groups of muscles rather than individual muscles. Bilateral movements of the jaws, upper face, neck, pharynx, larynx, thorax and upper abdomen are usually little affected although they may be impaired immediately following the onset of the lesion.

Ocular movements Immediately after a lesion of the internal capsule, the eyes may deviate to the side of the lesion in an unconscious patient. In the conscious patient there may be weakness of conjugate deviation to the opposite side (Chapter 4). This usually lasts for only a few hours or days and is rarely permanent.

Head and neck As with the eyes, there may be a deviation of the head or neck to the side of the lesion in the comatose patient.

Face The upper face is bilaterally innervated and is little affected. The lower face is weak but this may be apparent only as a filling-in of the nasolabial fold on the affected side, or a slight drooping of the corner of the mouth. Movements of the face following emotional stimuli, e.g. laughing or crying, may be quite normal because they are effected through extrapyramidal connections.

Jaw, palate, tongue Like other bilaterally innervated structures, these are only slightly affected. There may be transient weakness of these structures on the side opposite the lesion.

Limbs The side opposite the lesion is weak; fine skilled movements of the fingers and toes are most affected. In upper limbs, the abductors are primarily involved (deltoids, spinati, and finger abductors) and, in lower limbs, the flexors (hip flexors, hamstrings, dorsiflexors of ankle and toes).

Gait The upper limb on the affected side is held flexed and adducted. There is difficulty in flexing the lower limbs and it is necessary to circumduct the leg at the hip in order to bring the limb forward. The foot is plantar-flexed and the shoe drags along the ground.

Muscle wasting

Any muscular wasting results from disuse, except in the rare syndrome of wasting from a parietal lobe lesion, the mechanism of which is unknown.

Fasciculations

Fasciculations do not occur in pure upper motor neurone lesions.

Hypertonia

Immediately after a capsular lesion, the limbs may be completely flaccid. After 2–3 weeks, tone increases and the limbs are said to be spastic. Increased resistance to passive movement is most pronounced in the adductors and internal rotators of the shoulder, the flexors of the elbow, wrist and fingers, and the pronators of the forearm. In the lower limb the resistance is greater in the adductors of the hip, extensors of the hip and knee, and plantar-flexors of the foot and toes. The hemiplegic posture is the result of the abnormal distribution of muscle tone. It is influenced by tonic neck and labyrinthine reflexes, disinhibited from cortical control, and represents the antigravity posture (decorticate posture) of reflex standing in man. The resistance to stretch seen in spasticity is velocity-dependent; i.e. the resistance is increased with faster stretching movements. Therefore, in testing clinically for muscle tone, all limbs should be moved through a range of velocities.

An occasional accompaniment of spasticity of capsular hemiplegia is the clasp-knife phenomenon seen in the extensor muscles of the lower limbs. In this phenomenon muscle tension increases with velocity of stretch to about the mid-position of a joint. The subsequent sudden relaxation of tension is considered to be caused by inhibition arising from activation of Group II afferent fibres by increasing muscle length, although the Golgi tendon organs may initially cause some inhibition through Group Ib afferents (Fig. 5.4). The limb remains hypotonic as long as the extensor muscle is stretched beyond the clasp-knife point but spasticity becomes apparent again as soon as the limb is extended.

The increased muscle tone in upper motor neurone disorders is partly due to hyperexcitability of alpha motoneurones, which then become more readily excited reflexly by passive stretch. There is no direct evidence for hyperactivity of gamma motoneurones, which would theoretically cause the muscle spindles to become more responsive to stretch.

There is little increase in tone after section of the medullary pyramids in monkeys. The spasticity which follows upper motor neurone lesions in man is probably the consequence of damage to the extrapyramidal corticoreticulospinal pathway which has an inhibitory influence on the spinal motor neurone pool.

Reflexes

After the initial stages of an acute capsular lesion the deep tendon reflexes become exaggerated, and 'clonus', a rhythmical series of muscle contractions in response to maintained stretch, may be elicited.

Increased reflex activity can be explained on the basis of alpha motoneurone hyperactivity, which also accounts for the spread of reflexes (radiation) and clonus.

The finger flexion reflex may be increased, and Hoffman's sign (obtained by vibrating the tendons and muscles by flicking the terminal phalanx of a finger), which is merely another way of eliciting the thumb and finger flexion reflex, may also be positive. Abdominal and cremasteric reflexes which are polysynaptic are often, but not invariably, lost.

The plantar reflex

Babinski (1896) was the first to establish the plantar response as one of the most important signs in clinical neurology. Until the age of 18 months, the great toe extends (dorsiflexes) in response to stimulation of the lateral aspect of the sole as part of an uncontrolled protective response which involves all the flexors of the lower limb (including extensor hallucis longus and other dorsiflexors of the feet and toes since they act physiologically as flexor muscles). When the infant learns to stand, flexor reflexes are inhibited from the brain-stem by a reticulospinal pathway so that flexor pathways may be used for volitional movement such as walking. From this time on, the great toe then plantar-flexes in response to stimulation of the sole (flexor plantar response or 'down-going toe'). After damage to upper motor neurone pathways, flexor reflexes are released from their customary inhibition so that the toe again extends if the sole is stroked (extensor plantar response, 'up-going toe' or Babinski response). In addition, there may be abduction (fanning) of the toes. In such pathological states, there is an increase in the area in which stimulation will produce the reflex (receptive field); it can sometimes be elicited from the skin of the tibial surface of the leg. The release of flexor reflexes may also give rise to more widespread *flexor spasms* of the legs and trunk, particularly if brain-stem control of segmental mechanisms is impaired by a spinal lesion.

When testing for the presence of the Babinski response, the following important points should be noted:

- The outer border of the sole of the foot (S1 dermatome) should be stimulated with a light stroke. Traditionally a key is used but any mildly noxious pressure stimulus will suffice. The patient should be warned of the impending stimulus and asked to relax
- The Babinski reflex must be distinguished from a voluntary withdrawal response in which there is also extension of the big toe associated with hip and knee flexion
- The associated fanning of the toes may be of significance in confirming an isolated extensor plantar response
- The extensor plantar response indicates what is termed clinically 'pyramidal tract disease'. However, it does not correlate completely with lesions of the anatomical corticospinal tracts. In other words, one can have corticospinal tract damage without a positive Babinski sign, and a positive Babinski sign without any corticospinal tract damage. It is an oversimplification to equate absolutely a positive Babinski sign with corticospinal tract disease, since it is caused by damage to corticoreticulospinal fibres inhibiting flexor reflexes. Positive Babinski responses are found in the first 18 months of life, in sleep, in deep coma and after epileptic seizures. In these conditions there is functional rather than structural impairment of the pathways.

Contractures

Contractures are fixed shortenings of muscles and tendons that occur in any clinically shortened muscle and may develop in longstanding upper motor neurone disorders if adequate physiotherapy is not instituted.

Trophic changes

These are inconspicuous.

Electromyogram

There are no signs of denervation. On needle EMG, the recruitment pattern of motor units is characterized by low firing rates.

REFERENCES

Adams R. D. and Victor M. (1993) *Principles of Neurology*, 5th edn. McGraw-Hill, New York.

Alexander G. E. and DeLong M. R. (1992) Central mechanisms of initiation and control of movement. In: *Diseases of the Nervous System*, Eds A. K. Asbury, G. M. McKhann and W. I. McDonald. W. B. Saunders, Philadelphia. 285–308.

Brown P. (1994) The pathophysiology of spasticity. *Journal of Neurology, Neurosurgery and Psychiatry*, **57**, 773–777.

6 | Sensory system

The sensory system is usually considered and examined clinically as an entity separate from the motor system, but of course the two are closely related. Motor and reflex functions depend very much on the pattern of their sensory input. Clinical examples of this interdependence of the motor and the sensory system are inability to move a limb if all the dorsal roots are sectioned, and the disturbance of gait caused by an interruption of sensory pathways from the lower limbs. Most motor functions are ultimately an elaboration and integration of basic reflex mechanisms.

PATIENT HISTORY

The patient's history is of considerable importance. For example, he or she may complain of abnormal sensations (*paraesthesiae, dysaesthesia*) including 'pins and needles', numbness, burning, coldness or pain. Patients may notice a difference in temperature sensation in their legs when they sit in a hot bath or in their two hands when they place them in water. They often use descriptive terms such as 'numbness' in a different sense to the doctor and it is important to determine precisely what they mean. In cervical cord lesions, especially but not exclusively in multiple sclerosis, tingling electric shock-like sensations may be experienced down the spine on bending the neck (*Lhermitte's sign*). Band-like constrictions around the trunk or limbs are usually caused by spinal cord lesions and a feeling of the limbs being bloated or distended suggests a lesion in the dorsal columns.

When a patient complains of an abnormal sensation, one must determine its site, nature and quality, radiation, provoking and relieving factors, duration and time of onset and associated features, e.g. sweating, redness, dryness of skin, hyperalgesia.

EXAMINATION

Examination of the sensory system is the most difficult part of the neurological examination. Sensation is a purely subjective phenomenon and for accurate testing a fully conscious, alert, intelligent, cooperative patient (and doctor) is desirable.

Such an ideal combination of qualities may not be present. It is important to avoid suggesting to the patient sensory changes which may not exist since many patients are highly suggestible. The key point is to relate the sensory examination to the clinical history. For example, if the patient complains of numbness in the little and ring fingers, the examination starts by comparing sensation in the presumed numb area with that of the index finger and thumb; the numb area is then delineated precisely by moving the pin or other test object from the abnormal to the normal area so that a clear end-point is obtained and the distribution of sensory loss can be related to a peripheral nerve, spinal root, or central lesion. Similarly, if paraesthesiae are unilateral, one side of the body is compared with the other or, if the abnormal sensations are in the lower limbs, testing proceeds from below upwards to determine the upper level of sensory loss. As well as detecting loss of sensation, abnormal qualities of sensation may be elicited, such as excessive pain response to noxious stimuli (*hyperalgesia, hyperpathia*) or non-noxious stimuli (*allodynia*).

The sensations that are commonly tested clinically, as outlined in Chapter 2, are: (i) light touch, with a wisp of cotton wool; (ii) pain, with the point of a pin (the stimulus must be felt as sharp); (iii) temperature, with hot and cold objects; (iv) vibration sense, with a tuning fork of 128 Hz; (v) joint position sense; (vi) tactile discrimination, with compass points (usually < 3 mm on the fingers or < 3 cm on the feet; (vii) stereognosis, or the recognition of shape and form.

Quantitative tests of vibration, light touch, pain and temperature sensation have been devised, but are used mainly in research or in specialized laboratories.

SENSORY PATHWAYS

Human cutaneous nerves

Human cutaneous nerves contain myelinated (A) fibres which range in diameter from about 2 to 16 μm and unmyelinated (C) fibres, all having their cell bodies in the dorsal root ganglia. They terminate peripherally in the skin and deeper structures as free nerve endings or encapsulated endings such as Meissner's corpuscles and Pacinian corpuscles. Some of these encapsulated endings are specially adapted to respond to certain stimuli, e.g. Pacinian corpuscles respond to displacement and vibration. The free nerve endings also play an important role in sensory discrimination, and are divided into three groups: mechanosensitive, thermosensitive and polymodal receptors. Polymodal receptors respond to more than one type of stimulus e.g. mechanical and thermal changes.

Spinal cord

Pain fibres run for one or two segments in Lissauer's tract before entering the dorsal horn; small Aδ myelinated fibres synapse in Rexed laminae I and V and unmyelinated C fibres synapse in lamina II (substantia gelatinosa) where substance P and other neuropeptides are transmitters (Fig. 6.1). Fibres relaying pain sensation arise mainly from cells in lamina V and cross to the opposite side of the spinal cord to join the lateral spinothalamic tract (Fig. 6.2). Proprioceptive afferents enter the ipsilateral dorsal columns without synapsing. Tactile afferents pass through both ipsilateral dorsal columns and contralateral ventrolateral columns (Fig. 6.3).

Dorsal columns

The dorsal columns (i) transmit the sensation of light touch; (ii) are important in spatial discrimination of tactile stimuli (e.g. two-point discrimination); (iii) transmit

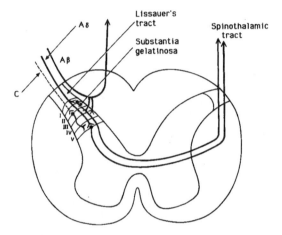

Fig. 6.1 Pathways of pain fibres in dorsal horn of spinal cord.

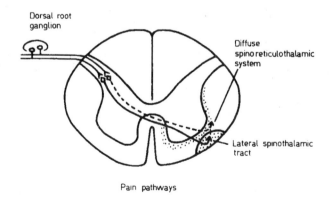

Fig. 6.2 Spinal pathways for pain. (From Lance and McLeod, 1981, with permission of Butterworths, London.)

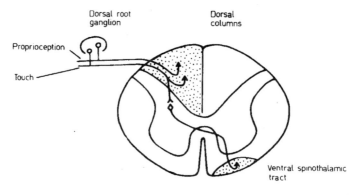

Touch and proprioceptive pathways

Fig. 6.3 Spinal pathways for proprioception and touch. (From Lance and McLeod, 1981, with permission of Butterworths, London.)

joint position and vibration sense, although transmission of these modalities may not be exclusively a posterior column function.

Ventrolateral columns

The ventrolateral columns transmit: (i) pain and temperature sensation; (ii) light touch sensation (the threshold for tactile sensation is raised after transection of the anterolateral columns); (iii) sensations of tickle and itch; (iv) sexual sensations; (v) vibration sense. The ability to perceive vibration may be impaired or lost in lesions of the lateral columns.

Thalamus and cerebral cortex

The dorsal columns and spinothalamic tracts project to the ventroposterolateral nucleus of the thalamus (VPL). The spinoreticular system projects to brain-stem reticular formation, and mid-line thalamic nuclei, centre median and lateral reticular nucleus.

All sensory modalities, with the possible exception of pain, project from the thalamus to the sensory cortex in the post-central gyrus (Brodmann areas 3, 2, 1; Figs 5.9, 6.4). Sensations are analysed in the sensory association areas of the parietal lobe (Brodmann areas 5, 7; Fig. 3.1). Disturbances of these areas, which may be physiological as in drifting off to sleep, or pathological as in migraine or epilepsy, may cause illusions of body parts growing larger or smaller, or sensory hallucinations. Parietal lobe lesions may cause neglect of, or inattention to, a contralateral stimulus if two stimuli are presented simultaneously to both sides of the body (tactile inattention; Chapter 3), or inability to recognize common objects (*tactile agnosia*). Two-point discrimination, position sense and stereognosis (recognition of the shape of objects) may be impaired if there is damage to the sensory cortex but will also be impaired by lesions of pathways at a lower level.

MODALITIES OF SENSATION

Light touch

Clinically, light touch is usually tested with cotton wool. Large myelinated fibres (Aαβ) are excited by light touch, but not exclusively so since Aδ and C fibres are also excited by stroking the skin with cotton wool. Human experiments indicate that tactile sensation may be induced by the excitation of only one or two large myelinated fibres.

Impulses excited in the periphery by light touch are conducted centrally in the spinal cord by way of the dorsal columns, through the medial lemniscal system to the opposite thalamus (VPL) and thence to the cerebral cortex (Figs 6.3, 6.4). Tactile sensation is also conveyed in the ventrolateral columns in an ill-defined tract, the ventral spinothalamic tract (Fig. 6.3).

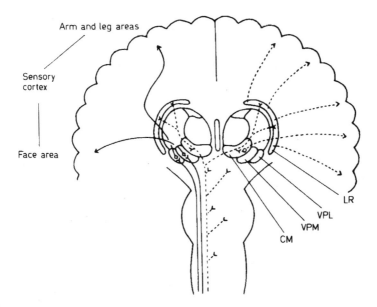

Fig. 6.4 Cerebral termination of sensory pathways. Specific afferent pathways are indicated as solid lines on the left of the diagram, fibres from the face synapsing in the postero-ventromedial nucleus (VPM) of the thalamus on their way to the cortex, while fibres from the rest of the body synapse in the posteroventrolateral nucleus (VPL). Diffuse spino-reticulothalamic pain fibres are shown as interrupted lines on the right side of the diagram, synapsing in the mid-line thalamic nuclei, centrum medianum (CM) and lateral reticular nucleus (LR) before projecting widely to the cerebral cortex. (From Lance and McLeod, 1981, with permission of Butterworths, London.)

Joint position sense

Information concerning the orientation of the body in space and the spatial relations between its parts is derived from input from the visual apparatus, vestibular receptors and somatic sensory system. The somatic sensory component, i.e. proprioception or the sense of position and movement of body parts, depends mainly upon receptor organs associated with joints that signal static position as well as changes in position. Muscle spindles also play a role in the signalling of movement of joints (*kinaesthesia*).

Afferent fibres from joint receptors project through the dorsal columns and the lemniscal system to the sensory cortex (Figs 6.3, 6.4). Destruction of the dorsal columns results in impairment of position sense.

Vibration

The testing of vibration is merely a specialized way of testing tactile receptors and their pathways; there is probably no specific modality of vibration.

The peripheral pathway consists of large afferent fibres which innervate one or two Pacinian corpuscles. Pacinian corpuscles rapidly adapt and are very sensitive to vibration. The central pathway is by way of the dorsal columns to the lemniscal system, but spinocerebellar pathways may also be involved.

Pain

In any clinical consideration of pain, the psychological aspects and the patient's reaction to the sensation are of the utmost importance. However, the present discussion will be confined to anatomical and physiological aspects.

The adequate stimulus for pain threatens tissue damage, and, in testing for painful sensation, it is important that the patient recognizes the feeling of sharpness and not simply the feeling of contact or pressure.

There do not appear to be any specialized receptors for pain in the skin or deep tissues; impulses giving rise to painful sensation are initiated from free nerve endings.

It is well established in man as well as in experimental animals that the small myelinated Aδ fibres (which conduct impulses at velocities of 10–20 m/s) and the unmyelinated C fibres (which conduct at velocities of 1–2 m/s) are required to be stimulated before painful sensations are aroused. Stimulation of the C fibres gives rise to a most unpleasant quality of pain sensation and, because of the slower rate of conduction, the phenomenon of 'second pain' which is felt 1–2 seconds after the initial stab of pain.

Impulses are transmitted in the spinal cord in the lateral spinothalamic tracts to the VPL nucleus of the thalamus. Pathways probably then project to the sensory cortex so that impairment of pain sensation may sometimes follow localized injury to the sensory cortex in man.

In addition to the direct spinothalamic pathway that enables painful stimuli to be localized, there is a second pathway, the spinoreticulothalamic system that is responsible for the transmission of diffuse, poorly localized pain; it travels to the reticular formation and mid-line thalamic nuclei (Fig. 6.4) and may play a role in the autonomic and affective reaction to pain.

Itching is closely related to pain in its physiological mechanisms and its anatomical pathways. Tickle is probably a combination of tactile and painful sensations.

The endogenous pain control system

The transmission of pain impulses from afferent fibres entering the dorsal horn to the second order neurones is inhibited by activity in large diameter low-threshold fibres and is also regulated by descending pathways from the brain-stem (Fig. 6.5).

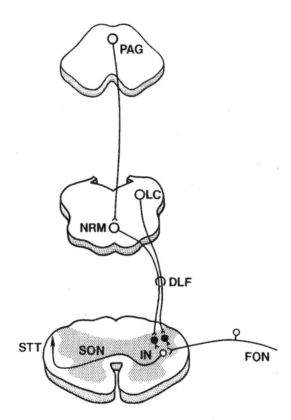

Fig. 6.5 Endogenous pain control system. The periaqueductal grey matter (PAG) of the mid-brain projects caudally through the nucleus raphe magnus (NRM) of the medulla to the spinal cord where 5-hydroxytryptamine (serotonin) is released as a neurotransmitter. A complementary noradrenergic pathway descends from the locus coeruleus (LC) through the dorsolateral fasciculus (DLF) to the spinal cord. First order neurons (FON) carrying pain impulses synapse in the dorsal horn with second order neurons (SON) that transmit impulses rostrally in the spinothalamic tract (STT). Transmission at this synapse is regulated by inhibitory interneurons (IN) which in turn are controlled by the descending pain control fibres in the DLF.

The nucleus raphe magnus of the medulla controls pain transmission in the spinal cord through a descending serotonergic pathway. The locus coeruleus and adjacent areas influence pain transmission through a noradrenergic pathway. The peri-aqueductal grey matter in the mid-brain contains opiate receptors and enkephalins, and descending pathways from this region to the brain-stem and spinal cord inhibit pain transmission.

Temperature sense

Specific warm and cold endings exist. Both small myelinated and unmyelinated C fibres respond to thermal stimulation. The central pathways are closely related to those subserving painful sensation.

REFERENCES

Lindblom U. and Ochoa J. (1992) Somatosensory function and dysfunction. In: *Diseases of the Nervous System*, 2nd edn. Eds A. K. Asbury, G. M. McKhann and W. I. McDonald. W. B. Saunders, Philadelphia. p. 213–228.

Maciewicz R. (1992) Organisation of pain pathways. In: *Diseases of the Nervous System*, 2nd edn. Eds A. K. Asbury, G. M. McKhann and W. I. McDonald. W. B. Saunders, Philadelphia. p. 849–857.

7 | Spinal cord

ANATOMY

The spinal cord in adults extends from the foramen magnum to the upper border of the second lumbar vertebra (L2; Fig. 7.1). The conus medullaris is the conical or inferior end of the cord from the apex of which a delicate filament, the filum terminale, extends and attaches to the first segment of the coccyx. The dura mater and arachnoid extend down to the level of the second sacral vertebra (S2) where they end as a blind sac. The spinal fluid is contained in the subarachnoid space, and since the spinal cord ends at the L2 level lumbar puncture can be safely performed at the L3 and L4 level (usually L3–4 interspace) to obtain a sample of cerebrospinal fluid.

Thirty-one pairs of roots (cervical, thoracic, lumbar, sacral and coccygeal) arise from the spinal cord, each with its ventral (anterior) and dorsal (posterior) root. The dorsal root ganglion is a swelling on the dorsal root which contains the cell bodies of afferent nerve fibres. The roots pass at an increasingly oblique angle at progressively lower levels of the spinal cord. In the lumbosacral region they descend almost vertically as the *cauda equina*. Ventral roots contain efferent fibres originating in anterior and lateral grey columns and also some afferent fibres. Dorsal roots contain afferent fibres originating in dorsal root ganglia.

When interpreting clinical signs of spinal cord disease it is important to remember the following anatomical points:

(1) The corticospinal tracts cross from the contralateral motor cortex to the opposite side in the lower medulla so that spinal cord damage will cause a motor deficit on the same side (Figs 5.1, 5.3).
(2) When sensory fibres enter the spinal cord from the dorsal roots:
   • Large diameter fibres conveying proprioceptive information pass up the dorsal columns on the same side (Fig. 6.3)
   • Small myelinated and unmyelinated fibres conveying pain and temperature sensation synapse in the dorsal horn of the grey matter within a few segments of their entry, and the second order neurones cross to the other side and ascend in the lateral spinothalamic tract (Fig. 6.2)
   • Most fibres conveying the sensation of light touch pass uncrossed up the dorsal columns but some cross and ascend in the ventral spinothalamic

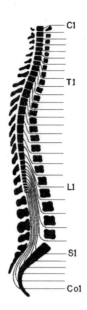

Fig. 7.1   Spinal cord and roots. (After Schadé, *The Peripheral Nervous System*, Elsevier Publishing Company, Amsterdam.)

tracts (Fig. 6.3). Because of this bilateral representation, unilateral spinal cord lesions do not usually completely destroy the sense of touch.

BLOOD SUPPLY

The largest arterial supply is the *anterior spinal artery* which is formed by the union of paired branches of the vertebrals and passes along the anterior surface of the cord, narrowing near the upper fourth thoracic segment at which level a watershed area exists. Below T4 there is a segmental supply from the intercostal arteries from the aorta; the longest of these branches, the great ventral radicular artery or artery of Adamkiewicz, enters about T10 (Fig. 7.2).

At the lumbosacral level radicular arteries are derived from larger regional vessels; the largest such vessel enters the intervertebral foramen at L2 to form the lowermost portion of the anterior spinal artery (the terminal artery) which runs along the filum terminale. Posterior spinal arteries are paired and considerably smaller than the anterior spinal vessels. They receive branches from the posterolateral plexus at various levels.

The anterior spinal artery supplies the anterior and lateral columns on either side. The posterior spinal arteries supply the posterior white columns and part of the posterior grey columns (Fig. 7.2).

Occlusion of the anterior spinal artery affects the corticospinal and spino-thalamic tracts but usually spares the dorsal columns (Fig. 7.2).

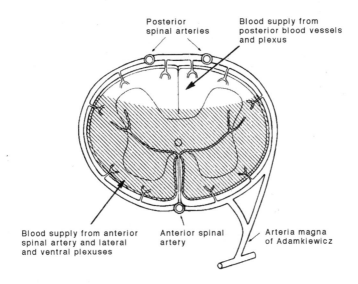

Fig. 7.2 Blood supply of the spinal cord. Shaded area is that supplied by anterior spinal artery (after Henson and Parsons, 1967).

GENERAL CLINICAL FEATURES OF SPINAL CORD LESIONS

Damage to the spinal cord may produce motor, sensory and autonomic signs.

Motor signs

Motor signs follow damage to corticospinal tracts or anterior horn cells, resulting in paralysis of the upper motor neurone type below the lesion (corticospinal tract) and of the lower motor neurone type at the level of the lesion (anterior horn cell). Damage below the conus medullaris, i.e. to the cauda equina, will cause only lower motor neurone signs.

Sensory signs

Sensory signs result from damage to the sensory pathways within the spinal cord or to the dorsal roots or ganglia. An anteriorly placed lesion, such as thrombosis of the anterior spinal artery, will affect the spinothalamic sensory pathways (pain and temperature) but not dorsal columns (joint position, two-point discrimination, vibration sense). This impairment of pain and temperature with sparing of other modalities is called 'dissociated sensory loss'. Because of the lamination of fibres entering the spinal cord, certain cutaneous areas may escape from sensory loss, since a compressive lesion affects mainly the outer layers. Thus it is common for sacral areas to be spared ('sacral sparing').

Compression of dorsal roots at the level of the lesion may result in a band of hyperaesthesia and hyperalgesia, but anaesthesia or analgesia may later follow.

The spine may be tender to pressure or percussion in disease of the vertebrae (e.g. inflammation), or after damage to the spinal cord or roots which innervate the same level as the vertebra.

Autonomic signs

Autonomic disturbances may occur below the level of a spinal cord lesion; the skin becomes warm and dry, and there is loss of pilomotor reaction and of vasomotor tone. Bladder, bowel and sexual function may be impaired.

CLINICAL APPROACH TO PATIENTS WITH SPINAL CORD LESIONS

The questions that need to be asked in a patient presenting with a spinal cord lesion are:
- What is the level of the lesion? Is the lesion localized, multiple or diffuse?
- What is the nature of the lesion?
- Is it surgically remediable?

These questions can usually be answered after a careful history has been taken, a systematic physical examination has been performed, and appropriate investigations have been carried out.

History

The patient may complain of girdle pains in thoracic lesions; of tingling in the spine, fingers and toes on flexing the neck (Lhermitte's sign) in cervical lesions; of pain in the shoulders and weakness in the hands in cervical cord lesions; or of weakness in the legs or difficulty in micturition at any level of cord lesion. An analysis of symptoms may help indicate the approximate level of the lesion. Root pain occurs especially with extramedullary lesions such as prolapsed intervertebral discs or neurofibromas.

Examination

A full examination with attention to distribution of muscle wasting or weakness, reflex changes, sensory levels and autonomic changes, will usually enable the level of the lesion to be localized. It is most important to determine accurately the level of the lesion. The spine should be palpated and percussed to elicit local or referred pain. Listen for a bruit if an angioma is suspected. Do not forget to look for signs on general examination which may reveal the nature of the underlying disorder, e.g. a hard prostate or lump in the breast (carcinoma with metastases), lymphadenopathy (reticuloses, carcinoma), smooth red tongue (pernicious anaemia), *café au lait* patches on the skin (neurofibromatosis), or cutaneous angioma.

Special investigations

Plain X-ray of the appropriate area of the spine   Reduction of intervertebral disc spaces, narrowing of intervertebral foramina and osteophyte formation indicate degeneration of the spine. Destruction or collapse of vertebrae may be seen with myeloma, metastases and infections; erosion of pedicles is a sign of an extramedullary tumour.

Chest X-ray   To exclude malignancy, lymphoma, tuberculosis.

CT scan of the spine, with or without myelography   Specify in the request the level at which the lesion is suspected. For myelography, a radio-opaque contrast medium is injected into the lumbar or cisternal subarachnoid space and tumours, disc protrusions and other causes of spinal cord or root compression can be delineated radiologically. Cerebrospinal fluid should be taken at the time of myelography and examined with particular regard to protein content, immunoglobulin G/albumin ratio and the presence of oligoclonal immunoglobulin G bands on electrophoresis if multiple sclerosis is suspected. Serological tests should be done if syphilis is suspected.

Magnetic resonance imaging (MRI)   This gives clear views of vertebrae, discs and cord that may obviate the need for myelography and may demonstrate intrinsic lesions such as syringomyelia.

Other routine investigations   These would include such tests as full blood count and erythrocyte sedimentation rate (ESR).

SPINAL CORD AND ROOT COMPRESSION

Compression of the spinal cord may be caused by:

Disease of the vertebral column   This could be a secondary carcinoma, tuberculosis, osteomyelitis or a prolapsed disc among others.

Lesions inside the spinal canal   The lesions may be extramedullary or intramedullary.

(1) *Extramedullary lesions* can be extradural or intradural.
   - Extradural. These often give rise to local pain and tenderness, are usually rapidly progressive and cause bilateral signs, e.g. secondary tumour, extradural abscess, haematoma, lymphoma, hydatid cyst.
   - Intradural. These are often benign and more slowly progressive. They may be predominantly unilateral, e.g. meningioma, neurofibroma, lipoma
(2) *Intramedullary lesions* These usually do not cause radicular pain, e.g. ependymoma, glioma, syringomyelia.

Symptoms and signs of spinal cord compression

The specific clinical features depend on the nature and extent of the spinal cord lesion. In general, clinical features of spinal cord compression at a given level consist of: (i) lower motor neurone lesion at the segmental level of compression;

(ii) upper motor neurone lesion below the level of compression; (iii) dorsal root irritation at the segmental level of compression; (iv) sensory loss below the level of compression with a distinct upper level; (v) autonomic changes (e.g. excessive sweating) below the level of the lesion.

This pattern of abnormal signs (upper and lower motor neurone signs and sensory abnormalities with a distinct upper level) is seen in various forms wherever the spinal cord is compressed.

Complete transection

This usually results from trauma. Initially there is a state of spinal shock with a flaccid paralysis and loss of all sensation and reflexes below the lesion (paraplegia, if lower limbs only are affected; quadriplegia [tetraplegia] if all four limbs are involved). The loss of reflexes and hypotonia are due to depression of alpha and gamma motoneurone activity. Reflex bladder and bowel function are suppressed and acute painless retention occurs. Below the level of the lesion autonomic changes may be seen; the skin is warm and dry and there is loss of pilomotor reaction and vasomotor tone.

The state of spinal shock passes after approximately 3 weeks and reflexes become brisk. Muscle tone is restored in the limbs especially in flexor muscle groups. A flexor withdrawal reflex may result from noxious stimuli applied to the skin below the level of the lesion. The reflexes are heightened because of recovery of gamma motoneurone function and alpha motoneurone hyperexcitability.

Incomplete or partial lesions

Partial spinal cord lesions may be due to trauma, tumours and other conditions. An early symptom of a spinal cord lesion is precipitancy or urgency of micturition which may later, in the case of expanding tumours and multiple sclerosis, progress to incontinence or retention of urine. Weakness of the lower limbs (spastic paraparesis) is usually present. Muscle tone and deep tendon reflexes in the lower limbs are increased, plantar responses become extensor, and a sensory level may be detected on the trunk.

Hemisection of spinal cord

Hemisection is rarely precise; an incomplete syndrome is more frequently seen. A pure hemisection causes *Brown-Séquard* syndrome (Fig. 7.3) which is characterized by:

- Ipsilateral paralysis of the upper motor neurone type below the lesion, with lower motor neurone signs at the level of the lesion
- Ipsilateral loss of joint position sense, two-point discrimination and vibration sense below the level of the lesion because of injury to the dorsal columns
- Contralateral loss of pain and temperature sensation below the level of the lesion as a result of damage to the spinothalamic tracts. Spinothalamic fibres cross to the opposite side within a few segments of entering the cord and thus it is usual to find that the level of contralateral spinothalamic sensory change is a few segments below the level of the causative lesion (Fig. 7.4).

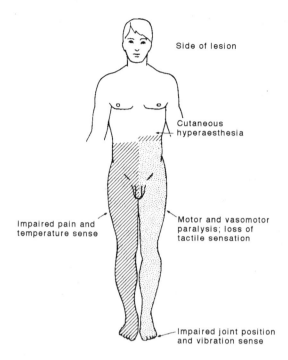

Side of lesion

Cutaneous hyperaesthesia

Impaired pain and temperature sense

Motor and vasomotor paralysis; loss of tactile sensation

Impaired joint position and vibration sense

Fig. 7.3 Clinical features resulting from hemisection of the spinal cord (Brown-Séquard syndrome). (After Walshe, 1963, *Diseases of the Nervous System*, 10th edn. E. & S. Livingstone, Edinburgh and London.)

There may be some ipsilateral impairment of pain and temperature sense at the level of the lesion because of interruption of the fibres at the dorsal root entry zone.

Cervical spondylosis

Cervical spondylosis is characterized by osteophyte formation, disc degeneration and disc protrusion (Fig. 7.5). These abnormalities cause compression of spinal roots and of the spinal cord and its blood supply. Although it may occur at other levels (particularly C4–5 and C6–7) the most common site of pathology is at C5–6, the clinical features of which are: (i) pain in neck and shoulders; (ii) wasting of deltoid, biceps or brachioradialis muscles (C5–6); (iii) exaggerated reflexes in lower limbs (corticospinal tract involvement); (iv) depression of C5–6 reflexes (i.e. biceps, brachioradialis), and exaggeration of triceps jerk (C7) and finger flexion (C8) reflexes. This combination of reflex changes is sometimes referred to as the 'inverted supinator reflex' (Fig. 7.6); sensory changes may not be prominent, but, if present, occur over the C5–6 dermatomes.

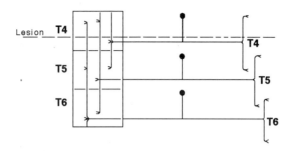

Fig. 7.4 Segmental overlap of pain fibres entering the spinal cord. A transverse lesion may result in sensory change over one or two segments below the level of the lesion.

Cauda equina and lumbosacral root lesions

One of the most common causes of compression of the *cauda equina* is a protruding lumbar disc. Other causes include neoplasms, arachnoiditis and cysts. Pain is usually a prominent feature. The most common cause of an isolated lumbosacral root lesion is an intervertebral disc protrusion, usually at L4–5 or L5–S1 levels. The main clinical features are:

Pain This is felt in the back and radiates down the back of the leg to: the heel and lateral border of the foot if the S1 root is compressed; the lateral aspect of the leg, lateral malleolus and dorsum of the foot if L5 is the main root involved and the thigh, knee and medial malleolus and sometimes the groin if the L4 root is compressed. The pain is made worse by coughing, sneezing, straining, bending and stooping.

Weakness and wasting L4 involvement results in wasting and weakness of quadriceps, tibialis anterior (dorsiflexion of foot) and tibialis posterior (inversion of

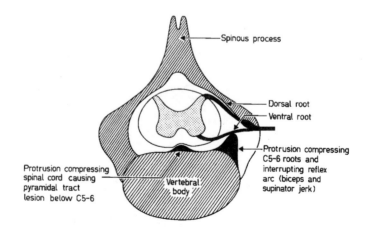

Fig. 7.5 Mechanism of reflex changes in cervical spondylosis at C5–6 level.

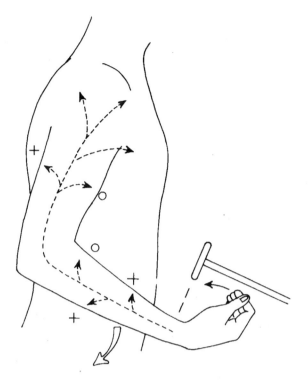

Fig. 7.6   The 'inverted supinator jerk'. Percussion of the radius sets up a vibration wave as in Fig. 5.6. When reflex arcs employing the fifth and sixth cervical segments are interrupted by disease, the biceps and brachioradialis responses to the vibration wave are absent (o). If the spinal cord is also compressed at the C5–6 level, reflexes below that level such as the triceps jerk (C7 segment) and finger jerk (C8 segment) may be enhanced so that the elbow extends while the fingers flex. (From Lance and McLeod, 1981, with permission of Butterworths, London.)

foot) and depression of the knee jerk. L5 lesions cause weakness of dorsiflexion of the foot (as well as L4 lesions), the extensor hallucis longus (dorsiflexion of the big toe) and internal rotation and abduction of the thigh and S1 lesions cause wasting of calf and extensor digitorum brevis muscles, intrinsic foot muscles, weakness of eversion (peroneus longus) and plantar flexion (gastrocnemius), and absent ankle jerk.

Larger disc protrusions or neoplasms can cause more extensive muscle wasting, weakness and sensory loss. There may be loss of sensation in the perineal region (saddle anaesthesia) when lower sacral roots are involved.

Disturbance of bowel and bladder function usually occurs later but may occasionally be the presenting symptom and is caused by direct involvement of S2–4 roots. Signs of an upper motor neurone lesion indicate that the spinal cord is involved above the conus medullaris.

Conus medullaris lesions

Tumours which invade the lowermost part of the cord (conus medullaris) may involve the roots as well as producing cord signs. Bowel and bladder function are affected early. The signs are similar to those of cauda equina lesions, although brisk ankle jerks and extensor plantar responses may also be present if the lesion extends above the conus.

OTHER CONDITIONS THAT MAY GIVE RISE TO SYMPTOMOLOGY RELATED TO THE SPINAL CORD

Acute lesions

Anterior spinal artery thrombosis

The blood supply to the cord may become impaired as a result of atherosclerosis, hypotension and emboli or surgical interference causing infarction most commonly · in the thoracic region (p. 108).

The symptoms can be acute in onset, or develop over several hours. There is usually weakness in the legs, sensory loss below the level of the lesion, and disturbance of bladder and bowel functions. Girdle pain may be associated.

Occlusion of the anterior spinal artery affects the anterior horns and the corticospinal and spinothalamic tracts, but usually spares the dorsal columns (Fig. 7.2).

Transverse myelitis

The onset is usually acute or subacute, often with pain. There may be a flaccid paralysis, a well defined sensory level and sphincter disturbance. The condition may be of viral or demyelinating aetiology.

Chronic lesions

The pattern of spinal cord degeneration in some chronic conditions is shown diagrammatically in Fig. 7.7.

Syringomyelia

This disorder is characterized by cystic dilatation in the spinal cord surrounded by gliosis, usually in the lower cervical and upper thoracic region. The cystic dilatation forms a cavity (syrinx) in the cord.

The anterior horn cells degenerate as a result of compression by the cyst causing muscle wasting and weakness, usually first seen in the small hand muscles. If the syrinx extends into the medulla, the nucleus ambiguus and hypoglossal nuclei are affected, resulting in wasting and weakness of the tongue, soft palate, pharynx and vocal cords. When the corticospinal tracts become involved, the lower limbs become spastic. Reflexes are lost over the affected segments of the cord.

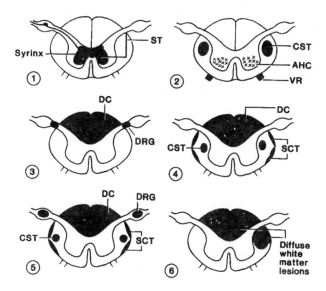

Fig. 7.7 Pattern of degeneration (black areas) in the spinal cord in (1) syringomyelia; (2) amyotrophic lateral sclerosis; (3) tabes dorsalis; (4) subacute combined degeneration; (5) Friedreich's ataxia; (6) multiple sclerosis. ST = spinothalamic tract; CST = corticospinal tract; AHC = anterior horn cells; VR = ventral root; DC = dorsal columns; DRG, = dorsal root ganglion; SCT = spinocerebellar tracts.

The crossing pain and temperature fibres destined for the lateral spinothalamic tracts become interrupted. This causes loss of pain and temperature sense in one or two segments in the upper limbs, often in a cape-like distribution across the back and shoulders. Touch and position sense are retained initially (*dissociated sensory loss*) but later the dorsal columns may also be involved. Patients often sustain burns without feeling them and scars may be seen on their hands. When the syrinx is in the upper cervical cord (C1, 2) loss of pain and temperature sense over one side of the face may result from involvement of the spinal tract of the fifth nerve. Trophic changes in the extremities give rise to a soft fleshy appearance of the fingers and Charcot joints.

Motor neurone disease (amyotrophic lateral sclerosis)

Also see pp. 277–278 for further reference. This disease commences most commonly between the ages of 40 and 60 years, and is characterized pathologically by degenerative changes most marked in the anterior horn cells of the spinal cord, the motor nuclei of the medulla and the corticospinal tracts. There is therefore degeneration of both the upper and lower motor neurones, but no involvement of sensory pathways.

Tabes dorsalis

Tabes dorsalis is a form of tertiary syphilis (Chapter 16). The patients commonly experience lightning (stabbing) pains mainly in the legs. The pathological changes are those of degeneration of dorsal roots and of fibres in the dorsal columns. Hypotonia and loss of reflexes result from damage to the dorsal roots and interruption of the stretch reflex arc.

There is often patchy loss of painful sensation over the sternum, tibial prominences and the bridge of the nose and impairment of position and vibration sense. Deep pain sensation may be lost and in about 10% of patients this results in a painless destruction of weight-bearing joints (Charcot joints). This arthropathy is seen in other neurological conditions in which central or peripheral pain pathways are damaged (e.g. syringomyelia, diabetes, hereditary sensory neuropathy). There is no primary motor involvement. Plantar reflexes are usually flexor. The gait is high stepping due to loss of proprioception. Retention of urine with a painless over-distended bladder is common. Argyll Robertson pupils (p. 63) are present in about 90% of cases.

Subacute combined degeneration

Subacute combined degeneration results from Vitamin B_{12} deficiency and is usually seen in pernicious anaemia and malabsorption states. The dorsal columns, corticospinal and spinocerebellar tracts degenerate and the peripheral nerves and brain may also be affected.

The condition usually presents with paraesthesiae, consisting of tingling sensations in fingers and toes, and the lower limbs become weak as a result of an upper motor neurone lesion combined with peripheral neuropathy. Position and vibration sense are usually markedly impaired. There may be a glove-and-stocking type of anaesthesia caused by the associated peripheral neuropathy. Romberg's sign may be positive as a result of loss of proprioception in the lower limbs resulting from degeneration of large diameter fibres in peripheral nerves and dorsal columns. Reflexes may be depressed or increased depending on the degree of corticospinal tract and peripheral nerve involvement. Plantar reflexes are often extensor because of corticospinal tract degeneration. Incoordination may be marked due to spinocerebellar tract degeneration. Lower motor neurone signs are absent, unless peripheral neuropathy is severe. Mental confusion, dementia and optic atrophy may occur.

There may be signs of glossitis, or anaemia, but it is important to remember that the neurological features may be present with a normal peripheral blood count. The serum Vitamin B_{12} level should always be measured if this diagnosis is suspected because the condition is potentially reversible.

Friedreich's ataxia

Friedreich's ataxia (p. 279) is a progressive degenerative disease with an autosomal recessive inheritance. It usually presents in the second or third decade of life with ataxia, dysarthria, and incoordination. Pathologically, there is degeneration of the dorsal columns, corticospinal and spinocerebellar tracts and dorsal root ganglia and peripheral nerves.

Clinically, slurred speech, nystagmus, ataxia, and incoordination are usually present. Reflexes are depressed or absent because of dorsal root involvement. Position and vibration sense are impaired. Plantar responses are extensor. In addition, there are usually associated skeletal deformities such as kyphoscoliosis and pes cavus. Cardiomyopathy is common.

Multiple sclerosis

Multiple sclerosis (Chapter 20), which usually starts in young adult life, is characterized by the occurrence of plaques of demyelination at different levels in the white matter of the central nervous system.

The lesions are disseminated in both time and space, and involvement of the optic nerves, spinal cord and brain-stem may occur at different times.

When a plaque of demyelination affects the spinal cord, it usually presents as a transverse lesion. There may be spasticity below the level of the lesion and sensory loss with a well-defined upper border. Bladder involvement is the rule.

To be sure of the diagnosis, one should have clinical evidence from history and examination of lesions elsewhere in the nervous system otherwise compressive spinal cord lesions must be excluded by appropriate investigations.

INNERVATION AND NERVOUS CONTROL OF THE URINARY BLADDER

THE STRUCTURE OF THE BLADDER

The bladder is composed of smooth muscle fibres in three layers; the outer and inner longitudinal layers and a middle circular layer. The fibres form a continuum and act as a functional whole called the detrusor muscle of the bladder. The smooth muscle fibres around the internal orifice of the urethra form the internal sphincter in the male. It is not a separate anatomical structure, but is simply part of the detrusor and has no separate innervation. On the other hand the external sphincter muscle is a separate structure and consists of striated muscle fibres.

INNERVATION OF THE BLADDER

The smooth muscle of the bladder is innervated by sympathetic and parasympathetic fibres, while the external sphincter receives only somatic innervation (Fig. 7.8).

Efferent

Parasympathetic innervation Preganglionic fibres arise from the intermedio-lateral columns of sacral cord segments S2–4, and travel in pelvic nerves to form a diffuse subserosal network in the bladder wall. Postganglionic fibres innervate the

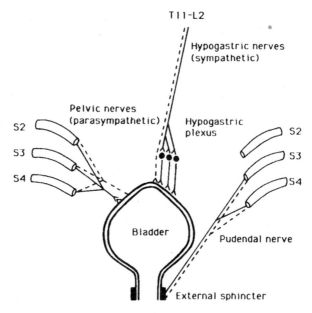

Fig. 7.8 Innervation of the urinary bladder. ——— Efferent fibres: ----- afferent fibres. (From Lance and McLeod, 1981, with permission of Butterworths, London.)

smooth muscle fibres. Parasympathetic efferent impulses cause the detrusor muscles to contract and the bladder neck to shorten thus allowing the passage of urine.

Sympathetic innervation Preganglionic fibres arise from the intermediolateral columns in the T11–L2 segments of the spinal cord and travel via the ventral roots and white rami to the hypogastric plexus. Postganglionic fibres join the subserosal plexus on the bladder wall and seem to go mainly to the trigone and the neck of the bladder rather than to the whole detrusor muscle. Sympathetic efferents may inhibit the detrusor but appear to play little part in the act of micturition. However, during ejaculation sympathetic activity causes the bladder neck to contract, preventing retrograde ejaculation.

Somatic innervation The pudendal nerve (S2–4) supplies the external sphincter of the bladder and also the anal sphincter; the cell bodies of the motor neurones lying in the conus. Its action is coordinated with the detrusor and it is relaxed during micturition. It can also be voluntarily contracted to terminate the act of micturition.

Afferent

Free and encapsulated nerve endings have been demonstrated in the bladder wall.

Parasympathetic fibres These fibres transmit sensations of bladder fullness and pain of overdistension and overcontraction. They also mediate the reflex for bladder contraction through S2–4 segments.

Sympathetic fibres These fibres convey painful sensation from the trigone area, and a vague sensation of bladder fullness. They play no part in the micturition reflex.

Somatic fibres The somatic fibres in the pudendal nerve innervate the sphincter and urethra. These fibres convey sensations of urine passing through the urethra and of bladder emptying, and urethral pain and temperature.

Afferent connections within the central nervous system

Impulses giving rise to sensations of bladder fullness and the desire to micturate, the sensation of pain from the bladder and pain and temperature from the urethra are mediated by lateral spinothalamic tracts. No thermal sensations can be elicited from the bladder.

Touch and pressure sense derived from the urethra and vague sensations of awareness of bladder fullness are mediated through the posterior columns (Fig. 7.9).

Supraspinal control of micturition

The higher centres inhibit the micturition reflex. Micturition is initiated by the removal of this tonic suprasegmental inhibition of the reflex arc. There are cortical centres in the region of the paracentral lobule of the frontal lobes and also centres of influence in the basal ganglia and pons. Descending pathways course in the lateral columns of the spinal cord medial to the corticospinal tracts (Fig. 7.9).

Bladder tone

This is a property of the smooth muscle of the bladder wall and is unrelated to the extrinsic innervation of the bladder. Thus spinal cord transection and spinal anaesthesia do not directly influence bladder tone. The 'atonic bladder' described in spinal cord and sacral nerve injury is due to chronic overstretching of the bladder consequent upon the loss of the micturition reflex and is only an indirect

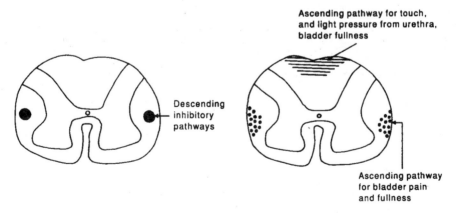

Fig. 7.9 Nervous control of the urinary bladder. Descending and ascending pathways in the spinal cord. (From Lance and McLeod, 1981, with permission of Butterworths, London.)

result of denervation. The hypertonic or small contracted bladder is the result of inflammatory changes in the bladder wall — chronic cystitis — rather than of damage to the innervation of the bladder.

Micturition reflex

When the bladder is distended to a critical level, the stretch receptors in the wall initiate impulses in the afferent limb of the sacral reflex arc, causing contraction of the detrusor muscle through the parasympathetic efferents from the S2–4 segments. The micturition reflex is normally inhibited through the descending cortico-spinal pathway and voluntary micturition is initiated by relaxation which removes this suprasegmental inhibition. Inhibition is maintained throughout micturition by a reflex triggered by passage of urine through the posterior urethra.

The *cystometrogram* records the relationship of urine volume to intravesical pressure. The usual technique is to fill the bladder through a urethral catheter measuring both the pressure and volume of fluid. As the bladder is filled, the pressure increases gradually. Low-level rhythmical contractions, associated with a transient sense of urgency, usually develop at a volume of 150–200 mL and a sense of fullness at about 150–300 mL. Reflex micturition then starts with rhythmic waves of increasing amplitude, developing into a sustained contraction of the detrusor muscle.

BLADDER DYSFUNCTION RESULTING FROM DISEASE OF THE NERVOUS SYSTEM

Cauda equina lesions

Afferent fibres of the micturition reflex arc may be selectively damaged by peripheral neuropathy, tabes dorsalis, subacute combined degeneration, herpes zoster, or compression by a prolapsed lumbar disc or neoplasm. Initially the sense of bladder fullness may be impaired and the sense of urgency becomes less clear-cut. The bladder becomes over-distended, because of lack of sensation and may contain huge volumes of urine (1500–2000 mL) with overflow incontinence. Abdominal compression may be necessary to empty the bladder. The cystometro-gram reveals loss of tone from overdistension, a high threshold for filling sensation, and elevation of the threshold or abolition of the micturition reflex.

If afferent fibres are preserved, bladder distension causes discomfort and pain. The pain eventually remits and thereafter the features are similar to those of afferent sacral lesions.

If the bladder is allowed to remain over-distended for long periods it may fail to regain significant autonomous activity. The patient should therefore be catheter-ized and the bladder decompressed as soon as possible. After decompression, the bladder usually regains contractility and may become hyperactive. After 2–3 months, autonomous contractions become sufficiently strong to contract the detrusor and open the internal sphincter. Emptying is incomplete but may be aided by abdominal compression. Usually significant residual urine remains and the bladder becomes prone to infections.

Spinal cord injury

In slowly developing and partial lesions of the spinal cord (such as multiple sclerosis and compression by spinal tumours) there may be loss of descending inhibition causing urgency and precipitancy of micturition with ejection of a small urine volume. As the lesion progresses, voluntary control of micturition may be totally impaired, causing retention of urine.

In acute spinal transection, descending nervous inhibition is overwhelming (spinal shock) and the micturition reflex is suppressed. Urinary retention and infection occur. After spinal shock has passed the micturition reflex may be facilitated.

Cerebral lesions

Loss of control of micturition may result from lesions of the motor cortex (paracentral lobules). Lesions of the frontal lobe may cause precipitancy and incontinence.

INNERVATION OF THE RECTUM

The nerve supply of the rectum is similar to that of the bladder, and micturition and defaecation are physiologically comparable.

SEXUAL FUNCTIONS

Erection of the penis is under parasympathetic control, mediated by the S2–3 segments. The reflex pathway may be tested by the bulbocavernosus response (squeezing the glans penis, or touching it firmly with a pin, which evokes a contraction of the bulbocavernosus muscle palpable at the base of the penis in the perineum). The reflex arc may be interrupted by any of the conditions discussed in relation to the micturition reflex and is particularly prone to damage in diabetes. Some cases of impotence are vascular or psychogenic in origin. The presence of the bulbocavernosus reflex, together with a history of nocturnal or morning erections, gives some reassurance that the reflex arc is intact.

Ejaculation into the urethra is a function of the sympathetic nervous system but ejaculation from the urethra requires activity of the bulbocavernosus muscle.

REFERENCE

Fowler C. J., Betts C. D. and Fowler C. G. (1992) Bladder dysfunction in neurologic disease. In: *Diseases of the Nervous System*, 2nd edn. Eds A. K. Asbury, G. M. McKhann and W. I. McDonald. W. B. Saunders, Philadelphia. 512–528.

8 | Cerebellum

The cerebellum is situated below the tentorium cerebelli in the posterior fossa of the skull, in close relationship to the pons and medulla, and forms the roof of the fourth ventricle (Fig. 8.1). Its chief functions are to control muscle tone, posture and movement.

The cerebellum is composed of a median vermis and two lateral hemispheres, but, functionally and phylogenetically, it has been divided into: flocculonodular lobe (archicerebellum), and corpus cerebelli which is in two parts: (i) anterior lobe (palaeocerebellum); (ii) posterior lobe (neocerebellum; Fig. 8.2).

The flocculonodular lobe is connected mainly with the vestibular nuclei, the anterior lobe mainly with spinal pathways and the posterior lobe predominantly with the cerebral cortex (Figs 8.3–8.5).

The cerebellar cortex has a uniform structure throughout the cerebellum and is divided into three main zones: (i) an outer molecular layer (basket cells, stellate cells, parallel fibres from granular cells and dendrites of Purkinje cells); (ii) Purkinje cell layer; (iii) a granular layer (granule cells, Golgi II cells).

Deep in the white matter lie the paired intracerebellar nuclei (the globose and emboliform, dentate and fastigial nuclei).

CONNECTIONS OF THE CEREBELLUM

Flocculonodular lobe

The flocculonodular lobe (archicerebellum) is intimately connected with the vestibular nuclei by way of the inferior cerebellar peduncle (restiform body; Fig. 8.3).

Posterior lobe

Descending fibres from the frontal, parietal and temporal lobes of the cerebral cortex project to the posterior lobe of the cerebellum (neocerebellum) and also to its anterior lobe by way of the pons and middle cerebellar peduncle. The efferent pathway from the Purkinje cells of the cerebellar cortex projects to the dentate nuclei, thence to the lateral ventral nucleus of the thalamus back to the frontal cortex. This cortico-ponto-cerebello-dentato-thalamo-cortical pathway

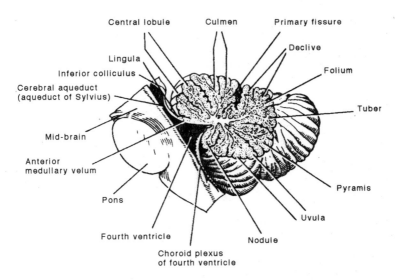

Fig. 8.1 Sagittal section of the cerebellum showing its relationship to the fourth ventricle and brain-stem. (Modified from Chusid, 1985, *Correlative Neuroanatomy and Functional Neurology*, 19th edn. With permission of Lange Medical Publications.)

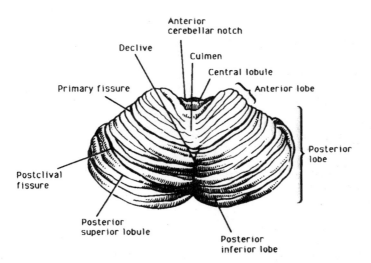

Fig. 8.2 Anatomical divisions of the cerebellum. (Modified from Chusid, 1985, *Correlative Neuroanatomy and Functional Neurology*, 19th edn. With permission of Lange Medical Publications.)

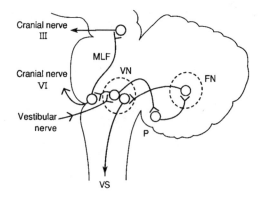

Fig. 8.3 Connections of the vestibular nerve and the flocculonodular lobe of the cerebellum. The vestibular nucleus (VN) projects to the flocculonodular lobe. Efferent fibres from Purkinje cells (P) pass directly or through the fastigial nucleus (FN) back to VN to influence the vestibulospinal (VS) tract. The vestibular nucleus also connects with the lateral conjugate gaze control centre to cause abduction of the ipsilateral eye through the sixth cranial nerve VI as part of the vestibulo-ocular reflex. Adduction of the contralateral eye is mediated through the medial longitudinal fasciculus (MLF) to the oculomotor nucleus and nerve III.

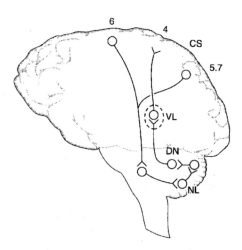

Fig. 8.4 Connections of the posterior lobe and cerebellar hemispheres.
The premotor area (6) and parietal areas (5, 7) project via pontine nuclei to the cerebellum. The output from Purkinje cells passes through the dentate nucleus (DN) to the ventrolateral (VL) thalamic nucleus and thence to the motor cortex (4), in front of the central sulcus (CS), thus completing a cerebro-cerebellar-cerebral circuit.

provides a feedback mechanism for the control of active movement, and also plays a part in the programming of movement (Fig. 8.4).

Anterior lobe

The anterior lobe (palaeocerebellum) receives an input from the spinal afferent system through the superior and inferior cerebellar peduncles and also via the inferior olive by way of the olivo-cerebellar tract (Fig. 8.5).

Muscle spindle afferents (Group Ia, II) and Golgi tendon organ afferents (Group Ib) project to the anterior lobe by way of the dorsal and ventral spinocerebellar tracts. Information derived from these proprioceptive sources is integrated in the cerebellar cortex, and efferent pathways from the cerebellum pass to the reticular formation, red nucleus and vestibular nuclei. The reticulospinal, rubrospinal and vestibulospinal tracts regulate posture and control movement by influencing activity in alpha and gamma motoneurones in the spinal cord segments (Fig. 8.5).

FUNCTION OF THE CEREBELLUM

The cerebellar cortex organizes information derived from a variety of afferent sources and each cerebellar hemisphere regulates motor activity on the ipsilateral side of the body.

The only efferent output from the cerebellar cortex is by way of the Purkinje cells, which have a purely inhibitory action on the subcortical intracerebellar nuclei and vestibular nuclei. By means of patterned inhibition, the cerebellum regulates

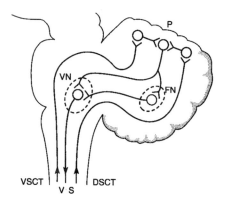

Fig. 8.5 Connections of the anterior lobe of the cerebellum.
The ventral spinocerebellar tract (VSCT) and dorsal spinocerebellar tract (DSCT) pass through the superior and inferior cerebellar peduncles, respectively, to the anterior lobe. Purkinje cells (P) project directly and via the fastigial nucleus (FN) to the vestibular nucleus (VN) to influence the vestibulospinal (VS) tract.

slow movements by feedback to the motor cortex. It controls ballistic movement by programming the timing and duration of contraction in antagonistic muscle groups so that a target is reached with precision. The lateral lobes of the cerebellum appear to compute the effort required to achieve a desired limb position based on the initial position of the limb, the position of the target and the inertia to be overcome.

The physiological role of the cerebellum becomes apparent when its normal function is impaired by disease or injury.

CLINICAL FEATURES OF CEREBELLAR DISORDERS

Hypotonia

Muscle tone is reduced on the ipsilateral side with unilateral cerebellar lesions; with more extensive lesions of the cerebellum, there is generalized hypotonia. The hypotonia may be demonstrated in several ways: (i) as a diminished resistance to passive movement; (ii) as a greater range of motion of the joints when the limbs are passively shaken; (iii) if the arms are held vertically and the hands allowed to fall loosely the hand may fall passively into a position of greater flexion on the affected side; (iv) if the arms are held outstretched and gently tapped there may be wider excursions of the affected limb; (v) with the patient lying supine, the heel on the affected side may be easily pressed against the buttock when the legs are flexed; (vi) if the knee jerk is tested with the leg hanging freely over the side of the bed, the leg may make several oscillations after the deep tendon reflex has been elicited — pendular knee jerks.

It seems that the hypotonia is caused by decreased muscle spindle responsiveness to stretch consequent upon a depression of fusimotor activity.

Tremor

Intention tremor   Intention tremor is an important sign because it occurs principally in disorders of the cerebellum or its connections. It is demonstrated in the upper limb by asking the patient to put his finger on his nose. There may be no tremor at rest or on commencement of the movement, but a coarse oscillating tremor develops as the finger approaches its target. Similar tests can be carried out on the lower limbs (see Chapter 2).

Static tremor   A slow, coarse tremor may be apparent when the arms are held outstretched.

Disturbance of posture

There may be a tendency to fall to one side or another (usually to the side of the lesion if there is unilateral cerebellar involvement), or forwards or backwards when standing with the feet together. This is not materially affected by eye closure. The head may be held in a rotated position.

Ataxia of gait

There is a wide based, staggering gait; with unilateral lesions, patients deviate and stagger to the affected side, and may rotate to one side when walking on the spot with the eyes closed.

Disorders of movement

There is delay in starting and stopping movements (which gives rise to the *rebound phenomenon*).

Dysmetria   There is a disorder of the rate, regularity, range and force of compound movements.

Decomposition of movements   The movements are jerky and broken up into their component parts instead of appearing smooth and free-flowing. Dysmetria and decomposition of movements may be demonstrated clinically by finger–nose and heel–knee tests.

Dysdiadochokinesis   There is an inability to carry out alternating movements with rapidity and regularity.

Speech

Speech is slurred and often broken up into syllables (scanning speech).

Nystagmus

The fast component of nystagmus is directed to the side of the lesion. It is due to involvement of the vestibular connections of the cerebellum.

LOCALIZATION OF LESIONS WITHIN THE CEREBELLUM

Lateral hemisphere lesions

Lesions of the neocerebellum result in hypotonia, dysmetria, dysdiadochokinesis, past pointing, pendular knee jerks on the side of the lesion and a tendency to stagger and to fall to the affected side. Primary tumours such as astrocytomas, metastatic tumours and abscesses are more common in the lateral hemispheres than in the mid-line of the cerebellum.

Anterior lobe lesions

Lesions of the anterior lobe cause ataxia of gait and of lower limbs and trunk, with relatively little involvement of upper limbs. The most common cause of this type of mid-line cerebellar lesion is alcoholic cerebellar degeneration, which affects the anterior superior surface of the cerebellum selectively.

Flocculonodular lobe

Lesions of the flocculonodular lobe (e.g. medulloblastoma) cause marked ataxia of gait and disturbance of balance or truncal ataxia.

CAUSES OF CEREBELLAR DISORDERS

Developmental anomalies

- Basilar impression: A deformation of the posterior fossa by invagination of the odontoid process through the foramen magnum, often associated with the Arnold-Chiari malformation (a tongue of cerebellum protruding through the foramen magnum and downward displacement of the medulla into the cervical canal)

Cerebellar atrophies

- Familial cerebellar degeneration
- Olivo-ponto-cerebellar atrophy
- Carcinoma: Cerebellar degeneration as a remote manifestation of a distant malignancy
- Chronic alcoholism

Infections

- Abscess
- Viral encephalitis, especially chicken pox

Toxins

- Anticonvulsants
- Acute alcohol intoxication

Metabolic

- Myxoedema
- Hypoglycaemia
- Heat-stroke

Vascular

- Occlusion of posterior inferior, anterior inferior or anterior cerebellar arteries
- Haemorrhage

Trauma

- Head injuries

Tumours

- Intracerebellar (e.g. astrocytoma, haemangioblastoma, medulloblastoma, metastases)
- Extracerebellar (e.g. meningioma, acoustic neuroma)

Demyelination

- Multiple sclerosis

REFERENCES

Gilman S. (1992) Cerebellum and motor dysfunction. In: *Diseases of the Nervous System*, 2nd edn. Eds A. K. Asbury, G. M. McKhann and W. I. McDonald. W. B. Saunders, Philadelphia. 319–341

Gilman S. (1994) Cerebellar control of movement. *Annals of Neurology*, **35**, 3–4.

9 | Autonomic nervous system

ANATOMY

The autonomic nervous system consists of two major divisions: the sympathetic (thoracolumbar division) and the parasympathetic (craniosacral outflow).

Sympathetic nervous system

Descending pathways from the hypothalamus and other regions of the brain synapse with cells of the preganglionic sympathetic efferents in the intermediolateral cell columns of the spinal cord which extend from T1 to L2. The axons emerge from the spinal cord through the anterior roots which they leave via the white rami communicantes to join the sympathetic chain that consists of a series of ganglia and nerve fibres extending from the base of the skull to the coccyx. The preganglionic fibres, which enter the chain through the white rami, may synapse in the nearest ganglion, pass up or down the sympathetic chain before making their synapse, or pass through the chain to synapse at more peripheral ganglia such as the coeliac or other mesenteric ganglia. Postganglionic sympathetic fibres are unmyelinated; those that arise from the ganglia of the sympathetic chain join the main nerve trunks by way of the grey rami communicantes and are distributed to the sweat glands and blood vessels of skin and muscles (Fig. 9.1). The preganglionic sympathetic fibres are myelinated and cholinergic. The unmyelinated postganglionic fibres are noradrenergic, except those cholinergic fibres that innervate the sweat glands and some cholinergic vasodilator fibres that innervate muscle blood vessels. The release of peptides may play a role in the control of vasomotor tone and in the regulation of regional blood flow. Afferent fibres in the sympathetic nervous system convey mainly painful sensation.

Ocular sympathetic fibres leave the spinal cord in the first thoracic root and synapse in the superior cervical ganglion. Postganglionic fibres follow the course of the internal carotid artery to the siphon, where they join the ophthalmic division of the trigeminal nerve for distribution to the pupil. Interruption of these fibres causes ptosis and miosis on the affected side. Fibres responsible for sweating and vasomotor control in the face accompany the second and third thoracic nerve roots. After synapsing in the superior cervical ganglion they are distributed along the carotid artery in the periarterial plexus before passing to the skin along

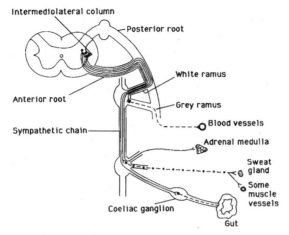

Fig. 9.1 Schematic diagram of sympathetic nervous system showing preganglionic myelinated cholinergic fibres (——), postganglionic unmyelinated noradrenergic fibres (- - - -) and postganglionic unmyelinated cholinergic fibres (•–•). (From Lance and McLeod, 1981, with permission of Butterworths, London.)

peripheral branches of the trigeminal nerve. Sympathetic deficit in the face is characterized by impairment of sweating and vasomotor control as well as ptosis and miosis (Horner's syndrome; p. 63).

Parasympathetic nervous system

The hypothalamus and other centres in the brain maintain control over the divisions of the parasympathetic nervous system. Parasympathetic fibres leave the brain-stem in the third, seventh, ninth and tenth cranial nerves, and the spinal cord in the second, third and fourth sacral nerves. Parasympathetic fibres in the third cranial nerve supply the pupillary and ciliary muscles; those in the seventh cranial nerve supply the lacrimal, submandibular and sublingual glands through branches of the greater superficial petrosal and chorda tympani nerves (Fig. 9.2). The parotid gland is supplied by parasympathetic fibres in the ninth cranial nerve; the vagus nerve innervates the thoracic and abdominal viscera; the sacral outflow supplies the bladder and genital system and the large bowel. The ganglia lie close to the innervated structures so that the postganglionic fibres are short. Both pre- and postganglionic fibres in the parasympathetic nervous system are cholinergic.

PHYSIOLOGY

The most important clinical functions of the autonomic nervous system are control of blood pressure and heart rate, sweating, bladder and bowel (Chapter 7) and pupillary reflexes (Chapter 4).

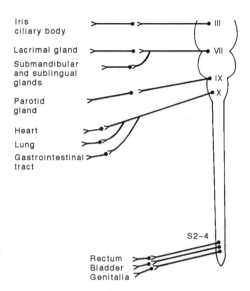

Fig. 9.2 Schematic diagram of parasympathetic nervous system. (From Lance and McLeod, 1981, with permission of Butterworths, London.)

Blood pressure and heart rate

Blood pressure and heart rate are controlled by baroreflex pathways (Fig. 9.3). Sensitive receptors in the carotid sinus, aortic arch and other thoracic regions respond to alterations in blood pressure. Afferent fibres from the baroreceptors in the carotid sinus run in the glossopharyngeal nerve and those from the aortic arch and thoracic low pressure receptors run in the vagus nerve; they synapse in the nucleus of the tractus solitarius and elsewhere in the brain-stem. Efferent fibres run in the vagus nerve to the heart and in the sympathetic nerves to the heart, mesenteric vascular bed and blood vessels in the skin and muscles. A rise in systemic blood pressure results in slowing of the heart and peripheral vaso-dilatation; a fall in blood pressure causes increased heart rate and peripheral vasoconstriction. The splanchnic vascular bed plays an important part in human blood pressure regulation. On standing, about 700 mL of blood leaves the chest and pools in the abdomen and legs, but as a result of reflex vasoconstriction in the splanchnic vascular bed and skeletal muscle vessels, blood is redistributed thus maintaining normal blood pressure.

Sweating

The sweat glands are innervated mainly by cholinergic postganglionic sympathetic nerve fibres and are under hypothalamic control.

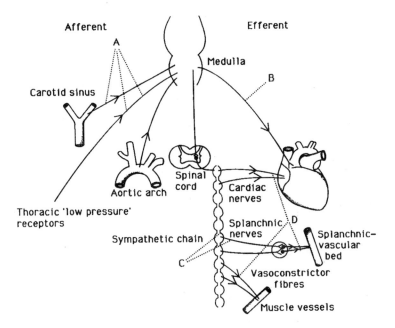

Fig. 9.3 Schematic representation of baroreflex pathways that control blood pressure and heart rate. (A) Afferent fibres from baroreceptors; (B) cardiac vagal efferent fibres; (C) preganglionic sympathetic efferent fibres; (D) postganglionic sympathetic efferent fibres. (From McLeod and Tuck, *Disorders of the Autonomic Nervous System*. Reprinted with permission from *Ann. Neurol.* **21**, pp. 419–430, 1987.)

CLINICAL FEATURES OF AUTONOMIC DYSFUNCTION

The most important clinical manifestations of autonomic dysfunction are postural (orthostatic) hypotension, impotence, disorders of bladder function, abnormalities of sweating and vasomotor disturbances.

Patients with postural hypotension feel light-headed, dizzy or faint or lose consciousness on standing upright. It is very important clinically to remember that postural hypotension may result from dehydration or loss of blood, effects of drugs and other causes, as well as diseases of the autonomic nervous system, which may affect central autonomic control or the peripheral autonomic pathways (Table 9.1).

Table 9.1 Classification of autonomic disorders

Diseases affecting central nervous system

Primary autonomic failure

Pure autonomic failure (PAF) or idiopathic orthostatic hypotension (IOH)

Autonomic failure with Parkinson's disease (AF-PD)

Autonomic failure with multiple-system atrophy (e.g. Shy-Drager syndrome; AF-MSA)

Spinal cord lesions above T6

Wernicke's encephalopathy

Miscellaneous diseases

Cerebrovascular disease

Brain-stem tumours

Multiple sclerosis

Adie's syndrome

Tabes dorsalis

Diseases affecting the peripheral autonomic nervous system

Disorders with no associated peripheral neuropathy

Acute and subacute autonomic neuropathy

- Pandysautonomia
- Cholinergic dysautonomia

Botulism

Disorders associated with peripheral neuropathy

Autonomic dysfunction which is clinically important

- Diabetes
- Primary and familial amyloidosis
- Acute inflammatory neuropathy
- Acute intermittent porphyria
- Familial dysautonomia (Riley-Day syndrome; HSAN III)
- Chronic sensory and autonomic neuropathy

Autonomic dysfunction which is usually clinically unimportant

- Alcoholism and nutritional diseases
- Toxic neuropathies (vincristine sulphate, acrylamide, heavy metals)
- Charcot-Marie-Tooth disease
- Malignancy
- Metabolic disorders e.g. Vitamin B_{12} deficiency, chronic renal failure, chronic liver disease
- Rheumatoid arthritis
- Systemic lupus erythematosus and other connective tissue diseases
- Chronic inflammatory neuropathy
- HIV infections

Drugs

Phenothiazines, barbiturates, antidepressants, anti-hypertensive drugs

---

Pure autonomic failure, or idiopathic orthostatic hypotension

This is a degenerative disorder affecting postganglionic sympathetic fibres. Males and females are affected, and the usual age of onset is between 40 and 60 years. The earliest symptoms are those of postural hypotension with dizziness and weakness on standing or walking. Impotence, bladder disturbances and loss of sweating are common features. There are no abnormalities on neurological examination other than postural hypotension. The condition is slowly progressive.

Autonomic failure associated with multiple system atrophy (MSA)

In this condition, which is more common than pure autonomic failure, abnormal neurological signs are associated with postural hypotension. One form is known as the Shy-Drager syndrome. There is degeneration of the cells of origin of the preganglionic fibres in the intermediolateral columns of the spinal cord, as well as pyramidal and extrapyramidal pathways. Patients usually have extrapyramidal features of rigidity and akinesia, pyramidal tract signs and cerebellar ataxia. The disease is steadily progressive (p. 280).

Autonomic failure associated with Parkinson's disease

Severe postural hypotension may rarely be associated with Parkinson's disease.

Peripheral neuropathy

Peripheral autonomic fibres may be damaged in peripheral neuropathies particularly those that affect small myelinated and unmyelinated fibres (e.g. diabetes, primary amyloidosis), or those which cause acute demyelination of the preganglionic sympathetic fibres and the vagal afferent and efferent fibres (e.g. Guillain-Barré syndrome). Postural hypotension, impairment of heart rate control, loss of sweating and impotence are the usual clinical manifestations. Autonomic neuropathy is particularly common in diabetes. Mild degrees of autonomic neuropathy manifested mainly by impairment of sweating, may be seen in most peripheral neuropathies, but are of little clinical importance.

Drugs

Many drugs, including antidepressants, phenothiazines and antihypertensive agents may cause postural hypotension and other autonomic disturbances.

TESTS OF AUTONOMIC FUNCTION

There are many tests of autonomic function. They include the following:

Alteration of blood pressure with posture

There is normally little alteration of blood pressure on changing from the supine to the standing position. A fall of greater than 30/15 mmHg is abnormal and indicates significant postural hypotension.

Change of heart rate with posture

The heart rate normally increases by about 11–29 beats/minute on changing from the supine to the standing position, reaching a maximum after 15 beats. There is then a reflex bradycardia which reaches its maximum at about the thirtieth beat. The ratio of the heart period, or R–R interval, on an electrocardiogram (EEG) corresponding to the thirtieth and fifteenth heart beats, is known as the 30:15 ratio; the normal ratio varies with age. In autonomic neuropathies affecting the afferent or efferent fibres of the reflex arc, the 30:15 ratio and the rise in heart rate with change in position are reduced. Heart rate changes with alteration in posture are reduced with increasing age.

Change of heart rate with respiration

During quiet respiration the heart rate increases during inspiration and decreases during expiration (sinus arrhythmia). The difference is less pronounced in older subjects. In autonomic disturbances affecting the vagus nerve the heart rate variation with respiration is impaired.

Isometric contraction

Sustained isometric contraction (e.g. a firm handgrip on a spring) for up to 5 minutes results in an increase in heart rate and systolic and diastolic blood pressure. The blood pressure rises because of increased cardiac output and peripheral vasoconstriction. The normal rise in diastolic blood pressure is 15 mmHg or more, and the response is impaired in diseases affecting sympathetic efferent fibres. It is not significantly reduced by ageing.

Response to emotional and other stimuli

Mental arithmetic, a loud noise, or cold or painful stimuli applied to the body, will all increase the arterial blood pressure due to peripheral vasoconstriction. The reflex response is impaired in lesions of the sympathetic efferent pathways but may also be absent in some normal people.

Valsalva manoeuvre

The heart rate and blood pressure normally change during and after the performance of a Valsalva manoeuvre (forced expiration against a closed glottis or mouthpiece; Fig. 9.4). The subject is asked to maintain a column of mercury at 40 mm pressure for 10–15 seconds while in a semi-recumbent posture. The ECG is monitored continuously and the blood pressure may be recorded through an intra-arterial catheter. The Valsalva ratio is the ratio of the longest pulse interval to the shortest pulse interval recorded on the ECG during the manoeuvre. In normal young adults it exceeds 1.45. It is reduced with increasing age and is impaired by diseases that affect the parasympathetic and sympathetic pathways.

Sweating

Sweating is usually impaired in autonomic disorders affecting the sympathetic efferent pathways. The usual test is to cover the skin with a powder such as quinizarin or alazarine red that changes colour when sweating occurs. The patient is warmed by radiant heat sufficient to raise the body temperature by 1°C. Local sweating may also be tested by injection or iontophoresis of acetylcholine which stimulates an axon reflex, or pilocarpine which stimulates the sweat glands directly.

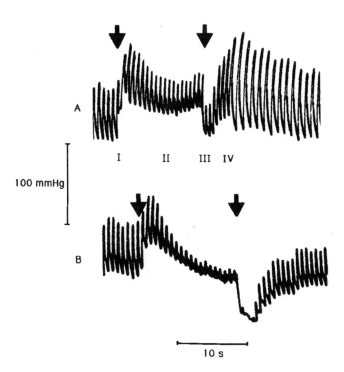

Fig. 9.4 (A) Valsalva response from control subject; (B) Valsalva response from patient with primary amyloidosis. Arrows indicate onset and cessation of the Valsalva manoeuvre. Note in (B) the pronounced fall in mean arterial pressure in phase II, absence of brady-cardia and absence of overshoot of blood pressure in phase IV. (From McLeod and Tuck, 1987.)

Pupillary responses

Instillation of 2.5% methacholine (Mecholyl) into the conjunctival sac does not affect the size of the normal pupil. It does however cause pupillary constriction if there are lesions of the parasympathetic innervation; this is because of the denervation supersensitivity of the constrictor muscle of the pupil.

Instillation of 0.1% adrenaline has no effect on the normal pupil but causes dilatation if postganglionic sympathetic innervation has been interrupted, again because of denervation supersensitivity.

Cocaine blocks the re-uptake of noradrenaline so that 4% cocaine eye-drops cause dilatation of the normal pupil. If there has been an interruption of the peripheral sympathetic innervation, pupillary dilatation does not occur.

Tyramine releases noradrenaline from peripheral nerve terminals so that 2% tyramine eye-drops produce pupillary dilatation. The reaction is impaired if there is noradrenaline depletion secondary to a sympathetic lesion.

Other tests of autonomic function

There are a number of other tests of vasomotor control and baroreflex sensitivity, as well as tests of bladder control, which are more difficult to perform. The tests referred to above can, for the most part, be performed simply at the bedside.

TREATMENT OF AUTONOMIC DISORDERS

Postural hypotension

General advice about rising slowly from the sitting and lying positions, avoiding straining and extremes of temperature and wearing light clothes should be given. Elevation of the head of the bed by 10–15 cm reduces renal arterial pressure and thus increases the secretion of renin resulting in sodium retention and increased blood volume. Elastic stockings with lower abdominal constriction reduce the volume of the venous capacitance bed.

The most useful drug is the mineralocorticoid, 9-α-fluorohydrocortisone (fludrocortisone, Florinef) which increases blood volume. The dosage commences at 0.1 mg/day and can be increased. The main side effects are supine hypertension, fluid retention and potassium depletion. Numerous other drugs can be used, but are less effective.

Bladder dysfunction

The drug treatment depends on the type of bladder dysfunction. Frequency of micturition can be helped by anticholinergic drugs such as propantheline bromide (Pro-Banthine) 15 mg 2–4 times daily, and penthienate bromide (Monodral) 5 mg 3–4 times daily, or tricyclic antidepressant drugs, e.g. amitriptyline 25–100 mg daily.

Distended bladder with incomplete emptying may be treated with cholinergic drugs such as bethanecol chloride (Urecholine, Urocarb) 10 mg 3–4 times daily.

REFERENCES

Appenzeller O. (1990) *The Autonomic Nervous System*, 4th edn. Elsevier, Amsterdam.

Bannister R. and Mathias C. J. (Ed) (1992) *Autonomic Failure*, 3rd edn. Oxford University Press, Oxford.

Low P. A. (ed.) (1993) *Clinical Autonomic Disorders*. Little, Brown & Co, Boston.

Part 2

NEUROLOGICAL DISORDERS

10 | Neuromuscular diseases

PERIPHERAL NEUROPATHY

The peripheral nervous system may be affected by injury or by disease processes. *Mononeuropathy* refers to a condition affecting a single nerve trunk, the most usual cause of which is trauma or entrapment. *Mononeuritis multiplex* is the term used to describe involvement by a disease process of several individual nerve trunks in an asymmetrical fashion. It is most often due to damage to the blood supply to nerves (*vasa nervorum*). *Polyneuropathy* or *peripheral neuritis* indicates a widespread symmetrical process affecting the peripheral nervous system.

STRUCTURE OF PERIPHERAL NERVES

The peripheral nervous system consists of motor and sensory neurones and autonomic nerves. It includes the dorsal and ventral spinal roots, dorsal root and other sensory ganglia, sensory and motor terminals, spinal and cranial nerves and the peripheral autonomic nervous system (Fig. 10.1). Nerve trunks contain fascicles or bundles of individual nerve fibres separated by connective tissue (endoneurium; Fig. 10.2). Each fascicle is surrounded by a fibrous connective tissue layer (perineurium); whole nerve trunks consist of a variable number of fascicles that are contained within a loose connective tissue sheath (epineurium). Nerve trunks receive their blood supply from branches of regional arteries; small nutrient vessels penetrate the epineurium and form anastomoses within the nerve trunk.

Single nerve fibres within fascicles may be myelinated or unmyelinated. The motor axons are extensions of motor neurones in the anterior horns; the sensory axons are derived from dorsal root ganglion cells. The postganglionic sympathetic efferent fibres are unmyelinated and arise from ganglia in the thoracolumbar sympathetic chain (Chapter 9).

Myelinated fibres range in diameter from 2 to 22 μm; unmyelinated fibres diameters range from 0.2 to 3 μm. The satellite cell of the peripheral nervous system is the Schwann cell which is associated with both myelinated and unmyelinated fibres.

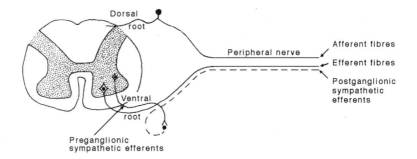

Fig. 10.1 Schematic representation of components of peripheral nerve trunks. (From Lance and McLeod, 1981, with permission of Butterworths, London.)

Myelinated fibres are characterized by their myelin sheaths which consist of alternating layers of protein and lipid and act as an insulating membrane around the axon. The myelin is interrupted at regular intervals by the nodes of Ranvier (Fig. 10.3). The segment of nerve between two successive nodes is an internode. Internodal length and myelin thickness are directly proportional to the external diameter of the nerve fibre. Myelin is the fusion of apposing layers of Schwann cell cytoplasmic membrane formed by the spiralling of the Schwann cell around the axon; myelin is thus not only formed by, but is actually a living part of, the Schwann cell. There is only one Schwann cell for each internode of the myelinated fibre, but by contrast there may be several unmyelinated fibres associated with a single Schwann cell.

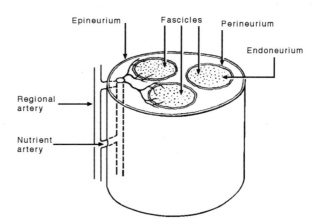

Fig. 10.2 Structure of peripheral nerve trunk and its blood supply. Regional arteries running longitudinally outside the nerve trunk supply nutrient arteries that penetrate the epineurium and form an anastomosis. Small arterioles perforate the epineurium of the fascicles and form an endoneurial capillary network. (Modified from P. J. Dyck *Postgraduate Medicine*, 1967, **41**, 279–289).

PATHOLOGICAL REACTIONS

Four major pathological processes may affect peripheral nerves (Fig. 10.3):
- Wallerian degeneration
- Axonal degeneration
- Segmental demyelination
- Neuronopathy or primary nerve cell degeneration

Wallerian degeneration

Wallerian degeneration is the process that follows mechanical injury such as transection or crush of nerve fibres, or it may follow ischaemic damage (e.g. vasculitis). Within a period of 4–5 days the axon and the myelin degenerate distal to the site of injury; the myelin forms linear arrays of ovoids and globules along the degenerating axon. The axon of the proximal segment then regenerates forming sprouts which grow distally, re-innervating the surviving distal neurilemmal tubes of the Schwann cell basement membrane inside which the Schwann cells have divided and arranged themselves in line. The regenerating axons are then myelinated by the Schwann cells but the nerve fibres are of smaller diameter and have disproportionately short internodal lengths compared with the original fibres. Some regenerated axons never reach their distal connections.

Axonal degeneration

Axonal degeneration is the most common pathological change in peripheral neuropathies and is seen in most nutritional, metabolic and toxic causes of peripheral nerve disease. The pathological appearances in nerve biopsy specimens

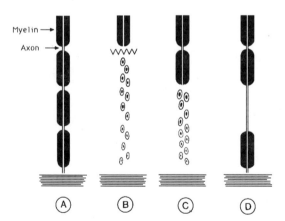

Fig. 10.3 Schematic representation of pathological changes in peripheral nerve fibres. (A) Normal myelinated fibre; (B) Wallerian degeneration following crush or section of nerve fibre. Axon and myelin degenerate; (C) axonal degeneration of distal portion of nerve fibre in 'dying-back' neuropathy. Axon and myelin are both degenerating; (D) segmental demyelination. Myelin has degenerated in one internode but axon remains intact.

are similar to those of Wallerian degeneration. The usual mechanism is that disturbance of the metabolism of the cell body, or perikaryon, results in impairment of fast axonal transport and other functions so that the most distal parts of the axon, which may be as far removed as 1 m from the cell body, are first affected and die back from the periphery ('dying-back neuropathy'). Because the longest and usually largest diameter nerve fibres are first affected, distal muscle wasting and glove-and-stocking sensory loss are the characteristic clinical manifestations.

Segmental demyelination

Segmental demyelination is the term applied to the process of primary damage of the myelin sheath while the axon remains intact. In inflammatory neuropathies (e.g. Guillain-Barré syndrome) it is caused by a direct immune-mediated attack on the myelin or possibly on the Schwann cell. It may also result from presumed disturbances of Schwann cell metabolism in some hereditary neuropathies (e.g. Déjèrine-Sottas disease) or toxic damage of the myelin sheath (experimental neuropathies produced with diphtheria toxin or triethyl tin). When demyelination is severe there may be secondary axonal degeneration. Demyelination usually commences paranodally and often affects proximal parts of the peripheral nervous system (e.g. roots) and the very distal portion at the neuromuscular junction to an equal or greater extent than the intervening regions. When remyelination occurs, Schwann cells divide and form new internodes of irregular length with thin myelin sheaths. Repeated episodes of demyelination will result in the formation of concentric layers of Schwann cell cytoplasm and endoneurial elements around the axon which are described as 'onion bulb' formations.

Neuronopathies

In neuronopathies there is primary destruction of the nerve cell body. Examples of motor neuronopathies in which anterior horn cells are primarily affected are the spinal muscular atrophies, amyotrophic lateral sclerosis and poliomyelitis. Sensory neuronopathies in which the dorsal root ganglion cell is primarily affected include Friedreich's ataxia, hereditary sensory neuropathies and some paraneoplastic neuropathies; there is distal degeneration of both peripheral sensory axons and the central processes ascending in the posterior columns and other spinal tracts. Since the cell bodies are destroyed in these disorders, there is no prospect of recovery.

DISEASES OF THE PERIPHERAL NERVOUS SYSTEM

The peripheral nervous system may be affected by localized injury to peripheral nerve trunks or roots, vascular occlusions in major nerve trunks (e.g. in polyarteritis or diabetes), or generalized disease processes affecting the function of peripheral nerves. Some of the causes of peripheral neuropathy are listed below. The most common are diabetes, alcohol, nutritional deficiencies, and, in many countries, leprosy.

Genetically determined neuropathies

Charcot-Marie-Tooth disease (peroneal muscular atrophy) usually has an auto-somal dominant inheritance and is the most common genetically determined neuropathy, with a prevalence of about 4:100 000 population. Symptoms usually begin at 10–30 years of age. The earliest signs are distal wasting of the lower limbs with foot-drop. The intrinsic hand muscles become affected later and mild distal sensory loss is usually apparent. Reflexes in the lower limbs are depressed or absent. The foot has a characteristic appearance with a high arch and retracted toes (pes cavus). The condition progresses very slowly over many years and most patients remain mobile into old age. Four major types are recognized:

Hereditary motor and sensory neuropathy type I (HMSN type I) or the hypertrophic type In this neuropathy the peripheral nerves are thickened and segmental demyelination is the underlying pathology. Most families with HMSN I (HMSN Ia) are linked to a gene locus on chromosome 17 (17p.11.2–12); this is the gene for peripheral myelin protein (PMP 22), where either mutation or duplication can cause expression of the disease. A rare type (HMSN Ib) is linked to the gene on chromosome 1 for Po myelin protein.

HMSN type II This is the neuronal type in which there is axonal degeneration without hypertrophic changes. A genetic linkage for HMSN II has not been established.

X-linked Charcot-Marie-Tooth disease This is due to a mutation of the gap-junction protein, connexin (Xq13).

HMSN type III (Déjèrine Sottas disease) This presents as a severe neuropathy in childhood. It is due to point mutations of the Po gene (chromosome 1) or PMP 22 (chromosome 17).

Other hereditary peripheral neuropathies include the familial and primary amyloidosis and hereditary sensory neuropathies in which mutilating deformities develop in the hands and feet. The peripheral nerves may be affected in a number of other hereditary diseases that also affect the central nervous system (e.g. Friedreich's ataxia, metachromatic leucodystrophy).

Drugs and other toxins

Heavy metals (arsenic, lead, mercury, thallium, gold), some organic industrial agents (acrylamide, hexacarbons, triorthocresyl phosphate), and some drugs (isoniazid, ethambutol, nitrofurantoin, vincristine, phenytoin, thalidomide, lithium carbonate, perhexiline, chloroquin, disulfiram, metronidazole) may cause a peripheral neuropathy. Generalized peripheral neuropathy or mononeuritis multiplex may sometimes follow as an allergic or immune response to vaccinations and injections of foreign proteins.

Metabolic and endocrine

Diabetes is a common cause of peripheral neuropathy, usually symmetrical and predominantly sensory. When there is severe sensory impairment, perforating ulcers of the feet and neuropathic joints (Charcot joints) may occur with associated sensory ataxia. Symptoms of autonomic dysfunction are common. *Diabetic amyotrophy* is a painful asymmetrical proximal motor neuropathy affecting predominantly the quadriceps, hamstring and gluteal muscles of the lower limbs. Isolated peripheral nerve lesions particularly the carpal tunnel syndrome and ulnar nerve lesions at the elbow are also common in diabetic patients.

Uraemia, porphyria, acromegaly, hypothyroidism and recurrent attacks of hypoglycaemia due to islet cell tumours of the pancreas may also be associated with peripheral neuropathies.

Vitamin deficiencies

Vitamin B_{12} deficiency, whether associated with pernicious anaemia or mal-absorption syndromes, results in a predominantly sensory neuropathy that may be accompanied by subacute combined degeneration of the spinal cord (p. 118). Vitamin B_1 (thiamine) deficiency is seen particularly in chronic alcoholism and severe nutritional disturbances and causes a painful, predominantly sensory neuropathy.

Alcoholism is one of the commonest associations with peripheral neuropathy in urban populations. Common symptoms are pains in the calves, burning feet and distal weakness. Distal muscle wasting, absent knee and ankle jerks and distal sensory impairment with tender calves are the usual physical findings. It is caused by Vitamin B deficiency rather than by the direct effects of alcohol.

Malignancies

Clinical peripheral neuropathy may be a remote (paraneoplastic) manifestation of malignancy in about 5% of patients with carcinoma and lymphoma. A pre-dominantly sensory ganglionopathy occurs in association with small-cell carcinoma of the lung. Paraproteinaemias and dysproteinaemias (e.g. multiple myeloma, macroglobulinaemia) are often associated with peripheral neuropathy.

Connective tissue diseases

Rheumatoid arthritis may be accompanied by a symmetrical sensory or sensori-motor neuropathy. Mononeuritis multiplex caused by arteritis and entrapment neuropathies are also well recognized complications of rheumatoid disease.

Polyarteritis nodosa classically causes a mononeuritis multiplex which may also be seen in systemic lupus erythematosus (SLE) and sarcoidosis. Sjögren's disease may also be associated with peripheral neuropathy.

Infections

Leprosy is the most common cause of peripheral neuropathy on a world-wide basis. *Mycobacterium leprae* invades the Schwann cell. The organism spreads intra-cutaneously so that a patch of numbness in leprosy may overlap peripheral nerve territories.

Inflammatory neuropathies

Guillain-Barré syndrome (acute inflammatory polyneuritis) has a rapid onset and is potentially fatal. The common initial symptoms of paraesthesiae or pain in the lower limbs are followed by weakness; because spinal roots are also involved in the inflammatory process, proximal muscles may be affected to the same or even a greater extent than the distal muscle groups. Facial and bulbar paralysis are common and there may be weakness of the extra-ocular muscles. Reflexes are usually depressed or absent and there is a variable degree of sensory loss. Within 3–4 weeks this predominantly motor neuropathy progresses to a maximum disability often with complete quadriparesis and respiratory paralysis. About 80% of patients recover without any significant disability, but some are left with long term disability due to secondary axonal degeneration. Typically the protein level in cerebrospinal fluid is elevated and the cell count is not increased. Circulating anti-myelin antibodies have been demonstrated during the acute phase of the disease and it is likely that the pathogenesis of the disorder is a combined humoral and cell-mediated immune response directed at myelin in peripheral nerve and spinal roots, that may be provoked by certain viral or bacterial infections (particularly *Campylobacter jejuni*) since these precede the onset of the condition in about 60% of cases. Chronic inflammatory neuropathy has a slower onset and may run a relapsing and remitting or progressive course.

Clinical features of peripheral neuropathy

Most chronic polyneuropathies are symmetrical, predominantly distal and have a mixture of motor and sensory manifestations. Motor symptoms are those of weakness of distal muscles; patients find difficulty in climbing stairs and difficulty in unfastening buttons or performing fine movements. Muscle wasting, foot-drop and wrist-drop are common. Sensory disturbances include numbness, tingling, pins and needles in the hands and feet, burning sensations, pain in the extremities, sensations of walking on cotton wool and band-like constrictions around the wrists or ankles, unsteadiness on the feet or stumbling. Autonomic dysfunction may be manifested as dryness or excessive sweating of the extremities, postural hypo-tension, impotence, diarrhoea and constipation.

The signs of peripheral neuropathy are usually those of distal muscle wasting and weakness and sensory impairment, often in a glove-and-stocking type of distribution. Two-point discrimination is the most sensitive test of mild degrees of sensory impairment. Reflexes are usually depressed or absent, but in mild cases the abnormalities may be confined to the ankle jerks since their pathway is longer than that of other reflexes. The clinical features of sensory impairment, distal muscle wasting and weakness and early loss of reflexes, distinguish peripheral neuropathies from myopathies (p. 157).

Onset and course

Most neuropathies have a gradual onset and slow progression. Acute onset of neuropathy is seen only in a limited number of conditions which include the Guillain-Barré syndrome, porphyria, diphtheria, acute toxic neuropathies and neuropathies that follow immunization.

Pattern of distribution

Most neuropathies have a symmetrical distribution and affect the lower limbs to a greater extent than the upper limbs. Some neuropathies have an asymmetrical presentation and these include the acute and chronic inflammatory neuropathies and those caused by disease of small blood vessels. Mononeuritis multiplex suggests a vascular cause (polyarteritis, rheumatoid arthritis, small vessel disease in diabetes) but other aetiological factors such as sarcoidosis, leprosy and autoimmune reactions to injections and vaccinations must be considered.

Brachial neuritis (neuralgic amyotrophy) is a condition characterized by the rapid onset of pain, weakness and wasting of the muscles of one shoulder and upper arm, although it is sometimes bilateral. Its onset may be related to an infection or immunization, but in most cases there are no recognized precipitating factors.

Most neuropathies characteristically have a distal distribution but proximal weakness may be a feature of acute and chronic demyelinating neuropathies, porphyria and Déjèrine-Sottas disease. Lower limbs are usually affected earlier and to a greater extent than the upper limbs; exceptions to the rule are acute and chronic demyelinating neuropathies, porphyria and lead poisoning.

Predominantly motor or sensory neuropathies

Some peripheral neuropathies affect mainly motor or mainly sensory fibres (Table 10.1), although most have manifestations of both. When large sensory fibres are predominantly affected (e.g. Friedreich's ataxia) light touch, vibration and position sense are characteristically impaired with sparing of pain and temperature sensations and loss of reflexes. In some other neuropathies (e.g. amyloidosis, diabetes) the small fibres are selectively involved causing autonomic dysfunction and burning pain associated with loss of pain and temperature sense whereas tactile sensation is relatively spared. Nerve conduction studies measure predominantly large fibre function and may be relatively normal early in the course of small fibre neuropathies.

NERVE INJURIES

In nerve injuries three main disorders of function are recognized.

Neurapraxia

Neurapraxia is transient loss of function of a nerve following compression or mild trauma; spontaneous recovery of function occurs within days or weeks. The underlying pathology is local demyelination; temporary localized block in conduction of the nerve impulse can be demonstrated at the affected site. The axon of the nerve remains intact.

Axonotmesis

Axonotmesis results from crush injuries that cause degeneration of the axon and its myelin sheath (Wallerian degeneration). The neurilemmal sheaths, consisting of tubes of basement membranes, are preserved and are repopulated by neural sprouts from the distal ends of the axonal stumps above the level of the lesion.

Table 10.1 Clinical types of peripheral neuropathy

Acute onset
Guillain-Barré syndrome
Porphyria
Toxic
Serum sickness (post-immunization)
Malignancy

Predominantly motor
Guillain-Barré syndrome
Porphyria
Diphtheria
Lead
Charcot-Marie-Tooth disease

Predominantly sensory
Leprosy
Diabetes
Vitamin B_{12} or thiamine deficiency
Malignancy
Hereditary sensory neuropathy
Amyloid disease
Uraemia
Friedreich's ataxia

Painful neuropathies
Alcohol, nutritional deficiencies
Diabetes
Hereditary sensory neuropathy
Arsenic
Cryoglobulinaemia
Vasculitis

Neurotmesis

This is the condition in which the whole nerve trunk is severed and continuity of the neurilemmal sheath is lost. The distal nerve trunk cannot be re-innervated effectively unless surgical repair is undertaken to approximate, as accurately as possible, the proximal and distal ends of the nerve trunk.

Entrapment and compression neuropathies

Isolated nerve trunks are frequently affected by entrapment or compression in anatomical compartments. The most common example is compression of the median nerve beneath the flexor retinaculum at the wrist causing the *carpal tunnel syndrome*. The condition is more common in women and is frequently bilateral. Narrowing of the carpal tunnel occurs in obesity, myxoedema, acromegaly, fluid retention caused by use of oral contraceptive pills or pregnancy, arthritis of the wrist or wrist trauma. The symptoms are numbness and tingling in the thumb and fingers supplied by the median nerve (index, middle and radial half of the ring finger), mainly at night. If the nerve has been entrapped for long periods of time there are signs of sensory loss over the median nerve distribution of the hand and wasting of the thenar muscles.

Other well-recognized entrapment syndromes are: (i) compression of the ulnar nerve at the elbow causing paraesthesiae and sensory loss in the little and ulnar half of the ring finger, and wasting and weakness of the interossei; (ii) compression of the peroneal nerve at the neck of the fibula resulting in foot-drop and numbness over the dorsum of the foot and lateral aspect of the leg; (iii) compression of the lateral cutaneous nerve of the thigh at the level of the inguinal ligament, which occurs particularly in people who are overweight and causes numbness and tingling over the outer aspect of the thigh (meralgia paraesthetica); (iv) radial nerve lesions at the lower end of the spiral groove of the humerus causing wrist-drop.

Predisposing factors to entrapment neuropathies are repetitive trauma, diabetes, alcoholism and other causes of peripheral nerve disease. Surgical decompression of the nerve may be necessary. The lower trunk of the brachial plexus may be compressed against a fibrous band or complete rib taking origin from C7 (cervical rib), causing wasting of the hand intrinsic muscles and sensory loss in the ulnar border of the hand.

INVESTIGATIONS

The basic investigations that should be performed on all patients with peripheral neuropathy of unknown cause include urinalysis, full blood count, measurement of erythrocyte sedimentation rate, fasting blood sugar, serum electrolytes, serum creatinine, serum proteins and immuno-electrophoresis, liver function tests and serum Vitamin B_{12} and folate levels. Serum lipoproteins, urinary porphyrins, heavy metals, amino acids and faecal fats should be studied in appropriate cases. Examination of the cerebrospinal fluid may be helpful in some cases (e.g. Guillain-Barré syndrome). Other investigations to exclude malignancy may include chest X-ray and other appropriate radiological and endoscopic investigations.

TREATMENT

Acute neuropathies

In the Guillain-Barré syndrome and other peripheral neuropathies with acute involvement of respiratory muscles, spirometry should be performed every 2–4 hours in the initial stages because tracheal intubation or tracheostomy and artificial ventilation may be necessary. Careful nursing is very important and particular attention should be paid to the care of the skin, bladder, bowels, mouth, pharynx and trachea. Lung and urinary tract infections require prompt treatment. Intravenous or intragastric feeding may be necessary. Physiotherapy should begin immediately and splints to prevent foot- and wrist-drop may be required. Plasmapheresis and intravenous human immunoglobulin hasten recovery and improve prognosis if commenced within days of onset of the Guillain-Barré syndrome. Corticosteroids do not have a beneficial effect.

Chronic neuropathies

Specific treatment for the underlying cause should be given when indicated. Corticosteroids, immunosuppressive therapy and plasmapheresis or intravenous immunoglobulin may be helpful in patients with chronic inflammatory neuropathy and in patients with vasculitic neuropathy. Treatment of other neuropathies is related to their underlying cause. Leprous neuropathy should be treated with the appropriate anti-microbial agents. There is some evidence that the progression of diabetic neuropathy may slow in response to good diabetic control. Heavy metal poisoning should be treated by appropriate chelation therapy and withdrawal of the source of intoxication. Drug related neuropathies may improve if the offending agents are withdrawn although disability in axonal neuropathy is often permanent. The neuropathies related to chronic alcoholism should be treated by institution of a diet replete in thiamin and in neuropathies related to vitamin B_{12} insufficiency patients should be treated with replacement therapy although recovery is often incomplete.

Physiotherapy is an important part of treatment. In severe cases splints, calipers and other walking aids will be necessary and occasionally surgical corrective procedures will be required. A programme of rehabilitation should be commenced.

DISEASES OF MUSCLE ——————————————

STRUCTURE OF MUSCLE

Muscles are composed of many parallel fibres, each of which is a large multinucleated cell enclosed by a sarcolemmal membrane. The sarcoplasm within the cell contains myofibrils which constitute the contractile machinery of the muscle as well as mitochondria that contain oxidative enzymes and other cellular constituents. Each myofibril is about 1 μm in diameter and is composed of precisely aligned thick (myosin) and thin (actin) protein filaments which alternate to form a repetitive band pattern, giving rise to the cross-striated appearance of muscle fibres that is apparent on light and electron microscopy (Fig. 10.4). The dark A band contains overlapping thick and thin filaments and the light I band contains only the thin actin filaments. At the centre of the A band is a dark H band composed only of myosin with the M line at its centre. The dense Z line at the centre of the I band represents the attachment of the actin fibres and is composed of desmin, alpha actinin and amorphin. The sarcomere is the unit between two successive Z lines and is about 2–3 μm in length. The myofibrils are closely embraced by the sarcoplasmic reticulum in which calcium is stored. The T system consists of tubules which run transversely, usually at the junction of the A and I bands. The T tubules arise as an invagination of the sarcolemmal membrane and are in direct continuity with the extracellular fluid.

When the muscle end-plate is depolarized, an action potential is propagated down the muscle fibre and along the T system leading to the release of calcium ions from the sarcoplasmic reticulum. The released calcium is bound by troponin, a protein associated with actin in the thin filament. When a muscle is at rest, troponin and tropomyosin are linked and prevent actin from binding to myosin. The binding of calcium to troponin breaks the linkage resulting in the interaction between actin and myosin that causes muscle contraction. The energy for the process is obtained from the breakdown of ATP. Muscle fibre relaxation results from active pumping back of calcium ions into the sarcoplasmic reticulum.

Muscle fibres may be classified according to their speed of contraction. Slowly contracting fibres are rich in mitochondria and derive their energy from oxidative metabolism. Fast contracting fibres are rich in glycogen and derive their energy mainly through the glycolytic pathway. Histochemical staining with ATPase, succinic dehydrogenase, and other stains, will differentiate the type I (slow contracting,

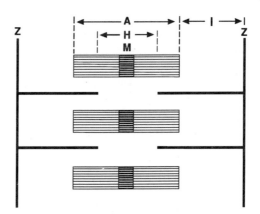

Fig. 10.4 Schematic representation of a myofibril. Thick myosin (thick band) filaments overlap thin actin (thin band) filaments. A sarcomere lies between two Z bands. A, I, H and M refer to bands seen on electron microscopy.

aerobic metabolism) from the type II (fast contracting, anaerobic metabolism) fibres. Histochemical analysis of muscle biopsies is very helpful in the diagnosis of muscle diseases.

CLINICAL FEATURES OF MUSCLE DISEASES

The onset is usually insidious. Proximal muscle groups tend to be affected first and patients may notice difficulty in walking, rising from a chair, climbing stairs, hanging clothes on a line or combing the hair. Facial weakness may be apparent in smiling and whistling, and weakness of bulbar muscles may be manifested by difficulty in chewing and swallowing. Pain is usually not a feature but may be present on exertion in McArdle's disease and polymyositis. A careful family history should always be taken in case there is a genetically determined disorder and the patient should be asked specifically whether there is any parental consanguinity. The distribution of weakness is variable and forms the basis for classification of muscular dystrophies. Usually proximal muscles are affected to a greater extent than distal muscles. Muscle tone and tendon reflexes are diminished in proportion to muscle weakness.

Clinical features that distinguish muscle diseases from peripheral neuropathies are their proximal distribution of weakness and wasting, the absence of sensory abnormalities and the relative preservation of reflexes.

CLASSIFICATION OF MUSCLE DISEASES

Diseases in which the muscle fibres are primarily affected are known as *myopathies*. They may be classified according to whether they are genetically determined or acquired. Genetically determined myopathies are known as *muscular dystrophies*. Myopathies must be distinguished from the neurogenic atrophies in which muscle wasting is secondary to disease of the anterior horn cells or peripheral nerves. In myopathies degenerative and metabolic changes occur primarily in the muscle fibres. In some conditions, there are distinctive morphological features.

Muscular dystrophies

Progressive muscular dystrophies
Duchenne muscular dystrophy   This is the commonest form of progressive muscular dystrophy. It affects 13–33/100000 live-born males and has a prevalence of about 3/100000 in the population. It is a sex-linked recessive disorder and, with rare exceptions, affects only males. Females are carriers of the disease. The disease becomes evident in the first decade of life and progresses to death from respiratory or cardiac failure usually in the second or third decade. Weakness usually begins in the proximal muscles of the lower limbs but soon spreads to involve the anterior

tibial group of muscles, trunk muscles and proximal muscles of the upper limbs. The calf muscles are unusually prominent, initially due to muscle hypertrophy but later to fatty infiltration of degenerated muscles (pseudohypertrophy). The heart is usually affected and intellectual retardation is common. The serum creatine kinase (CK) levels are very high in affected children and are also elevated in carriers. The genetic defect in muscular dystrophy has been localized to the short arm of the X chromosome (X p21.2) in the region of a gene that codes for *dystrophin*, a very large (427 kDa) cytoskeletal protein found on the sarcolemmal membrane. Patients with Duchenne muscular dystrophy have deletions within this gene. A milder form of X linked muscular dystrophy (Becker type) is also due to deletions within the gene for dystrophin but in these patients the defect produces a partially functional dystrophin molecule. Other rarer muscle diseases are also related to disorders in the dystrophin gene and the collective term *dystrophinopathies* is applied to them. Early detection of gene carriers is important for genetic counselling.

Facioscapulohumeral muscular dystrophy   This is autosomal dominant and has a later age of onset and slower progression than Duchenne muscular dystrophy. The muscles most affected are biceps, triceps and the muscles of the shoulder girdle. Scapular winging is prominent. Facial muscles are also involved early but pelvic muscles are affected later in the course of the disease. The gene is located on chromosome 4 (4q.35).

Limb girdle muscular dystrophy   This is probably a heterogeneous group of conditions in which the shoulder and pelvic muscles are predominantly involved but facial muscles are spared. Most cases are sporadic or have an autosomal recessive inheritance.

Scapuloperoneal muscular dystrophy   Shoulder girdle muscles and muscles of the anterolateral compartment of the leg are primarily affected. The condition may be X-linked or autosomal dominant.

Ocular myopathy (progressive external ophthalmoplegia)   Ocular myopathies are characterized by progressive external ophthalmoplegia, ptosis and often facial weakness. They are a heterogeneous group of disorders, many of which are related to disorders of mitochondrial function (*mitochondrial myopathies*).

Myotonic dystrophies

These are genetically determined muscle disorders, characterized by the presence of myotonia. *Myotonia* is the failure of the voluntary muscles to relax immediately after contraction and clinically it may be demonstrated by a slowness of relaxation of the hand grip or a prolonged dimpling of the muscle after being struck sharply with a percussion hammer (percussion myotonia). Electromyographically, myotonia is distinguished by prolonged spontaneous discharges from the resting muscle that commence at high frequency and then wane in both frequency and amplitude (Fig. 10.5). The myotonia is a manifestation of increased muscle cell membrane excitability due to reduced chloride conductance. Two main types are recognized: dystrophia myotonica and myotonia congenita.

Dystrophia myotonica   A relatively common form of muscular dystrophy affecting about 7/100 000 of the population. Inheritance is autosomal dominant

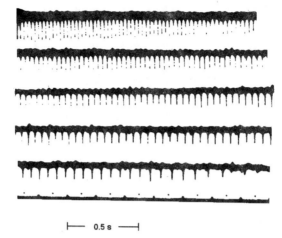

Fig. 10.5 Continuous electromyographic recording of myotonic discharge from muscle of a patient with dystrophia myotonica. Note that the amplitude of the action potential becomes progressively smaller and the frequency of the discharge becomes progressively reduced with time. (From Lance and McLeod, 1981, with permission of Butterworths, London.)

and the gene has been localized on chromosome 19 (19q3.2) where it codes for a protein kinase (*myotonin*). The onset is insidious, usually between the ages of 20 and 50 years, but it may be present in childhood or at birth, particularly when transmission is from the mother. The severity of the disease correlates closely with the number of trinucleotide repeats in the gene. There is progressive wasting and weakness of distal as well as proximal muscles, ptosis, weakness of facial muscles, weakness and wasting of sternomastoids, cataracts, gonadal atrophy, frontal baldness, cardiomyopathy and abnormalities of insulin secretion.

Myotonia congenita (Thomsen's disease) There are both autosomal dominant and recessive varieties of this disease. The onset is usually in early life with myotonia and muscle stiffness that normally improves with exercise, but when it is severe attempts to run or walk may cause the patient to fall. The muscles are hypertrophied and strong, in contrast to those in patients with dystrophic myotonia. The autosomal dominant form of Thomsen's disease has been demonstrated to be due to abnormalities in the gene for the chloride channel on chromosome 7 (7q35).

Mitochondrial myopathy

Mitochondrial myopathies are a group of disorders in which mitochondrial abnormalities are seen on muscle biopsy. The usual clinical manifestations are muscle weakness with fatiguability and progressive external ophthalmoplegia. Subsarcolemmal accumulations of mitochondria may be seen in appropriately stained muscle biopsies.

Specific mitochondrial enzyme deficiencies have been demonstrated in some cases. They may be associated with evidence of degeneration of other systems, e.g. cerebellar ataxia, myoclonus, strokes.

Many of the mitochondrial myopathies have been shown to be due to deletions in the small circular DNA molecules found in mitochondria (*mitochondrial DNA*). Because mitochondrial DNA comes from the maternal line, mitochondrial myopathies may demonstrate maternal inheritance. Many genes for mitochondrial peptides are coded in the autosomal DNA so that Mendelian dominant or recessive inheritance may also be seen.

Congenital myopathies

There are many genetically determined myopathies of unknown aetiology which are characterized by their muscle biopsy appearances, e.g. central core disease, nemaline myopathy, centronuclear myopathy. Some of these myopathies have a benign course with some improvement in strength as the child grows.

Familial periodic paralyses

Recurrent attacks of weakness lasting several hours may be related to changes in the serum potassium level. The most common form is *hypokalaemic periodic paralysis* which has an autosomal dominant inheritance. During the attacks, which may be precipitated by rest after exercise or by heavy carbohydrate intake, there is a low level of serum potassium due to an intracellular shift of potassium and other ions. One particular form of hypokalaemic periodic paralysis is associated with thyrotoxicosis. *Hyperkalaemic periodic paralysis*, which is also transmitted by an autosomal dominant gene, is associated with raised serum potassium during attacks. In this type myotonia may be a feature. This disease has been shown to be due to a mutation in the gene for the tetrodotoxin sensitive sodium channel on chromosome 17 (17q23.1-q25.3). In a third type, *normokalaemic periodic paralysis*, potassium levels remain normal during attacks.

Other genetically determined metabolic disorders

Some muscle disorders are associated with abnormalities of glycogen metabolism. The best known is McArdle's syndrome in which there is a deficiency of muscle phosphorylase. The symptoms are fatigue, cramps on exertion and sustained contraction of the muscles if exercise continues. In a similar disorder, an inherited absence of fructokinase has been identified.

Myopathies may also be associated with inherited disorders of muscle lipid metabolism, e.g. carnitine deficiency.

Acquired myopathies

Myopathies, usually presenting with proximal muscle weakness, may be secondary to a number of different causes:

Endocrine

- Thyrotoxicosis
- Myxoedema

- Cushing's disease
- Hyperparathyroidism
- Osteomalacia
- Acromegaly
- Steroid administration

Toxic

- Alcohol
- Malignancy
- Drugs (e.g. corticosteroids, chloroquine)

Metabolic disturbances

- Potassium loss from vomiting, diarrhoea or urinary excretion may cause profound generalized weakness or even complete paralysis. Hypokalaemia may reach dangerous levels in: (i) the recovery phase of diabetic coma; (ii) potassium-losing nephritis; (iii) hyperaldosteronism; (iv) long continued use of diuretic agents, adrenocorticosteroids or carbenoxolone sodium.

Polymyositis

Polymyositis is an inflammatory reaction of muscle which most likely has an autoimmune basis. Patients usually present with muscle weakness, affecting predominantly proximal muscles. This is usually painless although some patients may experience muscle pain and tenderness. In most cases of polymyositis no underlying cause is demonstrated, but it may be associated with connective tissue diseases (e.g. systemic lupus erythematosus, progressive systemic sclerosis, rheumatoid arthritis), malignancy and skin rash (dermatomyositis).

DISEASES OF THE NEUROMUSCULAR JUNCTION

The nerve terminals of motor fibres lie in grooves, or gutters, in the muscle end-plates. The cell membranes of nerve and muscle are separated by a space of about 50 nm (Fig. 10.6). At rest acetylcholine (ACh) is released spontaneously from synaptic vesicles in the nerve endings; it diffuses rapidly across the space to bind to acetylcholine receptors (AChR), partially depolarizing the muscle membrane and giving rise to miniature end-plate potentials (mepps) which may be recorded with an intracellular electrode in the end-plate zone. Spontaneous mepps have a frequency of about 1 Hz and an amplitude of about 0.5–1.0 mV. Each mepp represents the release of a single packet or quantum of ACh (about 10 000 molecules) from a synaptic vesicle. When a nerve impulse arrives at the nerve terminal there is an enormous increase in the number of quanta of ACh released;

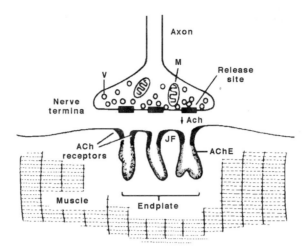

Fig. 10.6 Neuromuscular junction. V = vesicles; M = mitochondria; ACh = acetylcholine; JF = junctional folds; AChE = acetylcholine esterase. (Modified from Drachman, 1978, *New England Journal of Medicine*, **136**, with permission of the Editor.)

as many as 250–500 may be liberated by each nerve impulse. Depolarization of the muscle membrane which follows results in the production of an end-plate potential (about 30–40 mV in amplitude) and the initiation of a muscle action potential. Acetylcholine is broken down by cholinesterase and subsequently resynthesized in the terminal bouton of the axon.

Abnormalities of neuromuscular transmission occur in myasthenia gravis and in the myasthenic syndrome associated with malignancy.

MYASTHENIA GRAVIS

Myasthenia gravis is not a rare disease, having a prevalence of 5–12/100 000 population.

Clinical features

Patients with myasthenia gravis complain of rapid fatigue after muscular effort. Weakness is usually more pronounced at the end of the day and improved by rest. It may be confined to restricted muscle groups, such as the ocular muscles (ocular myasthenia) bulbar muscles or proximal limb muscles or it may become generalized. In severe cases respiratory muscles are involved. Patients often complain of double vision, drooping of the eyelids, alteration in speech, and difficulty in chewing and swallowing, as well as a weakness in the limbs. A snarling smile is characteristic of the myasthenic patient.

Thymic hyperplasia is present in the majority of patients with onset under the age of 40 years, and a thymoma is present in about 10% of all patients with myasthenia gravis. A computerized tomography (CT) scan may reveal the thymic enlargement in the anterior mediastinum. The diagnosis may be confirmed by diagnostic procedures, the most important of which is the detection of anti-ACh receptor (anti-AChR) antibodies which are present in about 80–90% of cases. Repetitive electrical stimulation of a motor nerve at rates of 1–30 Hz causes a rapid and marked decline in the amplitude of the compound muscle action potential in myasthenia gravis patients in contrast to normals (Fig. 10.7). Intravenous injection of a synthetic anticholinesterase, edrophonium hydrochloride (Tensilon; 2 mg test dose followed by 8 mg) improves muscle strength for a period of 2–5 minutes. Single fibre electromyography allows impairment of neuromuscular transmission to be recorded electrophysiologically as a variable latency of the individual single fibre potentials within a given motor unit ('jitter') and is useful in some cases where the diagnosis is in doubt.

Babies born to mothers with myasthenia gravis may have transient weakness due to the transplacental passage of maternal anti-AChR antibodies (*neonatal myasthenia*).

Pathogenesis

Anti-AChR antibody is an immunoglobulin G (IgG) antibody whose synthesis is predominantly controlled by thymic cells. These circulating antibodies become attached to, and inactivate, the muscle end-plate receptors, reducing the number of functioning ACh receptors so that mepps are reduced in amplitude although normal in frequency.

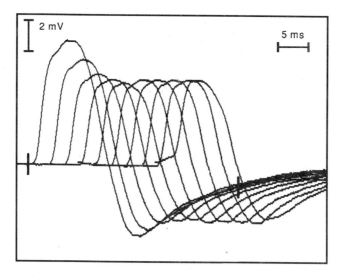

Fig. 10.7 Myasthenic response to repetitive electrical stimulation of a nerve. Ten successive muscle action potentials have been recorded with surface electrodes over the abductor digiti minimi muscle while stimulating the ulnar nerve at a rate of ·5 Hz. Note the progressive decrement in the amplitude of muscle action potential.

Myasthenia gravis is known to have an autoimmune basis because: (i) there are anti-AChR antibodies in 80–90% of patients; (ii) the disease can be passively transferred to mice; (iii) immunization with the antigen produces a model disease; (iv) reduction of the antibody ameliorates the disease. T cells play an important role in the auto-antibody response, and thymic hyperplasia or thymomas are present in many patients.

Treatment

Anticholinesterase drugs are useful in the treatment of myasthenia and act by increasing the local concentration of ACh in the synaptic cleft. Neostigmine (Prostigmine), 15 mg or more every 3 hours, or pyridostigmine (Mestinon), 60 mg or more every 4 hours, are the commonly used anticholinesterases.

Thymectomy should be considered, particularly in patients with onset less than 40 years of age, since it improves the long-term prognosis. It is not indicated in ocular myasthenia. Thymectomy is essential when a thymoma is present, and should be preceded or followed by radiotherapy if there is any evidence of invasion of adjacent tissues. Immunosuppression with corticosteroids and azathioprine plays an important role particularly in patients who do not respond to anticholinesterase drugs.

Plasmapheresis frequently produces a dramatic but relatively short-lived response by reducing circulating levels of anti-AChR antibodies. It is used in patients with acute relapses of the disease who are not responding to other forms of therapy.

Myasthenia may sometimes be induced by penicillamine. Some antibiotics, including neomycin, kanamycin, streptomycin, bacitracin, colistin, ampicillin and amoxicillin interfere with neuromuscular transmission and their use should be avoided in myasthenic patients.

Myasthenic syndrome

A myasthenic syndrome is present in about 3% of patients with small cell carcinoma of the lung (Eaton-Lambert syndrome) and some patients in whom no malignancy is found. The chief symptom is weakness of proximal muscles in the limbs, especially of the pelvic girdles and thighs. Muscle power may temporarily increase at the start of exercise, but weakness soon returns causing rapid fatigue. There may be a mild bilateral ptosis but ocular and bulbar muscles are rarely involved. Deep tendon reflexes are usually depressed or absent.

In contrast to myasthenia gravis the response to edrophonium and other anticholinesterase drugs is poor. Again, in contrast to myasthenia gravis the characteristic response to repetitive stimulation is an *increase* in size of an initially reduced compound muscle action potential. The mepps are of normal amplitude but reduced in frequency and the number of quanta of acetylcholine released by a nerve impulse is greatly reduced. There is an IgG antibody to a tumour antigen that cross-reacts with an antigen in the voltage-gated calcium channels in the presynaptic nerve terminals.

Anticholinesterase drugs are relatively ineffective in treatment. Drugs that increase acetylcholine release (e.g. calcium, guanidine and 3,4-diaminopyridine) may be effective. The syndrome may improve with treatment of the underlying malignancy.

REFERENCES

Drachman D. B. (1994) Myasthenia gravis. *New England Journal of Medicine,* **330**, 1797–1812.

Dyck P. K., Thomas P. K., Griffin J. W., Low P. A. and Poduslo J. F. (Eds) (1993) *Peripheral Neuropathy,* 3rd edn. W. B. Saunders, Philadelphia.

Aids to the Examination of the Peripheral Nervous System (1986) Baillière Tindall, London.

Martin J. B. (1993) Molecular genetics in neurology. *Annals of Neurology,* **34**, 757–773.

Newsom Davis J. (1992) Diseases of the neuromuscular junction. In: *Diseases of the Nervous System,* 2nd edn. Eds A. K. Asbury, G. M. McKhann and W. I. McDonald. W. B. Saunders, Philadelphia. 197–212.

Schaumburg H. H., Berger A. R. and Thomas P. K. (1992) *Disorders of the Peripheral Nervous System,* 2nd edn. F. A. Davis, Philadelphia.

Walton J. N. (1988) *Disorders of Voluntary Muscles,* 5th edn. Churchill-Livingstone, Edinburgh.

11 | Headache

PAIN PATHWAYS AND HEADACHE MECHANISMS

Pain sensitive structures

Headache may arise from intracranial or extracranial structures and may be referred to the head from the eyes, nasal sinuses or upper neck. The brain itself is insensitive to pain but the large intracranial arteries, veins, venous sinuses and parts of the dura may give rise to pain, referred to specific parts of the head. In general terms, structures in the anterior and middle cranial fossae refer pain to the anterior two-thirds of the head via the first division of the trigeminal nerve while pain from the posterior fossa is felt in the upper neck and occiput, being relayed by the second and third cervical roots. A dividing line between the anterior and posterior areas of referral may be drawn vertically above the ear. The external carotid artery and its frontal, temporal and middle meningeal branches also refer pain to the frontotemporal region via the first division of the trigeminal nerve. The occipital arteries and the joints of the upper cervical spine refer pain to the occiput through the C1–3 roots.

Referred pain

Pain referral is complicated by the fact that pain fibres from the head and face descend in the spinal tract of the trigeminal nerve to the upper three segments of the spinal cord where they synapse on the same second order neurones as afferent fibres from the C1–3 roots (Fig. 11.1). This means that pain originating from the upper cervical spine can be referred to the eye and forehead of the same side and that fronto-orbital headache may extend backwards like a bar of pain to the upper neck. The upper cervical cord can therefore be regarded as a centre for the transmission of head and neck pain.

Endogenous pain control system

Pain transmission in the cord is controlled by tracts descending from the brain-stem, a serotonergic pathway from nucleus raphe magnus of the medulla and a noradrenergic pathway from the region of the locus coeruleus, which act on the

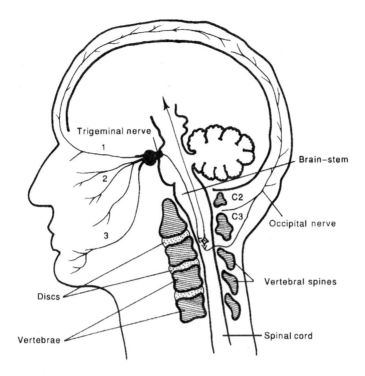

Fig. 11.1 Pain pathways from the head. The spinal tract of the trigeminal nerve descends to the upper three segments of the cervical cord where it synapses on second order neurones that also receive afferents from the second and third cervical roots. This convergence permits referral of pain from the head to neck and vice versa. (From Lance, 1975, with permission of Charles Scribner's Sons, New York.)

first order synapse indirectly through interneurones that employ enkephalins or GABA as a transmitter (Fig. 6.5). Failure of the endogenous pain control system could permit spontaneous aching to be felt in the head and neck on both sides. Depletion of monoamine transmitters in this system may be a factor in essential or idiopathic headaches such as tension headache and migraine.

Cranial nerves

Pain can also result from irritation of those cranial nerves (other than the trigeminal) carrying sensory fibres, such as the nervus intermedius of the seventh cranial nerve; the vagus nerve, which refers pain to the ear, and the glossopharyngeal nerve which refers pain to the pharynx and the base of the tongue (deep to the angle of the mandible).

CLASSIFICATION OF HEADACHE

Headache may be classified according to the presumed site of origin (Table 11.1) but the most useful working classification is to consider the way in which the headache presents; is it a single severe episode or does it have a progressive subacute onset?; is the headache continuous and long standing or recurrent and episodic? This helps to focus the mind on the differential diagnosis.

Acute severe headache

When a patient suddenly complains of severe headache for the first time, the presence or absence of fever and neck rigidity is of the greatest importance, since some of the more serious causes, namely the first and third listed below, are associated with these signs of meningeal irritation. The main causes of acute severe headaches are:

- Subarachnoid haemorrhage
- Cerebral haemorrhage or infarction
- Encephalitis or meningitis
- Systemic infections, such as influenza or the exanthemata
- Acute obstruction of cerebrospinal fluid (CSF) pathways
- Sudden gross elevation of blood pressure, such as in acute nephritis, malignant hypertension or other causes of hypertensive crisis
- Sinusitis, usually with tenderness over the frontal or maxillary sinuses; sphenoidal and ethmoidal sinusitis cause a mid-frontal headache
- Ocular disturbances, such as acute angle-closure glaucoma
- Injury to the head or upper neck
- The first episode of migraine or other conditions considered later as *recurrent episodic headaches*

Progressive subacute headache

This is a *sinister pattern of headache*, when the patient experiences a headache which may fluctuate in intensity but progressively becomes more severe over a period of days, weeks or months. If the headache is made worse by coughing, sneezing or straining, it suggests an intracranial origin with dilatation or displacement of intracranial vessels or obstruction of the ventricular system. If the headache is associated with drowsiness, mental changes, epileptic fits or any form of neurological deficit, the probability of an intracranial space-occupying lesion or chronic meningitis becomes greater. In the older age group, the possibility of temporal arteritis must always be considered. The progressive subacute headache always requires investigation. Possible causes include the following:

Space-occupying lesions: subdural haematoma, intracranial tumour and cerebral abscess

Infections of the ear may spread to the apex of the petrous temporal bone, causing pain in the first division of the trigeminal nerve and paralysis of the sixth cranial nerve (*Gradenigo's syndrome*). They may also cause thrombosis of the lateral venous sinus with resulting increase in the intracranial pressure *(otitic hydrocephalus)* or may form abscesses in the temporal lobe or cerebellum. Infections of the frontal sinus may cause an extradural or a cerebral abscess in the frontal lobe. Cerebral abscesses may also be embolic from infection in the lung or heart (acute or subacute bacterial endocarditis), or be caused by septicaemia.

Chronic meningitis

Chronic meningitis may result from:
- Tuberculous or cryptococcal (torula) meningitis
- Syphilis
- Meningitis carcinomatosa. Diffuse infiltration of the meninges by some tumours, such as primary lymphoma and secondary melanoma, which may simulate meningitis both in clinical presentation and in lowering CSF glucose levels below 2 mmol/L in the manner of a bacterial infection.

Benign intracranial hypertension (BIH)

If a space-occupying lesion or infectious process has been excluded in a patient presenting with progressive headache, papilloedema and elevated CSF pressure, the diagnosis of BIH must be considered (Chapter 18).

Temporal arteritis

Temporal arteritis affects women more than men in the ratio 3:1, mostly over the age of 50 years although one patient aged 35 years has been reported. The condition may affect intracranial arteries, particularly the ophthalmic artery, as well as extracranial arteries and occasionally branches of the aorta (coronary, renal and iliac arteries). In about half the cases it is associated with diffuse aching in the muscles and joints (polymyalgia rheumatica). The condition is probably an immune disorder and the characteristic pathological change is thickening of the intima, fibrosis and cellular infiltration of the media with giant-cell formation and thrombus formation in the lumen.

In classical cases, the extracranial arteries are palpable and tender but the condition should be suspected in any elderly patient with progressive headache, particularly if associated with generalized body aching and malaise. One pathognomonic symptom is claudication of the jaw muscles — aching of the jaw on repeated chewing caused by involvement of the branches of the external carotid artery.

Table 11.1   Classification of headaches according to presumed site of origin

---

Cranium
Expanding lesions within the cranial bones stretching the periosteum
Inflammation of cranium or scalp

Extracranial arteries
Temporal arteritis

Cranial nerves
Excessive stimulation of trigeminal or glossopharyngeal nerves (e.g. headache on eating ice-cream, diving into cold water)
Distortion or inflammation of cranial nerves
Tumour, aneurysm
Tolosa-Hunt syndrome (a recurrent granulomatous disorder affecting the region of the superior orbital fissure). Raeder's paratrigeminal neuralgia (lesions involving the pericarotid sympathetic plexus, thus producing a partial Horner's syndrome, as well as the first division of the trigeminal nerve)
Gradenigo's syndrome (lesions of the apex of the temporal bone involving the first division of the trigeminal and the sixth cranial nerve)
Postherpetic neuralgia
Trigeminal and glossopharyngeal neuralgia
Atypical facial pain

Referred pain
From eyes, ear, nose and throat, teeth, and neck

Intracranial sources of headache
Vasodilatation caused by one of the following:
- Concussion
- An epileptic fit (postictal)
- Pressor reactions
    Phaeochromocytoma
    Tyramine ingestion by a patient taking monoamine oxidase inhibitors
    Sexual excitement at orgasm
    Malignant hypertension
- Toxic effects
    Systemic infections of intoxications
    'Hangover' headache after alcohol intoxication
    Foreign protein reactions
    Withdrawal of caffeine after excessive intake
    Some medications such as indomethacin

Table 11.1 (continued)

- Metabolic disturbances
    Hypoxia
    Hypoglycaemia
    Hypercapnia
- Vasodilator agents
Meningeal irritation
- Subarachnoid haemorrhage
- Meningitis, encephalitis
Displacement of intracranial vessels
- Space-occupying lesions — tumour, haematoma, abscess
- Increased intracranial pressure — obstructive hydrocephalus, cerebral oedema, benign intracranial hypertension
- Reduced intracranial pressure — post-lumbar puncture headache
Exertional and cough headache of benign aetiology

Episodic headaches of uncertain mechanism
    Migraine
    Cluster headache
    Acute cerebral vascular insufficiency

Tension headache
    Primary muscle overcontraction
    Secondary to other factors such as eye strain, temporomandibular joint dysfunction (Costen's syndrome), cervical spondylosis
    Idiopathic chronic tension headaches
    Tension-vascular headache

Psychogenic headache
Secondary to a delusional, conversion or hypochondriacal state

---

The erythrocyte sedimentation rate (ESR) is elevated above 40 mm/hour in two-thirds of patients but note that a normal ESR does not exclude the condition. If the index of suspicion is high, one temporal artery should be biopsied since it is important to make the diagnosis with certainty. If the index of suspicion is high, corticosteroid therapy should be started before temporal artery biopsy and may have to be continued for months and possibly years. The importance of early diagnosis and treatment is that the ophthalmic artery becomes involved in 20–50% of cases in various reported series and causes rapid loss of vision in the affected eye. The chance of this complication is reduced to half by the use of steroids.

Chronic continuous headache

A constant headache, present most of the time for most days of the week over a long period of time is unlikely to be caused by any structural abnormality and is often closely linked with the emotional state of the patient. The following forms of chronic continuous headache may be encountered.

Tension-type headache

This is a tight, pressing or band-like sensation felt on top of or around the head, and is usually bilateral. It affects women about twice as often as men and may start at any age. Fifteen per cent of patients recall their headaches starting under the age of 10 years.

Tension-type headache may result from constant overcontraction of the frontal, temporal and occipital muscles in some patients who are helped to overcome their symptoms by learning to relax the appropriate muscles. Some authors have considered tension headache to be one end of a spectrum with migraine at the other end and have postulated that a defect in monoamine neurotransmitters and in the endogenous pain control system are common factors in all headaches not associated with a structural lesion. The frequency of migraine attacks may increase until it develops into chronic daily headache (*transformed migraine*), often as the result of stress or the over-use of ergotamine or analgesics. In other patients, chronic daily headache may follow infections such as glandular fever, or start without obvious cause. Chronic tension-type headache is usually, but not always, related to or exacerbated by, anxiety or depression. Although the basic cause is unknown, treatment is directed at the following factors:

Physical abnormalities   (i) Imbalance of the bite. Some patients have an uneven bite which throws strain on one temporomandibular joint, with the development of a clicking noise in the joint and pain radiating over the face and head from the affected joint (*Costen's syndrome*). Dental attention is required to correct the bite, but equally important is the reduction of excessive jaw clenching (bruxism) and the underlying anxiety state which is often present; (ii) cervical spondylosis. Spasm of cervical muscles may be secondary to degenerative changes in the cervical spine and may respond to manipulative or other therapy for the neck problem; (iii) eye strain. Ocular imbalance or refractive errors may be a source of tension and should be corrected. The subject should sit in a comfortable chair at work or school, adjusted to the height appropriate for the desk to ensure good posture, with lighting adjusted to the correct angle for comfort.

Psychological factors   In some patients exacerbations of headache may clearly be linked with sources of stress and may be helped by psychological counselling, alteration of life-style or readjustment of stresses. In other patients problems may be either inapparent or insoluble.

Other forms of treatment consist of muscle relaxation or pharmacotherapy. A course in relaxation training may be highly beneficial in a well-motivated patient. Various forms of biofeedback may assist relaxation but do not substantially improve the result. Courses of relaxation training are now conducted by many hospitals, community health centres and physiotherapists or psychologists.

Pharmacotherapy involves the use of tricyclic antidepressants, particularly amitriptyline, which are particularly helpful in those who tolerate them well. It is advisable to start with one half of a 25 mg tablet of amitriptyline at night then gradually increase to 3 tablets (75 mg) as a single nocturnal dose if there are no untoward side effects such as drowsiness or confusion. Improvement is usually noted within two weeks and the treatment can be continued for 6 months before slowly weaning off medication to see whether improvement can be maintained by relaxation alone. Tranquillizers such as the benzodiazepines should be used for short periods only because of the risk of habituation. Sodium valproate 200–400 mg three times daily has been reported to be helpful in the control of chronic tension-type headache.

Atypical facial pain

This is a constant pain, usually described as tight or boring, that starts in a localized area of the lower face, particularly the nasolabial angle but may spread across the cheeks, bridge of the nose or other areas. It may come on after minor trauma such as dental extraction and persist indefinitely, defying all surgical measures including section of the trigeminal nerve. The aetiology is unknown. Management is along the same lines as for tension-type headache. The combination of amitriptyline and thioridazine (Melleril) will usually reduce the intensity of the pain and monoamine oxidase inhibitors such as phenelzine may be helpful in patients not responding to tricylic antidepressants.

Post-herpetic neuralgia

This complication of herpes zoster is more common as age advances. Once it has developed, it tends to persist but may be suppressed by the medications recommended above for atypical facial pain.

Post-traumatic headache

There are many varieties of post-traumatic headache, often complicated by the anxiety (and sometimes desire for financial gain) engendered by legal proceedings which are often protracted for many years. The following syndromes are recognized:

Post-concussional headache   This affects only about 40% of patients and clears up rapidly.

Post-traumatic migraine   A migraine which may be limited to the vascular distribution of the area of scalp injured and is managed along the same lines as migraine.

Episodic unilateral headaches   This type of headache resembles cluster headache and follows a blow to the carotid artery ('dysautonomic cephalgia'). This is very rare and is said to respond to propranolol.

Whiplash syndrome   This is an 'upper cervical syndrome' which results from disruption of soft tissues and zygapophyseal joints in the upper cervical spine which has been caused by a rapid acceleration of the body with passive extension of the neck, e.g. when the patient is sitting in a car hit from the rear. Pain is referred to the occiput. Treatment includes the application of heat, wearing of a surgical collar and the injection of a local anaesthetic agent and hydrocortisone into tender areas.

Tension-type headache This is often seen in conjunction with the other varieties, commonly associated with a state of anxiety and depression following head injury.

Recurrent episodic headaches

These have been called *vascular headaches* in the past because scalp arteries and veins dilate in some patients and the pain may be throbbing in character and relieved by pressure over the appropriate vessels. This may be too simplistic a view as there are many other factors involved.

Migraine

Migraine is the most common of the episodic headaches and affects some 10% of males and 20% of females at some time of their lives. Some 25% of sufferers date the onset of their attacks from childhood, the incidence progressively increasing and remaining equal in both sexes until puberty, after which age women are affected twice as often as men.

Migraine is preceded in about 20% of cases by an aura of neurological symptoms such as blurred vision, flashes of light, jittering zig-zags of light (*fortification spectra*) or, less commonly, paraesthesiae and dysphasia. Migraine with aura is often termed *classical migraine*. The aura persists for 10–60 minutes and then commonly fades away as the headache starts, although it may continue into the headache phase. There may be vague premonitory symptoms of elation ('feeling on top of the world'), hunger, thirst or drowsiness for up to 24 hours before the migraine attack.

More commonly the headache appears without any prodromal symptoms (*migraine without aura* or *common migraine*). If the neurological symptoms develop and subside slowly without a headache ensuing, they are called *migraine equivalents*.

Variations on the theme of migraine include:

Vertebrobasilar migraine The association of visual, brain-stem and cerebellar disturbances, often leading to syncope, preceding or accompanied by headache. It is attributed to vasospasm in the vertebrobasilar circulation and resembles a slow-motion episode of the vertebrobasilar insufficiency encountered as a form of cerebral vascular disease.

Retinal migraine A rare disorder in which loss of vision is limited to one eye as a result of retinal ischaemia, rather than to one or both homonymous visual fields as commonly encountered with the occipital lobe ischaemia of classical migraine.

Ophthalmoplegic migraine A transient Horner's syndrome or, conversely, dilatation of one pupil, is not uncommon during a severe migraine attack. The term *ophthalmoplegic migraine* is reserved for the appearance of paralysis of one or more of the cranial nerves supplying the extra-ocular muscles, usually the third nerve, at the height of migraine headache. It is probably a transient ischaemic neuropathy, which may persist after repeated episodes.

Facial migraine   Recurrent episodes resembling migraine in which pain affects the eye, cheek and chin rather than the head.

Hemiplegic migraine   Hemiplegia may develop before or during a migraine headache. This form usually affects families as a dominant characteristic. The gene has been located on chromosome 19.

Migrainous infarction   Neurological symptoms may persist more than 24 hours after the end of migraine headache. A permanent deficit may result from vascular thrombosis, particularly in young women taking a contraceptive pill.

Characteristics of migraine headache

Migraine is characteristically episodic, separated by intervals of freedom. It is unilateral in two-thirds of patients, commonly affecting the frontotemporal region, radiating to the occiput. The headache is usually accompanied by nausea (90%), vomiting (60%) or diarrhoea (20%). Most patients (80%) become sensitive to light and many are acutely aware of noise and smells during the headache. Fluid retention is common at the onset of headache and polyuria is noticed as the headache subsides. The scalp becomes tender on the affected side in two-thirds of patients.

The migraine personality

Migrainous patients are not more intelligent than their peers or more subject to stress but react more strongly to stress. There is a family history of migraine affecting close relatives in 55% of patients.

Precipitating factors

Intrinsic   Many patients with migraine have attacks with a regularity that suggests that the episodes are being triggered by some internal biological clock. Such rhythms may be: monthly, linked with the menstrual cycle (the trigger for menstrual migraine is probably the drop in oestradiol level); weekly, associated with weekends or a particular week-day; or nightly, awakening the patient in the phase of rapid eye movement (REM) sleep. These internal rhythms may be altered by metabolic factors such as hypoglycaemia or by external triggers.

Extrinsic   Some patients state that their attacks are brought on by: (i) excessive afferent stimulation, such as flickering light, loud noise, strong perfumes or compression of scalp nerves (e.g. 'swim-goggle migraine'); (ii) a sharp blow to the head, such as heading the ball in soccer ('footballer's migraine'); (iii) certain rich foods such as chocolates and other fatty foods. The specificity of food factors is dubious; (iv) stress or sudden relaxation after stress; (v) the ingestion of vasodilators such as alcohol, monosodium glutamate or drugs used in the management of angina pectoris and peripheral vascular disease. Physical exertion may have the same effect in producing vasodilatation and triggering a migraine headache.

Pathophysiology

Migraine is commonly associated with a diminution of cortical blood flow of about 20% which starts in the occipital region and slowly moves forward, accompanied by a spreading depression of cortical function. Transcranial Doppler studies have shown that the headache phase is accompanied by dilatation of the large intracranial arteries. Extracranial arteries also dilate in about one-third of patients.

There is evidence that migraine attacks are associated with fluctuation in the levels of monoamines in the blood, possibly as a reflection of their neurotransmitter function within the central nervous system. Serotonergic and noradrenergic pathways project from the brain-stem to the cortical microcirculation as well as projecting to the spinal trigeminal nucleus and spinal cord as part of the endogenous pain control system.

Blood platelets discharge serotonin (5-hydroxytryptamine, 5-HT) at the onset of the migraine headache. It is postulated that hyperactivity followed by diminished activity in central monaminergic transmission could produce the vascular changes of migraine and at the same time diminish inhibition of incoming afferent impulses, thus causing sensitivity to pain (and to light, sound and smells). Platelet aggregation takes place in migraine, associated with release of serotonin from platelets, which may underlie the tendency to vascular thrombosis causing the neurological deficits of complicated migraine. Vasodilator peptides probably play a role in vascular dilatation during migraine headache as the level of calcitonin gene-related peptide (CGRP) increases in external jugular venous blood at that time.

General management

Psychological counselling and relaxation therapy are employed as in the management of tension headache and may reduce the frequency of headache to half or less before any medication is used.

Treatment of acute attacks

The objective in the drug treatment of each attack as it comes is to abort the development of headache or to shorten its severity and duration. The vasoactive agents ergotamine tartrate and sumatriptan are used to prevent the dilatation of cranial vessels that is largely responsible for the pain of migraine headache. The action of ergotamine tartrate on blood vessels depends upon the intraluminal pressure, tending to dilate constricted vessels and constrict dilated vessels. It should therefore be given as early in the attack as possible during the aura or headache phase. Sumatriptan constricts cranial vessels through a specific subtype of serotonin receptor, the 5-HT_{1D} receptor. It is ineffective when given during the aura phase but should be administered early in the headache phase although it is usually still effective when the headache is fully developed.

Ergotamine tartrate   This can be given as a 1 mg capsule (Ergodryl Mono); combined with caffeine 100 mg (Cafergot); as a 2 mg tablet combined with caffeine and an anti-emetic (e.g. Migral); or as a Cafergot suppository containing 2 mg ergotamine and 100 mg caffeine. Dihydroergotamine acts on venous capacitance vessels rather than arteries and is administered in a dose of 1.0 mg, i.m. or 0.5 mg, i.v.

Sumatriptan (Imigran) A serotonin analogue that may be given orally as a tablet of 100 mg or as a subcutaneous injection of 6 mg. Sumatriptan or ergotamine should not be prescribed for patients with suspected coronary artery disease, Prinzmetal angina or uncontrolled hypertension.

Aspirin, naproxen and ibuprofen These drugs may also be effective if given early in the attack, particularly if preceded by the injection or ingestion of meto-clopramide 10 mg.

Preventive therapy

Those patients subject to two or more migraine headaches each month are suitable for prophylactic medication (interval therapy).

Beta-noradrenergic antagonists Those beta blockers without any agonist activity have proven useful in the prevention of migraine. These include the non-selective beta-blockers propranolol and timolol and the relatively selective $beta_1$-blocking agents atenolol and metoprolol. Propranolol (Inderal) can be introduced in a dose of 10–20 mg twice daily and increased to full beta-blocking doses if necssary. Beta blockers should not be given to asthmatic patients since they may aggravate bronchospasm. Other side effects include fatigue, postural hypotension and vivid dreams.

Pizotifen The antiserotonin, antihistamine agent pizotifen (Sandomigran) is a $5\text{-}HT_2$ antagonist. Dosage is started as a single nocturnal dose of 0.5 mg to avoid drowsiness, increasing slowly from one to six tablets at night until migraine is controlled or side effects (drowsiness, increased appetite and weight gain) limit its use.

Methysergide The antiserotonin agent methysergide (Deseril) is a partial $5\text{-}HT_1$ agonist as well as a $5\text{-}HT_2$ antagonist. It may give rise to side effects (indigestion, peripheral vasoconstriction, muscle aches) in one-third of patients if the full dose is started immediately. The patient should be advised to cut a tablet in half (an intricate procedure as the tablets are small and coated) and take one half tablet twice daily. The dose is then progressively increased to two tablets three times daily if necessary to control headache. Medication should be continued for 4 months, then discontinued for 1 month before starting again, to minimize the possibility of pleural or retroperitoneal fibrosis developing. Such fibrotic side effects are extremely rare (less than 5/1000) even when medication is continuous but patients should be advised to have a regular medical check-up and blood urea test every 3 months and to report if they experience chest or abdominal pains.

Other drugs of use in migraine (i) Amitriptyline, a drug which prevents re-uptake of serotonin and is also helpful in interval therapy of migraine; (ii) non-steroidal anti-inflammatory drugs may also be useful; (iii) the calcium channel-blocking agent flunarizine 10 mg daily has proven effective in preventing migraine. Since it also has anti-dopamine activity, Parkinsonian side effects may develop with long-term use.

Cluster headache (migrainous neuralgia)

Cluster headache is an unusual unilateral headache syndrome (only 3% as common as migraine), affecting males in 85% of cases, which gains its name from the tendency to occur in bouts or clusters, lasting from weeks to months at a time, separated by months or years of freedom. During a bout, the patient is subject to brief attacks of severe pain, usually lasting 15 minutes to 2 hours, which recur once or more in each 24 hour period, often at night.

The pain usually affects one eye and radiates upwards over the fronto-temporal region or downwards over the face. It is commonly associated with redness and watering of the eye and blockage of the nostril on the same side. In one-third or more of cases, a partial Horner's syndrome (ptosis and miosis) is noted on the affected side.

Treatment of episodic cluster headache consists of regular (interval) medication during the susceptible period.

Ergotamine tartrate During a bout, 1–2 mg are given daily. It may be sufficient to give a nocturnal dose if the attacks occur only during the night. This is usually adequate to control the first or second bout.

Methysergide This is given 1–2 mg three times daily, as for migraine. It is used if ergotamine tartrate is ineffective.

Prednisone Given 50 mg daily, for 3 days and then reduced rapidly to a dose just sufficient to prevent the attacks (usually about 25 mg daily). This dose is then maintained for the duration of the bout before weaning off slowly. This is effective in suppressing a bout in approximately 80% of cases. In the acute episode, the inhalation of **100% oxygen** or the subcutaneous injection of **sumatriptan** 0.6 mg stops the pain rapidly in most cases.

There are two variations on the theme of cluster headache:

Chronic cluster headache In chronic cluster headache, the pain recurs regularly without remission, in the manner of migraine. This form usually responds to medication with verapamil in large doses or lithium carbonate, 250 mg two or three times daily, the dose being adjusted to provide a blood level of 0.5–1.2 mmol/L. Side effects include tremor and confusion.

Chronic paroxysmal hemicrania Brief attacks of pain recur six or more times daily. This form is usually controlled rapidly by indomethacin, 25 mg three times daily.

Trigeminal neuralgia

Definition and pathophysiology Trigeminal neuralgia is a degenerative condition of the trigeminal pathways, commonly caused by branches of the anterior or superior cerebellar arteries impinging on the root of the trigeminal nerve where it enters the pons, which causes severe stabbing pains in the distribution of one or more divisions of the trigeminal nerve. Other causes include a small angioma or neuroma overlying the trigeminal root, or a plaque of multiple sclerosis at the root entry zone in the pons (which accounts for some 2–3% of cases of trigeminal neuralgia). Partial demyelination is thought to cause repetitive synchronous discharges of nerve fibres.

The condition is known as *tic douloureux* (a painful spasm) because of the lightning-like jabs of pain which are typical of the condition. It affects females more than males in the ratio 1.6:1 and usually starts after the age of 40 years, most commonly in the fifties. Most start in the second or third divisions, only 5% starting in the first division. Trigger factors include talking, chewing, swallowing, shaving, cleaning the teeth and wind blowing on the face. Trigger points are usually areas around the nose or lips which evoke a paroxysm if touched.

Episodic pattern   The pain may recur many times a day for weeks and months, and then may remit for months or years. This episodicity bears a superficial resemblance to cluster headache from which trigeminal neuralgia can be distinguished on every other ground (character and distribution of pain and lack of the autonomic features associated with cluster headache).

Examination   No abnormality is found on examination in idiopathic trigeminal neuralgia. If sensory loss is found, if the corneal response is depressed, if there is associated deafness on the side of pain, or if an aching pain persists between the characteristic stabs, some underlying lesion must be sought since acoustic and trigeminal neuromas and other posterior fossa tumours as well as intrinsic lesions such as multiple sclerosis may present with tic-like pains.

Management   The pain can usually be subdued by the use of carbamazepine (Tegretol), 200 mg three times daily, phenytoin (Dilantin), 100 mg three times daily, or baclofen (Lioresal), 10–20 mg three times daily.

If the pain persists in spite of medical management, one of three surgical procedures can be undertaken:

(1) *Posterior fossa exploration* with separation of compressing arteries or veins from the trigeminal root. This is called the Jannetta procedure, but was first advocated by Dandy in 1932. It is appropriate for the younger patient as it preserves normal facial sensation.

(2) *Thermocoagulation* (radiofrequency lesion) of the Gasserian ganglion. This is relatively simple since the probe is inserted into the foramen ovale under local anaesthesia without the need for craniotomy. General anaesthesia is administered only during the process of coagulation which is otherwise very painful. This procedure is effective in most cases and preserves some sensation but troublesome dysaesthesiae develops in 17% of cases.

(3) *Intracranial section* of the appropriate divisions of the trigeminal nerve.

Other episodic syndromes

Recurrent sinusitis   This rarely presents any diagnostic difficulty in genuine cases. Most patients claiming to have episodic sinus headache suffer from migraine or one of its variants.

Paroxysmal hypertension   Phaeochromocytoma may cause 'funny turns', accompanied by headache in 80% of cases.

Transient ischaemic attacks   Transient ischaemic attacks of thrombo-embolic origin are associated with headache in about 25% of cases but the headache is usually overshadowed by the neurological symptoms.

Intermittent obstruction of CSF pathways This is more likely to present as a subacute progressive headache with fluctuations in intensity.

Recurrent meningitis This may be caused by a communication between CSF and nasopharynx or middle ear as a result of a fracture, most commonly through the cribriform plate. Cerebrospinal fluid rhinorrhoea may be observed as the patient bends forwards and the fluid can be distinguished from sinus secretions by the fact that it contains glucose. There is a recurrent aseptic meningitis known as Mollaret's meningitis in which there is probably a susceptibility to viral infections (possibly herpes simplex) in patients with deficient immune mechanisms.

Recurrent subarachnoid haemorrhage Recurrent subarachnoid haemorrhage from an angioma (which, as a low pressure venous bleed, presents less hazard to life than haemorrhage from an aneurysm) may escape diagnosis on the first occasion, the bleed being labelled as 'viral meningo-encephalitis'. Beware of recurrent 'meningo-encephalitis'!

Benign syndromes Headache during sexual intercourse, or on coughing or on exercise is benign only if an intracranial lesion has been excluded.

INVESTIGATION OF HEADACHE

Patients with chronic continuous headache or episodic headaches usually require no more investigation than a careful history to establish the pattern of headache, followed by a physical examination of all systems.

Patients with an acute or subacute progressive pattern of headache usually require a computed tomography (CT) scan of the brain as the initial investigation. Plain radiographs of the skull have little point if a CT scan is available but an X-ray of the chest should always be taken to exclude a carcinoma of the lung or other relevant condition. Bilateral cerebral angiography may still be required if the index of suspicion is high even if the CT scan is negative since it may demonstrate bilaterally symmetrical subdural haematomas or an aneurysm which has escaped diagnosis by the other investigation.

A full blood count and ESR should always be obtained since temporal arteritis, collagen diseases, subacute bacterial endocarditis, multiple myeloma, leukaemia, anaemia and polycythaemia may all cause headache and may not be suspected on other grounds.

An electroencephalogram is rarely necessary if CT scanning and other diagnostic measures are available but can give valuable localizing information in cerebral abscess, herpes simplex encephalitis and some cases of cerebral tumour.

A lumbar puncture may be necessary to confirm the presence of encephalitis, meningitis, subarachnoid haemorrhage or benign intracranial hypertension. A CT scan of the brain is strongly advised to exclude a space-occupying lesion before lumbar puncture is attempted, since herniation of the brain through the tentorium or foramen magnum can be caused by withdrawal of CSF from below, with serious and possibly fatal consequences.

If a headache history suggests one of the more sinister causes, immediate referral to a neurological unit is advisable.

REFERENCES

Dalessio D. J. and Silberstein S. D. (1993) *Wolff's Headache and Other Head Pain*, 6th edn. Oxford University Press, New York.

Lance J. W. (1993) *The Mechanism and Management of Headache*, 5th edn. Butterworths, London.

Olesen J., Tfelt-Hansen P. and Welch K. M. A. (Eds.) (1993) *The Headaches*. Raven Press, New York.

12 | Epilepsy

Epilepsy is a recurring disturbance of cerebral function caused by paroxysmal neuronal discharges, usually (but not always) accompanied by loss of consciousness. Attacks may consist of the sudden onset of sustained muscular contraction, producing an abnormal posture (*tonic seizure*), rhythmic jerking of the face, trunk or limbs (*clonic seizure*), or one phase followed by the other (tonic–clonic or *grand mal* seizure). Epilepsy may also take the form of a transient loss of consciousness (*petit mal* absence), a muscular jerk (*myoclonus*) or the sudden impairment of postural tonus, causing a falling attack (*atonic* or *akinetic epilepsy*). Some epileptic attacks, known as *partial* or *focal seizures*, reflect the function of the cortical area from which they arise and may be characterized by unilateral motor or sensory symptoms, or more complex states in which impaired awareness is accompanied by hallucinations of the special senses and disturbances of memory or emotion (*complex partial seizures*), that usually originate in one temporal lobe.

PREVALENCE

Some 5% of children under the age of 6 years are liable to convulsions (tonic–clonic seizures) when body temperature becomes elevated, usually with an infection. These are known as febrile or infantile convulsions and, unless they cause severe hypoxia, have a good prognosis since only 10% of such children continue to have any form of epilepsy over the age of 6 years.

The prevalence of epilepsy in the community is generally estimated at 0.5% but the true prevalence is probably closer to 1%.

CLASSIFICATION

Epilepsy may be regarded as *symptomatic* or *idiopathic* depending on whether or not a cause (such as metabolic disturbance or a cortical lesion such as angioma or tumour) can be demonstrated.

The International Classification of Epileptic Seizures divides epilepsy into two main categories: *generalized epilepsy*, in which both hemispheres are involved virtually synchronously in the epileptic process and *partial epilepsy*, in which the disturbance remains localized to one cortical area until the paroxysm ceases or becomes generalized.

Generalized epilepsy

Absences (petit mal)

An absence is a brief lapse of consciousness in which the patient, usually a child, stares blankly for a few seconds. The attack can be so transient that it may escape notice by patient and observer. It may be associated with any one or more of the following signs: fluttering of the eyelids, rolling upwards of the eyes, simple actions (automatism) such as fumbling with clothing, slight jerking of the limbs (myoclonus), passing urine, falling to the ground (akinetic attack).

The child who day-dreams, appears inattentive in class, 'switches on and off' all the time or falls without obvious cause, should be suspected of having *petit mal* absences. The electroencephalogram (EEG) is very helpful in diagnosis, the characteristic abnormality being paroxysmal discharges of rhythmic 3 Hz spike-and-wave activity (Fig. 12.1). About 80% of children with absences lose their attacks by the end of the second decade of life.

Myoclonus

Myoclonus is jerking of the face, limbs or trunk, commonly affecting muscles asymmetrically, in which case it is usually made worse by voluntary movement (action myoclonus) or by sensory stimulations such as a flash of light, sudden

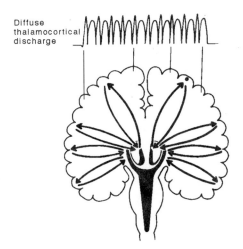

Fig. 12.1 3 Hz spike-wave discharge of generalized epilepsy, most commonly associated with *petit mal* absences. The paroxysms may arise in the reticular formation of the thalamus and mid-brain as indicated, or may spread via associated fibres from one area of cortex to another. (From Lance and McLeod, 1981, with permission of Butterworths, London.)

sound or touch (stimulus-sensitive myoclonus). A second variety is a rhythmic contraction of muscles which may cause symmetrical flexion of the limbs or trunk. This is usually seen in progressive cerebral disorders such as subacute sclerosing panencephalitis (SSPE) — a slow virus infection (p. 247), or in infants with brain damage when the movements may become violent (infantile spasms). Rhythmic jerking of the palate (palatal myoclonus) may be seen in disease of the lower medulla but here the term is misleading since it is a tremor rather than a manifestation of epilepsy.

Myoclonus is often seen in association with other forms of generalized epilepsy and a series of jerks may precede tonic–clonic seizures (*grand mal* fits). It may be of genetic origin in various forms of familial myoclonic epilepsy or may be acquired as the result of diffuse brain damage such as hypoxia, encephalitis or metabolic disturbances. It is caused by a loss of normal inhibitory influences so that any afferent input to the nervous system leads to a synchronous motor response. Myoclonus may be confined to one limb in partial epilepsies or focal cerebral lesions (*segmental myoclonus*).

Myoclonic jerks may be associated with lapses in contraction of postural muscles (*negative myoclonus*) which can cause the patient to fall (*akinetic attacks*).

Akinetic attacks

An akinetic or atonic attack is a sudden unexpected fall, with or without loss of consciousness, caused by inhibition of the normal postural mechanisms. The *petit mal* absence is a temporary failure of the arousal mechanism responsible for consciousness, the upstream projection of the reticular formation (reticular activating system). The akinetic attack is a comparable disruption of the downstream projection of the reticular formation, the reticulospinal pathways. It is not surprising therefore that absences and akinetic attacks may occur together. The child who frequently falls without warning at home or in the school playground ('trips over his shadow') should be suspected of having akinetic attacks.

If absences and akinetic attacks are associated with tonic seizures and mental retardation (Lennox-Gastaut syndrome), the EEG usually shows atypical spike-wave paroxysms of 2–2.5 Hz and the prognosis for control of seizures is poor.

Infantile spasms (West's syndrome)

These are seizures, occurring in the first year of life, consisting of muscle contractions. Characteristically, the child flexes forwards with outstretched arms (*salaam attacks*). The EEG is grossly abnormal (*hypsarrhythmia*). Most of these children are mentally retarded. The seizures may respond favourably to treatment with ACTH or corticosteroids.

Tonic–clonic seizures (major fits, grand mal epilepsy)

Before an attack, some patients have premonitory symptoms of elation, depression, irritability or headache. The classical epileptic seizure comprises a tonic phase, in which facial, jaw, limb and trunk muscles contract, followed by a clonic phase with jerking of the limbs (Fig. 12.2). At the beginning of the tonic phase, which usually

Grand mal seizure

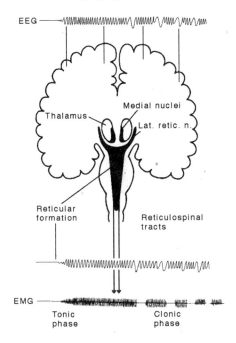

Fig. 12.2 Tonic–clonic seizure. The tonic phase, seen in muscle recordings (EMG), is associated with a high-frequency discharge in the EEG and reticular formation, which is later interrupted by inhibitory slow waves to give rise to EMG silent periods characteristic of the clonic phase. (From Lance and McLeod, 1981, with permission of Butterworths, London.)

lasts for about 15–30 seconds, patients may utter a cry as air is forced out of their lungs, bite their tongue, then become cyanosed as apnoea continues in a position of forced expiration. The misguided insertion of a finger or firmer object into the mouth at the onset of the seizure serves only to amputate a phalanx or chip a tooth, each being a poor exchange for an unbitten tongue.

As the tonic phase passes into the clonic phase, patients may pass urine or occasionally open their bowels. The rhythmic jerking of the clonic phase gradually subsides, leaving patients in a state of stupor or confusion for some minutes or hours, after which they may complain of headache (or a painful back if a vertebral body or the paravertebral muscles have been injured during the tonic spasm).

If the seizure is preceded by focal neurological symptoms or signs (an *aura*), these indicate a focal origin for the epileptic episodes with secondary spread to other cortical areas. The attack is then called a *secondary generalized seizure* and attention is paid to the site of origin. A succession of tonic–clonic seizures, without the patient regaining consciousness, is known as *status epilepticus*.

Partial (focal) epilepsy

The term partial implies that the seizure involves a limited area of cortex and its thalamic connections (Fig. 12.3).

Elementary (simple) partial seizures

Focal motor seizures These attacks usually start with twitching of the face or thumb since the largest area of the motor cortex is devoted to control of facial and hand muscles. Rhythmic jerking may then extend down one side of the body as the epileptic 'march' progresses over the contralateral motor cortex (*Jacksonian epilepsy*, named after Hughlings Jackson, an English neurologist,1835–1911, who made many contributions to the understanding of epilepsy).

Versive seizures Turning of the head and eyes, usually to the side opposite an irritative lesion which is situated in the frontal eye-fields (area 8) or occasionally in the occipital lobe. When the lesion is in the supplementary motor area, as well as head turning, there is flexion of one arm and extension of the other.

Focal sensory seizures These may arise from the primary sensory cortex, causing contralateral paraesthesiae, or from the primary receptive areas for the special senses, causing unformed hallucinations of vision (flashes of light), or hallucinations of smell or hearing. Since the centres for smell and hearing are part of the temporal lobe, hallucinations derived from these areas are usually part of the syndrome known as *complex partial seizures.*

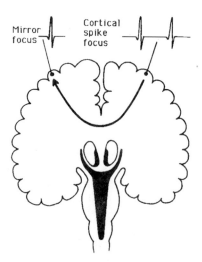

Fig. 12.3 Partial (focal) epilepsy. A potentially epileptic discharge may remain localized to one area of cortex or propagate via the corpus callosum to form a mirror focus in the opposite hemisphere. The discharge may spread over one or both hemispheres to produce a partial or generalized seizure. (From Lance and McLeod, 1981, with permission of Butterworths, London.)

Complex partial seizures

Seizures arising from the temporal lobe may include the following symptoms, associated with impairment of consciousness.

Hallucinations of smell (olfactory) or taste (gustatory)   Such hallucinations are usually acrid or otherwise unpleasant, often associated with a dreamy state (called *uncinate fits* by Hughlings Jackson because they arise from the region of the uncus in the anterior temporal lobe).

Hallucinations of hearing and vision   Abnormal sounds, such as buzzing, crackling or popping, or a transient sensation of movement (vertigo) may arise from the primary auditory receptive area in the superior temporal gyrus. More complicated hallucinations of conversation or music may originate in the auditory association cortex. Visions of animals, people or objects are derived from the visual association area or, rarely, a complete memory trace combining visual, auditory and sometimes olfactory sensations may provide a play-back of some past event.

Memory disturbances   Memory disturbances include transient amnesia, a false feeling of familiarity as though a place or conversation has been experienced previously (*déjà vu*) or the converse, the sensation of everything being strange and unfamiliar (*jamais vu*). There may also be illusions of time passing unduly rapidly or slowly.

The rapid onset of emotions   Commonly an inexplicable ghostly fear, or more rarely an elevation of the mood to ecstasy, may arise from the temporal lobe. A child suddenly running to his or her mother in unreasoned terror should be suspected of having complex partial seizures.

Automatisms   The combination of impaired consciousness with the execution of relatively simple movements is known as an automatism. Automatisms may last up to 15 minutes and may consist merely of chewing movements, smacking of the lips and fumbling with objects but can be as intricate as driving a car through several sets of traffic lights without disaster.

PATHOPHYSIOLOGY

Since most of us are subject to occasional *déjà vu* experiences or 'night starts' (resembling myoclonus) on drifting off to sleep, it is apparent that we all dwell on the rim of the epileptic volcano. Those who are engulfed by the eruption are victims of their genetic background, metabolic disturbances or some localized source of cortical irritation.

The epileptic neurone

The functional characteristics of neurones are altered in epilepsy so that dendrites are readily depolarized. Epileptic neurones may develop high frequency discharges because of failure of the normal modulation from surrounding cells, either as a result of gliosis or of diminution in inhibitory neurotransmitters. In the hippocampus, deafferented granule cells sprout mossy fibres which send collaterals to denuded granule cell dendrites, thus setting up recurrent excitatory circuits. The repeated synchronous firing of epileptic neurones renders them more likely to discharge in the future, a phenomenon known as *kindling*.

The spike-wave complex

Neurones are arranged radially with respect to the cortex, their dendrites ramifying in the superficial layer and their cell bodies lying deeply in layers 5 and 6 (Fig. 12.4). Waves of depolarization (paroxysmal depolarization shift) affect the dendrites, causing current flow from cell bodies to dendrites, which are recorded as negative spike discharges from the surface of the cortex or in scalp recordings (EEG). The spike discharge may be followed by a surface-negative slow wave because, while dendrites recover from depolarization, their cell bodies become hyperpolarized as the result of inhibitory feedback circuits activated by the epileptic discharge (Fig. 12.4).

A spike-wave complex may therefore be recorded in the EEG from a localized abnormality in the cortex or may spread over the cortex through association fibres or to the opposite hemisphere via the corpus callosum. Such spread may cause a 'mirror focus' in the opposite hemisphere or cause generalized epilepsy without involving the reticular formation (Fig. 12.3).

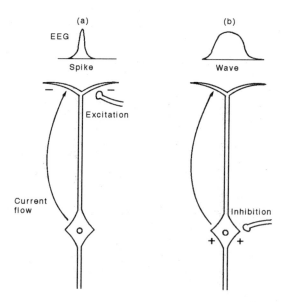

Fig. 12.4 Cortical origin of spike-wave discharge. Dendrites ramifying in superficial layers of the cortex are first depolarized so that current flows from the neutral cell body toward the cortex to form a surface-negative EEG spike. Following excitation of the neurone, the cell body becomes hyperpolarized by inhibition from recurrent fibres. Current thus flows from cell body to neutral dendrites, causing a negative slow wave in the EEG. (From Lance and McLeod, 1981, with permission of Butterworths, London.)

Causes of generalized epilepsy

There is experimental evidence that *petit mal* absences may arise from the reticular formation of the mid-brain and medial thalamus since they may be induced by stimulation of these central areas in young animals (Fig. 12.1). Major tonic–clonic seizures probably always arise from the cerebral cortex, either as spread from a focal cortical lesion or as a virtually simultaneous discharge throughout the cerebral cortex. Some forms of myoclonus, such as post-hypoxic myoclonus, are associated with deficiency in serotonergic transmission. Changes in other neurotransmitters such as gamma aminobutyric acid (GABA) have been postulated as factors in the causation of epilepsy.

Genetic factors

The 'spike-wave trait' is the genetic tendency to develop paroxysms of spike-wave complexes, usually at 3 Hz, which may not be associated with overt clinical seizures. It is inherited as a dominant characteristic, but fortunately clinical expression in the form of minor or major seizures is low. Some forms of temporal lobe epilepsy may be inherited as a dominant trait and some rare conditions such as progressive myoclonic epilepsy may be recessively inherited. There is also a family tendency to seizures, apart from any recognizable genetic pattern, to which many factors contribute.

Metabolic factors

Seizures may be caused, or their frequency increased, by: hypoxia; hypocapnia; hypoglycaemia; electrolyte disturbances, especially hypocalcaemia; fluid retention, e.g. at menstruation; hyperthermia; pyridoxine deficiency; withdrawal from sedative drugs or alcohol; drugs, heavy metals, insecticides, toxins; fatigue; pregnancy.

Local disturbances of cortical function

An epileptic focus may arise in an area of cortical gliosis or where part of the cortex has been isolated from its normal afferent inflow. Causes include the following:

- Cortical gliosis, due to: birth trauma or hypoxia; head injury (the risk of epilepsy increases from 2% after a moderately severe closed head injury to 40% in cases where the cortex is lacerated); meningitis, brain abscess, neurosyphilis
- Prolonged febrile convulsions in childhood
- Congenital abnormalities and inherited disorders. These include arteriovenous malformations (angiomas); hamartomas; tuberous sclerosis; cerebral lipidosis
- Cerebral tumours, primary and secondary
- Cerebral oedema e.g. hypertensive encephalopathy
- Vascular disease, cortical ischaemia or infarction. The risk of epilepsy after stroke is 10% if no seizure occurs at the time of the stroke but increases to 32% if there are early fits.
- Cortical atrophy, e.g. the pre-senile dementia known as Alzheimer's disease.

Reflex precipitation of epilepsy

Some patients may have epilepsy induced by a specific form of afferent stimulation, the commonest being flickering light, e.g. on changing television channels 'television epilepsy'). Other rarer types of epilepsy are reading epilepsy and musicogenic epilepsy.

DIFFERENTIAL DIAGNOSIS

Fainting (syncope)

Fainting almost invariably occurs when the subject is standing or sitting and is usually preceded by a feeling of faintness, dimness of vision, nausea and sweating. Loss of consciousness can usually be forestalled by lying down promptly or putting the head between the knees.

Syncope may be caused by a primary failure of cardiac output as the result of heart block (Stokes-Adams attacks), paroxysmal dysrhythmias or valvular defects such as aortic and mitral stenosis. More often it is due to failure of venous inflow to the heart, for example, after prolonged standing on a hot day (*vasovagal syncope*), standing up suddenly (*postural hypotension*) or passing urine while standing after getting out of bed in the middle of the night (*micturition syncope*). Autonomic failure and other causes of postural hypotension are considered in Chapter 9.

The diagnosis of syncope may be made more difficult by the fact that some fainting attacks cause cerebral hypoxia sufficient to trigger epileptiform manifestations such as the eyes rolling upwards and stiffening or jerking of the limbs. Such attacks can clearly be distinguished from epilepsy by their premonitory symptoms and the circumstances in which they occur.

Non-epileptic drop attacks

Apart from myoclonus and epilepsy, drop attacks may be caused by brain-stem ischaemia as the result of vertebrobasilar insufficiency or sudden failure of cardiac output. They may be symptomatic of mid-line cerebral or posterior fossa lesions, hydrocephalus, spinal cord ischaemia, multiple sclerosis or various neurodegenerative diseases.

Narcolepsy

Narcolepsy is a recurrent irresistible desire to sleep at inappropriate times or places. After a brief sleep of 10–15 minutes, the subject usually awakes refreshed. It is commonly associated with physical weakness brought on by amusement or anger (*cataplexy*), inability to speak or move usually on awakening or falling asleep (*sleep paralysis*) or visual hallucinations (*hypnogogic hallucinations*) while drifting into or out of sleep. It is genetically determined being associated in almost all cases with the HLA DR2 antigen.

Non-epileptic focal cerebral symptoms

Intermittent disturbance of specific areas of the brain may occur suddenly in transient ischaemic attacks (TIA; Chapter 13), or evolve and resolve slowly as a migrainous aura (Chapter 11). A structural lesion, such as a tumour or arterio-venous malformation, may also give rise to episodic focal symptoms without any definite epileptic manifestations.

Movement disorders

Paroxysmal choreoathetosis may present as transient unilateral tonic muscular spasms or involuntary movements that simulate partial seizures (Chapter 15).

Metabolic disturbances

Hypoglycaemia, uraemia, hepatic encephalopathy, hypocalcaemia, inappropriate secretion of anti-diuretic hormone and drug overdosage can produce transient toxi-confusional states that could be mistaken for complex partial seizures.

Breath-holding attacks

Breath-holding attacks may occur in infants or young children usually as a mani-festation of rage or frustration. They may become cyanosed (or less commonly pale, generally after a head injury), lose consciousness and have minor clonic jerking of the limbs. Calm reassurance and soothing of the infant and parents is the best management although the child must remain subject to normal discipline so that he or she will not employ the attacks to manipulate domestic situations.

Psychological disturbances

Pseudoseizures may be a feature of hysteria or may develop in a patient who has been subject to genuine epileptic seizures. In doubtful cases, recording the EEG during an attack will generally establish the diagnosis. Acute anxiety attacks with hyperventilation may simulate epilepsy.

THE INVESTIGATION OF EPILEPSY

When the patient is seen at the time of the first fit, life-threatening conditions such as hypoglycaemia and meningitis must be considered. It never does any harm to take a blood sample for glucose estimation and then to inject glucose intravenously in an unconscious patient; on some occasions it may be life-saving. Unless there are clinical signs suggestive of meningitis or subarachnoid haemorrhage, lumbar puncture is not usually necessary.

When the patient is seen in less urgent circumstances, the most useful diag-nostic test is the EEG but it is a worthwhile routine to arrange a full blood count and erythrocyte sedimentation rate (ESR), blood glucose, calcium and electrolytes (and serological tests for syphilis, and HIV infection, if indicated) as well as chest X-ray.

If the EEG demonstrates a diffuse spike-and-wave discharge, whether typical or atypical, the epilepsy is classified as generalized and the likelihood of a focal cerebral lesion is small, although focal lesions may sometimes be associated with secondary generalized discharges.

If the EEG shows a localized spike, sharp wave, or spike-and-wave discharge, it indicates a partial seizure originating from a focal cortical lesion, irrespective of the clinical manifestation of the seizure.

Any other EEG abnormality, such as asymmetry of normal rhythms, local or generalized slow activity, may indicate an underlying cerebral disturbance but is not specifically epileptogenic. A normal EEG does not exclude epilepsy. The record may remain normal even when some attacks, such as tonic seizures or some form of myoclonic jerking, are in progress. If epilepsy is still suspected when the EEG is normal, a sleep recording may be helpful in unmasking epileptic activity suppressed in the waking state. Since a routine EEG lasts only for about 20 minutes, intermittent irregular epileptic discharges may be missed; prolonged telemetric EEG recording over 12–24 hours is undertaken in many laboratories in such circumstances.

If the clinical description of the attack or the nature of any EEG abnormality indicates a focal disturbance, further investigation is usually necessary, particularly in adults, to exclude cerebral tumour or other potentially remediable conditions.

Computed tomography (CT) scanning demonstrates most cerebral tumours and also shows the cerebrospinal fluid pathways clearly so that it is the technique of choice for demonstrating hydrocephalus, a porencephalic cyst or cortical atrophy. It demonstrates acute extradural or subdural haematomas, but may miss subacute haematomas as the density of the haematoma then approaches that of the adjacent cerebral tissue. Areas of gliosis, hippocampal atrophy and small hamartomas are better demonstrated by magnetic resonance imaging (MRI) than by CT scanning.

Further investigations such as angiography may be required in some cases but these are the prerogative of a specialized neurological/neurosurgical department.

A child or young adult in whom the clinical features and EEG suggest generalized epilepsy does not usually require any of the organ-imaging techniques since it is unlikely that they will contribute to diagnosis or management.

MANAGEMENT OF EPILEPSY

The aim of managing epilepsy is to prevent the seizures entirely if possible so that the patient can lead a completely normal life. If the various metabolic and local causes of epilepsy have been excluded, or if the family history and EEG indicate that the epilepsy is idiopathic, then anticonvulsant medication can be started provided that the patient has had more than one seizure. Care must be taken that epileptiform movements during profound syncope are not mistaken for a primary epileptic disturbance. With present treatment about one-third of patients remain liable to seizures in spite of medication.

Isolated seizures

The chance of recurrence within two years after a solitary fit is 12% if the EEG is normal, about 40% if there are non-specific abnormalities and around 80% if the EEG discloses epileptic discharges. Although anticonvulsant medications will lower the risk of another seizure, the usual practice is to withhold treatment after a single episode.

Psychological and social factors in management

It is important to place oneself in the position of a person who has previously been perfectly well and is suddenly told that he or she is suffering from epilepsy. Considerable time must be spent in explaining that many eminent people in the community have been subject to seizures but have succeeded in achieving their goals in their vocation and in their family lives.

Questions that commonly arise concern the following:

School

It is advisable for the child's school teacher and peer group to know the type of seizure to which the child is subject so that an attack does not lead to a panic reaction, and that reasonable supervision can be maintained. It is most important to ensure that an epileptic child is not singled out, teased or bullied by other children. The better educated the child, the more chance of his or her obtaining a suitable job later on, so that epilepsy should not be a reason for leaving school prematurely unless there is some associated condition such as mental retardation.

General activities

The patient should be encouraged to join in all normal activities with as few restrictions as possible. There are some common sense precautions to be taken. The patient should swim only in the company of some responsible person; a child should not climb trees to a great height or ride a bicycle on a busy road.

Driving

The practice varies in different places but in general no-one may hold a driving licence until 2 years have elapsed from the date of the last fit. Some exceptions are made; e.g., a patient whose seizures have occurred only during sleep for a period of at least 2 years.

Occupation

The teaching and nursing professions, airlines, and the armed services do not usually accept anyone with a history of epilepsy. Julius Caesar, whose seizures before a battle were regarded as a good omen, would not be admitted to the ranks of a modern army. Any occupation that requires working at heights, electrical wiring or using moving machinery should be avoided. One of the professions or a trade or business in which the patient is self-employed gives the best opportunity for fulfilment.

General advice

Patients should be advised to avoid excessive fatigue, missing meals and taking more than the most modest amount of alcohol. There are many other questions that will arise, concerning marriage, having children and other life decisions which must be handled sympathetically with the knowledge of the particular patient and the most recent information available to guide the patient.

Anticonvulsant medication

Seizures can be controlled by medication in about two-thirds of patients. The appropriate drug must be selected and increased slowly to a dose which maintains a blood level in the therapeutic range without blunting the intellectual ability of the patient. Ideally, only one drug should be used (monotherapy), but if seizures are only partly controlled a second medication may be added. However, addition of a second drug benefits only about 15% of cases. The patient should understand the importance of taking medication regularly and continuing for at least 5 years from the date of the last seizure. Even then, if treatment is discontinued, 40% of patients will relapse and have further attacks.

Mode of action of anticonvulsant drugs

Many antiepileptic drugs interact with GABA inhibitory mechanisms although this may not be relevant to their anticonvulsant action. The newly introduced agents GABApentin, vigabatrin (gamma-vinyl-GABA) and piracetam are GABA analogues. Benzodiazepines and barbiturates modulate the GABA-A receptor complex; sodium valproate increases GABA synthesis and slows its breakdown, whereas vigabatrin exerts only the latter effect by irreversibly inhibiting GABA transaminase. Tiagabine blocks GABA re-uptake. Milacemide is broken down in the body to glycine, another inhibitory neurotransmitter.

Phenytoin, carbamazepine and lamotrigine tonically inhibit voltage sensitive sodium channels in the neuronal cell membrane and gate release of the excitatory agent, glutamine. These agents impair the passage of a rapid train of impulses but do not interfere with isolated impulses or slow trains of neuronal discharge occurring physiologically. Felbamate is similar in structure to the anxiolytic agent meprobamate, but the mechanism of its antiepileptic action is unknown.

Tonic–clonic and partial (focal) seizures

The most commonly used drugs for the control of generalized and focal (partial) seizures are phenytoin and carbamazepine, but sodium valproate is as effective as phenytoin in preventing generalized seizures when used as monotherapy.

Phenytoin (Dilantin) Phenytoin is a hydantoin, first used for epilepsy in 1938. It is safe and effective but may cause coarsening of the features, excess body hair and swelling of the gums, particularly in children and adolescents. It is available as capsules of 100 mg and 30 mg, chewable tablets of 50 mg and a suspension for paediatric use of 6 mg/mL. The usual adult dose is 200–400 mg daily, given in divided doses twice daily, to maintain a blood level of 40–80 mmol/L. Dosage for children starts at 5 mg/kg daily. The half-life is about 24 hours. Overdosage causes nystagmus, dysarthria and ataxia. Phenytoin may cause a skin rash, lymphadenopathy and hepatomegaly as an idiosyncratic reaction. Long-term use may cause fall-out of Purkinje cells in the cerebellum, mild peripheral neuropathy and osteomalacia.

Carbamazepine (Tegretol) Carbamazepine is structurally related to tricyclic antidepressants and was introduced for the management of epilepsy in 1964. Tablets contain 200 mg or 100 mg carbamazepine, and the usual maintenance dose varies from 600 to 1200 mg daily, given in two or three divided doses. Treatment is started with a low dose, e.g. 100 mg three times daily, since vertigo and ataxia are not uncommon initial side effects. Leucopenia is common during carbamazepine therapy but rarely is severe enough to warrant cessation of treatment. Initially, the half-life of carbamazepine is 24–48 hours, but this is reduced to about 9 hours after continued use. The therapeutic range of blood levels is 20–50 mmol/L.

Sodium valproate (Epilim, Valpro) The anticonvulsant properties of sodium valproate were discovered in 1961 but it was introduced into general use only in the 1970s. It is effective in major and focal seizures as well as in petit mal absences and myoclonus. It is available as crushable tablets of 100 mg, 200 mg and 500 mg enteric-coated tablets, and as a syrup for paediatric use containing 40 mg/mL. The usual starting dose is 200 mg morning and night, given after meals to minimize gastric irritation since the tablets liberate valproic acid in the stomach. The dose is slowly increased to 400 mg three times daily or even to 1000 mg three times daily if necessary. With doses of more than 1000 mg daily, the 500 mg enteric-coated tablets are more convenient to use than the smaller tablets. The drug has a short half-life in the plasma (6–9 h) so it is better given as three divided doses. It usually makes patients brighter rather than drowsier and may sometimes cause tremor and insomnia. It may increase appetite and cause weight gain. Prolongation of pro-thrombin time may be found but does not appear to be of clinical significance. Hepatic damage, fatal in some instances, has been reported, particularly in young children and when combined with other drugs. For this reason the drug should be stopped if there is continued nausea, weight loss or abnormal liver function tests (except for gamma glutamyl-transpeptidase [GGT] which is usually slightly elevated in patients on anticonvulsant medication). Like all drugs, it should be used with caution but it can give satisfactory seizure control without sedation.

Barbiturates Phenobarbitone has been used as an anticonvulsant since 1912. It is cheap and effective but has the disadvantage of causing sedation and irritability in some patients, particularly children. The usual dosage varies from 90 to 300 mg/day to maintain a blood level of 45–75 μmol/L. It has a long half-life in adults of 3–4 days, and can therefore be taken as a single daily dose. Methylpheno-barbitone (Prominal), which is broken down to phenobarbitone in the body, is given in double the dose of phenobarbitone but confers no special advantage. Primidone (Mysoline) breaks down to phenobarbitone and another metabolite, phenylethylmalonamide, in the body. It is probable that all three substances have an anticonvulsant action, so that primidone may be more effective than phenobarbitone although hard evidence is lacking. Dosage of primidone is usually 250 mg two or three times daily but a small dose (quarter to half a tablet) is advisable to start with as it may cause vertigo when first used.

Clonazepam (Rivotril) Clonazepam is one of the benzodiazepine series that has a more effective and sustained anticonvulsant action than diazepam (Valium), although both these drugs can be given intravenously in cases of status epilepticus. Clonazepam is useful for tonic–clonic, partial seizures and petit mal epilepsy but has the disadvantage that it may cause sedation, irritability and aggression. It is available as tablets of 0.5 mg and 2.0 mg, and the dose varies from 0.5 mg to 4.0 mg three times daily according to its clinical effect and the tolerance of the patient. It has a long half-life of about 20–40 hours.

Vigabatrin (Sabril) Vigabatrin (gamma-vinyl GABA) is available for severe epilepsy that is not controlled by other anticonvulsants. It is available as 500 mg tablets and is added to previous medication as one tablet twice daily, increasing at weekly intervals 2–4 g/day. Seizure frequency is decreased to less than half in about 50% of patients. It may cause the side effects of drowsiness, weight gain and depression with occasional psychotic reactions.

Lamotrigine (Lamictal) The action of lamotrigine resembles that of phenytoin and it is currently available as an 'add-on' drug. The drug has to be introduced slowly, particularly if the patient is already taking sodium valproate which reduces its catabolism in the liver. For this reason, it is presented as tablets of 25 mg, 50 mg and 100 mg. Patients on valproate start with 25 mg on alternate days for 2 weeks, then 25 mg daily for two weeks with progressive increases to a maintenance of 50–100 mg twice daily. Those patients not taking valproate may tolerate double this dosage schedule, progressing up to 100–200 mg twice daily if necessary. Seizure frequency has been reduced by about 30% in add-on trials. A skin rash develops in some 10% of patients, requiring withdrawal of medication.

GABApentin (Neurontin) GABApentin is used as an 'add-on' drug and is presented as capsules of 300 mg and 400 mg. The effective dose range is 1200–2400 mg/day. It has reduced the frequency of complex partial seizures to less than half in about 40% of patients and secondarily generalized tonic–clonic seizures in about 60% in doses of 1800 mg/day in clinical trials. It is not effective for absence seizures. Side effects include somnolence, fatigue and ataxia. It is usually administered three times daily as it has a half-life of 5–7 hours.

Other medications Tiagabine, felbamate, piracetam and milacemide are currently under trial.

Petit mal absences, myoclonus and akinetic attacks

These minor forms of generalized epilepsy are associated with a 3 Hz spike-wave pattern in the EEG and usually respond satisfactorily to treatment with sodium valproate. If not, ethosuximide can be prescribed in combination with one of the anticonvulsants mentioned above since it has little action on major seizures, which may develop once the absences have been controlled. Clonazepam can be used for resistant cases.

Ethosuximide (Zarontin) Ethosuximide is used only for the control of petit mal absences, 250 mg capsules being introduced twice daily and the dose then being increased to three or four capsules daily if necessary. It may cause drowsiness and bone marrow depression.

Status epilepticus

Patients with status epilepticus should be treated in an intensive care ward as the condition is potentially fatal. Diazepam, 5–10 mg, should be given intravenously over 2 minutes and repeated in 10 minutes if seizures persist. Intravenous therapy may be given continuously at the rate of 5–10 mg/hour (50 mg in 500 mL saline). Side effects are hypotension, bradycardia and respiratory depression. Clonazepam (1–2 mg intravenously) may be more effective than diazepam in the treatment of status epilepticus.

Sodium amylobarbitone, 50–100 mg, i.v. over 10 minutes, or phenobarbitone sodium, 200 mg by intramuscular injection, may be used if diazepam is ineffective, but these drugs produce respiratory depression and hypotension.

Slow intravenous infusion of 250 mg phenytoin in an adult who has been taking the drug, or of 1000 mg over several hours in an adult previously untreated, may help control seizures. Phenytoin is of no value if given intramuscularly. Regular anticonvulsant medication must be continued subsequently. Paraldehyde (5–10 mL, i.m.) is also useful if diazepam and phenytoin are not effective.

If other treatment is unsuccessful, general anaesthesia and muscle relaxants may be necessary. The important principle of management is to keep the patient well oxygenated at all times to prevent further cerebral damage.

Interaction between anticonvulsants

Sodium valproate increases blood levels of barbiturate. There are many possible interactions between anticonvulsants and it is sensible to obtain a new estimation of blood levels if a drug is added to or subtracted from the patient's medication.

Pregnancy

Most epileptic mothers will have normal pregnancies and babies. The risk of foetal malformations, many of which are minor, has been assessed in various published series as being between 5 and 10% in the pregnancies of epileptic mothers, compared with 3.6 to 5% in non-epileptic controls. Spina bifida and other neural tube defects are more common in the babies of epileptic women than in those of women without epilepsy. The risk is highest in those patients taking sodium valproate (1–2%) or carbamazepine (0.5–1.0%). There is evidence that increasing maternal intake of folate or a supplement of 0.4–0.8 mg daily reduces the incidence of neural tube defects without adversely affecting control of epilepsy. Patients maintained on valproate during pregnancy should be warned of the possibility of spina bifida and offered monitoring of foetal development by ultrasound imaging. Phenytoin and barbiturates increase the risk of hare-lip, cleft palate and ventricular septal defect. The general consensus of opinion is that the patient should be maintained on the most appropriate monotherapy during pregnancy since there is not sufficient evidence that any one anticonvulsant is more teratogenic than another. Polytherapy increases the risk of anomalies.

Seizure frequency increases in pregnancy in about one-third of patients, usually because the dose of anticonvulsants has been reduced or blood levels have not been monitored. Enzyme-inducing anticonvulsants reduce the activity of vitamin K-dependent clotting factors in the foetus which can cause a haemorrhagic syndrome. Oral supplements of vitamin K, 20 mg/day, during the last month or pregnancy and vitamin K, 13 mg, i.m., during delivery have been recommended.

The surgical management of epilepsy

When a focal cerebral lesion has been demonstrated in a site consistent with the nature of the seizure and the EEG discharge, it may be removed surgically. Even if the causative lesion cannot be visualized by CT scanning or MRI, it may be localized by EEG techniques, sometimes involving intracerebral electrodes or recording at the time of operation (electrocorticography). Speech and memory are tested before operation by the intracarotid injection of amylobarbitone to determine hemisphere dominance for language and the ability to register memory in each half of the brain (Wada test). The most common operation is anterior temporal lobectomy with complete remission from seizures in 65%, improvement in 25% and no response in 10%. Operation is usually reserved for patients not responding to anticonvulsant therapy.

REFERENCES

Blum D. and Fisher R. S. (1994) Advances in epilepsy. *Current Opinion in Neurology*, **7**, 96–101.

Delgado-Escuata A. V. and Janz D. (1992) Consensus guidelines: preconception counseling, management, and care of the pregnant woman with epilepsy. *Neurology*, **42** (Suppl. 5), 149–160.

Eadie M. J. (1992) Epileptic seizures. In *Drug Therapy in Neurology*. Ed. M. J. Eadie. Churchill Livingstone, Edinburgh. 97–171

Engel J. (1989) *Seizures and Epilepsy*. F. A. Davis, Philadelphia.

Yerby M. S., Leavitt A., Erickson D. M., McCormick K. B., Loewenson R. B., Sells C. J. and Benedetti T. J. (1992) Antiepileptics and the development of congenital anomalies. *Neurology*, **42** (Suppl. 5), 132–140.

13 | Cerebral vascular disease

The term 'cerebral vascular accident', is as non-specific as the term 'heart attack'. The cerebral vessels are branches of the internal carotid and vertebrobasilar arteries and are not subject to 'accidents': regional cerebral blood flow may be compromised by reduction in filling pressure, embolism, thrombosis or haemorrhage, causing symptoms and signs referable to a specific vascular territory, and should be diagnosed precisely whenever possible. The term 'stroke' is commonly used to describe any cerebrovascular event that causes a neurological disability.

DEFINITIONS

Transient ischaemic attack (TIA)

Neurological symptoms or signs lasting less than 24 hours (usually 1–30 min).

Reversible ischaemic neurological deficit (RIND)

Symptoms or signs persisting more than 24 hours but clearing over days or weeks.

Stroke

Permanent deficit from cerebral infarction or haemorrhage.

PREVALENCE

Approximately 14% of the population die of stroke, the third most common cause of death. Transient ischaemic attacks occur as a warning in only 10–30% of stroke patients. Complete strokes are caused by thrombosis with or without embolism in 80% of cases, by cerebral haemorrhage in 10% and by subarachnoid haemorrhage in most of the remainder.

PATHOGENESIS

Risk factors for stroke

Most cerebral vascular disease is directly or indirectly attributable to atheroma. Risk factors include:

Hypertension

Mortality from thrombotic and haemorrhagic stroke is twice as high in patients whose diastolic blood pressure is greater than 110 mmHg as it is in normotensive controls.

Cigarette smoking

Cigarette smoking is a more potent risk factor than hyperlipidaemia for carotid artery stenosis.

Hyperlipidaemia

Elevation of cholesterol and triglyceride levels is significantly associated with the onset of stroke under the age of 50 years.

Diabetes

Atheroma and stroke are more prevalent in diabetic patients.

Age

Cerebral vascular disease is more common with advancing years but may affect people in any decade of life. About 20–25% of all strokes affect people under the age of 65 years.

Changes in the arterial wall

Atheroma

The extracranial vessels may be narrowed (stenosed) at their origin. The most common sites of stenoses are the bifurcation of the carotid artery, the origin of the vertebral arteries and the basilar artery. These stenoses are common in people of middle or old age and are frequently symptomless; blood flow in the internal carotid artery is decreased only when the lumen is 2 mm² or less, and symptoms may then result if the blood pressure drops. The vessel may become completely occluded by thrombosis resulting in a cerebral infarction. Ulcers in an atheromatous plaque may be the site of platelet accumulation or the source of cholesterol crystals, either of which may embolize the distal cerebral circulation.

Arteritis

Temporal arteritis may cause vascular occlusion in patients aged 55 years or older. Arteritis may also rarely be the cause of unexplained stroke in the first three decades of life. 'Moya moya' is a Japanese term (meaning mist, smoke or haze) used to describe the copious collateral circulation seen on angiography after occlusion of the distal part of the carotid siphon in young people. The collateral circulation fills the middle cerebral artery distal to the point of occlusion.

Sudden lowering of filling pressure

A fall in arterial pressure may reduce cerebral perfusion, particularly in the presence of stenosis of the carotid and vertebral arteries. Causes include:
- Cardiac dysrhythmias or myocardial infarction with fall in cardiac output
- Postural hypotension or a sudden fall in blood pressure from the use of hypotensive drugs
- Blood loss or severe anaemia
- Functional narrowing of extracranial portion of the arteries by neck turning

Increased platelet aggregation or blood viscosity

- Polycythaemia vera
- The use of oral contraceptive pills or other female hormonal preparations
- Pregnancy, postpartum or postoperative states
- The oligaemic phase of classical migraine (which is associated with increased platelet aggregation)

Strokes in young people

Treatable and rarer causes of stroke should be diligently sought in people under age of 45 years. Cardiac causes, trauma and dissection of carotid and vertebral arteries, drug abuse, blood coagulopathies and dyscrasia, collagen vascular diseases, antiphospholipid syndrome, fibromuscular dysplasia, homocysteinuria, and venous sinus thrombosis should be excluded.

TYPES OF CEREBRAL VASCULAR DISEASE

Transient ischaemic attacks

Carotid circulation

Please refer to Figs 13.1 and 13.2. Approximately 50% of carotid TIA are caused by thrombo-embolism from an atheromatous ulcer in the extracranial portion of the internal carotid artery, usually at the bifurcation of the common carotid artery. Emboli consist of platelets and fibrin, or occasionally of cholesterol crystals, and can sometimes be seen passing through the retinal arteries during a TIA. The source of platelet emboli may also be intracranial, commonly at the carotid siphon or the origin of the anterior or middle cerebral arteries.

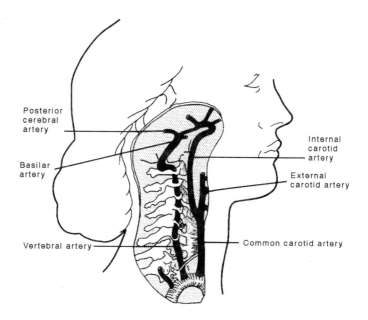

Fig. 13.1   The vertebrobasilar and carotid arterial systems, showing their course in the neck and communication through the circle of Willis. (Modified from Lance, 1975, *Headache*, with permission of Charles Scribner's Sons, New York.)

Less commonly, emboli may arise from atheromatous plaques in the aorta or from the heart in atrial fibrillation, from mural thrombi following myocardial infarction, and possibly from prolapsed mitral valves in young women. Septic thrombi from subacute bacterial endocarditis may lodge in distal branches of the cerebral vessels and produce mycotic aneurysms. Very rarely, fragments of atrial myxoma may embolize cerebral vessels.

Symptoms   (i) Amaurosis fugax. Transient loss of vision in the ipsilateral eye, described as a curtain or shutter descending over the eye, caused by retinal embolization from a plaque in the internal carotid artery, is a symptom in 30% of carotid TIA. Unilateral blindness may also be caused by insufficiency of the posterior ciliary artery supplying the optic nerve head (ischaemic papillopathy; Fig. 4.7); (ii) contralateral paraesthesiae or hemiparesis (each in 60% of cases); (iii) transient dysphasia if the dominant hemisphere is involved (17% of cases); (iv) headache, usually ipsilateral, in approximately 20% of cases.

Physical examination   A harsh mid-systolic bruit may be audible at the angle of the mandible opposite the carotid bifurcation. A bruit may sometimes be heard on the side opposite the more severe stenosis because of increased blood flow on the relatively unaffected side.

Vertebrobasilar circulation

Please refer to Figs 13.1 and 13.2. Transient ischaemic attacks in vertebrobasilar territory are referred to as vertebrobasilar insufficiency (VBI) and, in contrast to

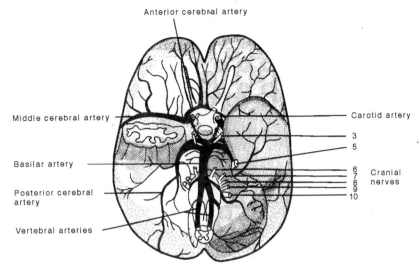

Fig. 13.2 Intracranial course of carotid and vertebrobasilar arterial systems. The basilar artery gives off the superior cerebellar arteries before terminating as the posterior cerebral arteries that supply the medial part of the temporal lobes and occipital cortex. The third cranial nerve emerges from the mid-brain between the superior cerebellar and posterior cerebral arteries, close to the posterior communicating artery. (From Lance, 1975, *Headache*, with permission of Charles Scribner's Sons, New York.)

carotid TIA, are only rarely caused by thrombo-embolism from atheromatous plaques. Most cases appear to result from loss of normal autoregulation in the hind-brain circulation which leaves the patient vulnerable to any diminution of filling pressure. An atheromatous plaque is sometimes found at the origin of one or both vertebral arteries. Particular attention must be paid to causes of hypotension as described above. Two specific but rare causes of VBI should be sought:

(1) *Cervical spondylosis* Osteophytes project laterally from the neurocentral joints so that rarely, twisting of the neck may obliterate the lumen of the vertebral artery where it runs through the foramina transversaria of the cervical spine (Fig. 13.1).

(2) *Subclavian steal syndrome* This is a rare but interesting cause of vertebro-basilar insufficiency (VBI). Stenosis of one subclavian artery proximal to the origin of the vertebral artery may lower the filling pressure sufficiently to cause reversal of blood flow so that blood flows up the vertebral artery on the normal side and down the vertebral artery on the side of subclavian stenosis, thus 'stealing' blood away from the hind-brain circulation (Fig. 13.3). Symptoms of VBI may become apparent when the arm on the affected side is exercised, thus dilating the peripheral vascular bed and reducing pressure distal to the stenosis. Subclavian stenosis is not uncommon although the symptoms are rare. The condition is surgically remediable, but treatment is indicated only if it is causing symptoms.

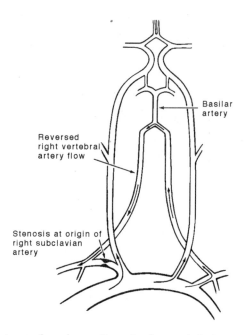

Fig. 13.3 Subclavian steal syndrome. Stenosis of one subclavian artery converts the distal part of the artery (and the vertebral artery arising from it) into a low pressure system. Blood may thus flow up one vertebral artery and down the other, lowering basilar artery filling pressure and 'stealing' blood away from the brain-stem to cause symptoms of vertebro-basilar insufficiency.

Symptoms of vertebrobasilar insufficiency (i) Brain-stem symptoms and signs. Vertigo (50% of cases), diplopia (40%), circumoral or unilateral paraesthesiae (40%), weakness of one or both sides of the body (33%) and falling or 'drop attacks' in 3% of cases (caused by ischaemia of the reticular formation); (ii) cerebellar symptoms and signs. Dysarthria, ataxia or incoordination (33% of cases); (iii) impairment of vision in one or both visual fields, i.e. right, left or bilateral homonymous hemianopia (from ischaemia of occipital cortex, supplied by posterior cerebral arteries which derive their blood supply from the basilar artery). Visual symptoms occur in about 60% of cases; (iv) there may be transient amnesia because the medial temporal lobe is also supplied by the posterior cerebral circulation; (v) occipital headache in about 20% of cases.

Physical examination The radial pulses are asymmetrical in subclavian stenosis, the blood pressure being lower on the affected side. Blood pressure should always be taken in both arms of patients with VBI. A systolic bruit is usually heard above the clavicle over the site of the stenosis.

Prognosis of transient ischaemic attacks

Of patients with TIA, some 36% will suffer a complete stroke within 5 years, about 13% in the first year. Thereafter, the stroke rate is 5–6% per year (16 times that of control subjects who have never experienced TIA). Ten year survival is 40%, compared with 60% for age-matched controls. It should be noted that death from myocardial infarction is twice as common as death from stroke. If hypertension is controlled, the mortality rate of patients with TIA approximates that of normal controls.

Investigation of transient ischaemic attacks

All patients warrant a full blood count and erythrocyte sedimentation rate (ESR), since the ESR is greater than 40 mm/hour in two-thirds of patients with temporal arteritis. Other routine investigations comprise blood glucose, serum lipids, chest X-ray, electrocardiogram (ECG; plus echocardiogram if embolization from the heart is suspected). A computed tomography (CT) scan of the brain will confirm cerebral haemorrhage immediately and will help to exclude a cerebral tumour which may sometimes cause intermittent symptoms resembling those of TIA. Cerebral infarcts may not be seen clearly for several days.

The most cost-effective screening technique for carotid stenosis is carotid ultrasound scanning (carotid Doppler Duplex). If this shows significant abnormalities, patients with unilateral carotid TIA should be assessed by bilateral carotid angiography or digital subtraction angiography, both performed by femoral catheterization. These demonstrate ulceration, stenosis or occlusion of extracranial and intracranial portions of the carotid circulation. Arteriography carries a risk of causing transient neurological deficit in 13% of such patients and permanent deficit in 0.65%. Angiography should therefore be carried out only if endarterectomy or some other surgical procedure is being considered, and it may be inadvisable in patients with evidence of generalized atheroma (angina, intermittent claudication). Magnetic resonance angiography (MRA) is a non-invasive technique that gives accurate information about the presence of carotid artery stenosis.

In patients in whom there is a reasonable suspicion of a cardiac source of embolism, echocardiography (transthoracic or transoesophageal) should be considered.

Patients with VBI require an X-ray of the cervical spine and careful observation for postural hypotension or intermittent cardiac dysrhythmias (Holter monitoring of the ECG may be useful if attacks of VBI are recurring daily). Angiography is usually undertaken only if there is a localized bruit at the base of the neck or evidence of subclavian steal since the chance of showing a surgically correctable lesion is otherwise remote.

Present evidence in patients with an *asymptomatic carotid bruit* is that the risk of stroke is sufficiently low not to warrant angiography or endarterectomy. Some develop TIA but the death rate is not much different from that of the general population, most deaths being from myocardial infarction and not from stroke.

Treatment of transient ischaemic attacks

General management Hypertension, hyperlipidaemia and diabetes should be controlled in appropriate patients. It is advisable for patients not to smoke tobacco or to use the contraceptive pill. Cardiac dysrhythmias, polycythaemia, anaemia or other underlying conditions should be controlled.

Specific management This may be surgical or medical.

(1) Surgical intervention includes:

- Carotid endarterectomy in patients with severe unilateral disease (greater than 70% stenosis) on the side appropriate to symptoms improves expectation of life as well as reducing risk of stroke. The combined mortality and morbidity rate of the procedure should not exceed 3%. In patients with a lesser stenosis, or disease of more than one vessel, operation may not improve the natural history of the disorder.

    Bear in mind that life-expectancy depends on coronary rather than cerebral vessels. If coronary bypass surgery and carotid endarterectomy are both to be undertaken, results are better if the operation is done in two stages, the carotid surgery being done first. Either way there is a stroke rate of 3%, but this doubles if both procedures are done together.

- Symptomatic subclavian steal syndrome is uncommon but is readily repaired surgically

- Operations on the cervical spine (removal of osteophytes or anterior interbody fusion) may rarely be indicated in some patients with VBI

- Anastomosis of the superficial temporal branch of the external carotid artery to the middle cerebral artery (EC/IC bypass) has been evaluated for the treatment of internal carotid and middle cerebral artery occlusion and found to be of no benefit in most cases.

(2) Medical treatment includes:

- Prevention of platelet aggregation in TIA. Aspirin therapy (the optimal daily dose has yet to be determined but 300 mg/day is as effective as 1200 mg/day) reduces the risk of stroke and death by 25%. The platelet anti-aggregant ticlopidine 250 mg twice daily is at least as effective as aspirin and reduces the risk of cerebral infarction but has side effects of gastrointestinal disturbance (20%), rash (10%) and neutropenia (2–4%). Aspirin acts by irreversibly inhibiting the enzyme cyclo-oxygenase, thus preventing the formation of thromboxane A2 from arachidonic acid for the life of the platelet (5–10 days). Sulphinpyrazone (Anturan) and dipyridamole (Persantin), other agents for preventing platelet aggregation, have not been proven to be useful in preventing stroke

- Anticoagulants. The administration of warfarin to patients with TIA with careful monitoring of prothrombin times, reduces the risk of stroke but does not reduce mortality since more patients die of cerebral haemorrhage and other conditions. However, it is indicated when the TIA are definitely due to cardiac emboli and when atrial fibrillation is present

- Antispasmodics or vasodilators. These are of use *only* if the attacks are caused by migrainous vasospasm (migraine equivalents or transient migrainous accompaniments; TMA), in which case the inhalation of isoprenaline spray as used for asthma, or oral administration of glyceryl trinitrate or nifedipine may be effective

- Intravenous heparin is given in many centres to patients with a recent TIA, but its efficacy is unproven

Thrombotic cerebral infarction

The factors in the pathogenesis of cerebral infarction are the same as those discussed for TIA as platelet aggregation can lead to thrombosis and infarction.

Since 90% of strokes occur without warning, the most effective long-term measure in prevention is the control of hypertension and hyperlipidaemia at an early age and avoiding smoking, particularly in those people with a family history of cerebral vascular disease. In 20% of cases, the stroke has a stuttering onset caused by the gradual occlusion of a major vessel and is known as a *progressive stroke* or *stroke-in-evolution*.

Clinical features

In 80% of cases, the patient presents with a completed stroke, the symptoms and signs of which depend upon the vascular territory affected. *Internal carotid occlusion* may be symptomless but commonly results in infarction in the ipsi-lateral hemisphere producing a contralateral hemiplegia, hemi-anaesthesia (and sometimes hemianopia) with the head and eyes turned to the side of the lesion, i.e. away from the hemiplegic side. Speech and other intellectual functions may be impaired, depending on whether the dominant or non-dominant hemisphere is infarcted. If infarction is extensive the patient may be obtunded or stuporose. The symptoms of *middle cerebral artery occlusion* are much the same as described above. Flow in the ophthalmic artery may rarely be impaired sufficiently by internal carotid occlusion to cause ipsilateral blindness. Obstruction of the distal branches of the *anterior cerebral artery* which supplies the 'leg area' of the cortex can cause a monoparesis of the contralateral leg, while occlusion of the recurrent branch of the anterior cerebral artery (Heubner's artery) infarcts the part of the internal capsule carrying descending motor pathways for movement of the lower face and arm on the opposite side of the body. Blockage of the parent trunk of the anterior cerebral causes hemiparesis by the combination of these effects.

A circumscribed infarction may result from occlusion of a small perforating vessel with localized brain softening and subsequent formation of a cyst or *lacune*. These usually occur in hypertensive patients. *Lacunar infarction* in the internal capsule or pons may cause a pure hemiplegia or, in the thalamus, may produce a pure hemi-anaesthesia which recovers in a few days. Some capsular or upper pontine lacunes may cause 'ataxic hemiparesis' in which weakness is accompanied by cerebellar signs on the same side because of involvement of corticoponto-cerebellar pathways. In hypertensive patients multiple lacunes can lead to pseudo-bulbar palsy (pp. 39, 78).

Basilar artery occlusion causes brain-stem infarction with bulbar palsy and quadriparesis so that the patient may be able to communicate only by eye movements ('locked-in syndrome'; p. 217). Various regions of the brain-stem may be selectively infarcted by occlusion of the vertebral artery or branches of the basilar artery; e.g., lateral medullary infarction from obstruction of the posterior inferior cerebellar artery or the vertebral artery which gives rise to it (Fig. 4.29).

Homonymous hemianopia, cortical blindness and amnesia may also be features of basilar artery obstruction because the posterior cerebral arteries, which supply the medial part of the temporal lobes and the occipital lobes of the brain, arise from it (Fig. 13.2).

Diffuse hypertensive cerebral vascular disease   In sustained hypertension the small perforating arteries of the brain may be obstructed, causing small areas of softening (lacunes), which may be symptomless or cause small strokes. When many such softenings develop bilaterally in the putamen, head of the caudate nucleus and internal capsule (*état lacunaire*), the signs of *pseudobulbar palsy* appear with bilateral spastic quadriparesis, upper motor neurone lesions of the lower cranial nerves, inappropriate and excessive laughter or crying, and dementia (multi-infarct dementia; pp. 78, 266). If ischaemic changes affect the white matter diffusely the condition is known as *Binswanger's subcortical encephalopathy.*

Prognosis

If hemiplegia develops within 3 hours and persists for 36 hours there is a 90% chance that deficit will be permanent. Of patients with hemiplegia *and* impaired consciousness, 41% die. Of patients conscious on admission to hospital, more than 80% survive. Most patients can walk again and move the shoulder and elbow but not the hand. Unfortunately about one-third remain disabled and dependent.

Investigations

A CT scan is the most useful investigation in completed stroke, since it distinguishes infarcts from haemorrhages. However, an infarct may not be clearly seen on the first day and the scan should be repeated if necessary at 5–7 days. Computed tomography scans do not invariably exclude subdural haematoma or some cerebral tumours; if these conditions are strongly suspected the scan should be repeated (with injection of contrast medium) and consideration given to magnetic resonance imaging (MRI) or arteriography (MRA). Magnetic resonance imaging is not used in the investigation of most strokes, but demonstrates structures in the posterior fossa better than CT.

Routine investigation includes full blood count, ESR, blood glucose and lipids, serum electrolytes and creatinine, chest X-ray and ECG. If cardiac emboli are suspected, echocardiography must also be performed.

In young people with strokes, the following additional tests should be considered: MRI, MRA, serological tests for syphilis and HIV screen, lupus anti-coagulant, anti-cardiolipin antibodies antinuclear factor, screening for homo-cysteinuria and muscle biopsy since mitochondrial myopathy may present with stroke-like episodes (Chapter 10).

Treatment

There is no evidence that the use of heparin, steroids, intravenous dextran, sympathetic block, CO_2 inhalation or hyperbaric oxygen has any effect on a completed stroke. There is some evidence that intravenous mannitol may reduce mortality in the first week by reducing cerebral oedema. The emphasis at present is on maintaining normal blood pressure, treating hyperglycaemia if present and early rehabilitation.

The effects of early administration of thrombolytic agents (recombinant tissue plasminogen activator [rTPA], urokinase, streptokinase) and the calcium channel antagonist nimodipine are currently being evaluated.

A progressive stroke may be treated by intravenous heparin but a CT scan should always be performed first since there is difficulty in distinguishing a stroke-in-evolution from a TIA or a small cerebral haemorrhage.

Embolic cerebral infarcts

As discussed under the heading of TIA, many strokes begin as cerebral emboli which may arise from the heart, carotid arteries or other great vessels.

Management is similar to that of cerebral thrombosis causing infarction but, in the case of suspected embolism, early heparinization is usually commenced provided there is no evidence of haemorrhage on the CT scan. The underlying cause of embolism should be sought and treated; anticoagulant therapy is usually indicated to prevent recurrence of emboli and progressive thrombosis at the site of embolization. Patients with atrial fibrillation should be treated with warfarin indefinitely.

Intracerebral haemorrhage

Intracerebral haemorrhage almost always occurs in hypertensive patients. Bleeding originates from micro-aneurysms on small vessels (Charcot-Bouchard aneurysms). The blood clot may remain localized or it may infiltrate and destroy the surrounding brain. The most common sites are the putamen, thalamus, cerebellum and pons.

Clinical features

The onset may be rapid or gradual over a period of hours, often accompanied by headache. With the most common cerebral haemorrhage, that in the putamen and internal capsule, contralateral hemiplegia is the earliest symptom, followed by sensory loss, hemianopia and aphasia if the dominant hemisphere is affected. On examination there is usually a dense hemiplegia and the head and eyes are deviated away from the hemiplegic side. If bleeding continues the patient becomes drowsy and unconscious.

In pontine haemorrhage, the patient usually loses consciousness and dies within a matter of hours. In cerebellar haemorrhage, occipital headache, vertigo and vomiting usually occur at the onset.

Investigation

A CT brain scan demonstrates the haemorrhage in almost all cases. The cerebro-spinal fluid (CSF) is blood stained in about 90% of cases but lumbar puncture is rarely indicated. Routine investigations are similar to those used in cerebral infarction.

Management

Careful attention to the airway, oxygen therapy, care of bladder and skin, the use of intravenous or intragastric fluids, followed by physiotherapy, is the supportive treatment required for most patients. Patients with intracerebellar haemorrhages (10% of cases) require urgent surgical evacuation of the blood clot. Only occasionally is surgical treatment of value in the other cases of cerebral haemorrhage.

Subarachnoid haemorrhage (SAH)

Subarachnoid haemorrhage is haemorrhage into the subarachnoid space, the most common cause of which is a ruptured aneurysm of one of the major vessels at the base of the brain. Other causes of subarachnoid haemorrhage include angiomas, trauma, infections (mycotic aneurysms), and haemorrhage secondary to haemorrhagic diseases. The ratio of aneurysm to angioma as a cause of SAH in various Western series varies from 5:1 to 25:1, but in Asia angioma is a more common cause than aneurysm.

Clinical features

The most common symptoms of SAH are the sudden onset of headache, stiff neck, photophobia, vomiting and loss of consciousness. Pain in the back and legs may follow SAH after some days because of blood descending in the CSF to irritate the cauda equina. On examination, the neck is usually rigid and Kernig's sign (p. 17) may be present. Cranial nerves, commonly the third nerve, may be compressed by an enlarging aneurysm of the internal carotid or posterior communicating arteries (see Figs 4.10 and 13.2 for anatomical relations) and focal neurological signs may be caused by rupture into the cerebral substance or by the extensive vasospasm which usually follows SAH. Subhyaloid haemorrhages are observed in the fundi in some 7% of patients and papilloedema in 13%. Fever, albuminuria, glycosuria, hypertension and ECG changes may be found in the acute phase. The possibility of spinal SAH must be considered if weakness has a paraplegic rather than hemiplegic distribution. About one third of patients experience a minor leak (sentinel haemorrhage) hours or days before a major bleed.

Investigations

A CT scan will usually show blood in the subarachnoid space or ventricles and may also demonstrate an aneurysm or angioma. A lumbar puncture may be required to confirm the presence of uniformly blood-stained CSF. Xanthochromia of the supernatant CSF becomes apparent after 4 hours, is maximal at 7 days, and persists for several weeks after SAH. A lymphocytic cellular reaction and increase in CSF protein to 0.7–1.3 g/L usually follows SAH. If the patient is conscious, four vessel cerebral angiograms should be obtained as soon as possible. If the patient is obtunded, extensive vasospasm is likely to prevent the demonstration of any aneurysm so that angiography is best deferred until the patient's mental state improves.

Some 80% of aneurysms are found on the anterior (30%) and posterior (30%) communicating arteries or the middle cerebral artery near its division into branches within the Sylvian fissure (20%). Fifteen per cent of aneurysms arise from the hind-brain circulation. Multiple aneurysms are found in 10–15% of cases.

Prognosis

About one-third of patients die with the first haemorrhage within 24 hours, and, of the survivors, about one-third have a further SAH within the first four weeks if the aneurysm cannot be clipped surgically.

Management

Aneurysms should be operated on as soon as practicable after demonstration by angiography because of the danger of recurrent haemorrhage. If no aneurysm is demonstrated or surgery is not feasible, the patient is usually kept at rest in bed for several weeks with the room darkened as long as the photophobia persists. The use of epsilon aminocaproic acid (an antifibrinolytic agent, given to prevent re-bleeding by inhibiting lysis of the clot surrounding the aneurysm), and the calcium channel blocker nimodipine (intended to diminish vascular spasm) remain controversial.

Unnecessary exertion should be avoided and the bowels kept loose by aperients to prevent straining during defaecation. The use of a bedside commode is usually preferable to the gymnastics required to use a traditional bedpan. Hypertension should be controlled.

Carotico-cavernous fistula

Trauma, or rupture of a saccular aneurysm of the internal carotid artery within the cavernous sinus, may form a fistula that increases intra-orbital pressure with the development of a pulsating exophthalmos, periorbital oedema, conjunctival injection, ophthalmoplegia (because of involvement of nerves III, IV and VI in the wall of the cavernous sinus; Fig. 4.12), pain around the eye and noises in the head and an orbital bruit. The fistula may be occluded by a balloon inserted by a catheter through the femoral artery and floated into place under angiographic monitor. Internal carotid blood flow is thus preserved.

Extradural haemorrhage

Extradural haemorrhage is usually caused by laceration of the middle meningeal artery by a fracture of the parietal or temporal bones. There is a history of head injury which may or may not be followed by a brief period of unconsciousness. Classically there is a lucid interval for some hours or even days after the injury before the patient becomes drowsy, usually with headache and vomiting. As the haematoma extends, consciousness is progressively impaired and the pupil on the side of the haematoma dilates because the third nerve is compressed in the tentorial notch by displacement downwards of the temporal lobe (p. 218). Urgent surgical treatment is required to evacuate the haematoma and prevent further bleeding. X-ray of the skull may show a fracture line but the diagnosis is most readily confirmed by CT scan of the brain. If the condition is advancing too rapidly for any investigation to be done, the placement of burr holes on the same side of the skull as the dilated pupil can be a life-saving procedure.

Subdural haematoma

Acute subdural haematoma

This presents after head injury in the same manner as an extradural haematoma and is dealt with in the same way.

Chronic subdural haematoma

This condition may develop slowly over days, weeks or months after a relatively minor head injury which tears one of the veins running from the cortex to a venous sinus. The head injury may be so trivial as to be forgotten, particularly if it took place during a bout of excessive alcohol intake. Subdural haematoma should be suspected in any patient with progressive impairment of intellect or memory, recent onset of headache or drowsiness or any other symptom suggestive of a space-occupying lesion. The diagnosis can usually be confirmed by a CT scan of the brain but, after some days, the density of the haematoma approaches that of the surrounding tissue and it may escape detection. If the index of suspicion remains high after CT is normal, MRI or bilateral carotid angiography should be undertaken as the definitive investigation. It must be remembered that mid-line structures may not be displaced if subdural haematomas are bilateral. Once diagnosed, the haematomas are evacuated surgically.

VENOUS SINUS THROMBOSIS

Thrombosis of cerebral veins or venous sinuses most commonly presents as headache, hemiplegia, focal epileptic seizures or symptoms and signs of raised intracranial pressure. Predisposing factors include sinus or ear infections, dehydration, coagulopathies, polycythaemia, connective tissue disease, trauma and homocystinuria. The diagnosis can be confirmed with CT, MRI or angiography. The treatment is to reduce intracranial pressure, prevent seizures and anticoagulants are sometimes indicated, although their use is controversial.

REFERENCES

Bousser M. G., Chiras J., Bories J. and Castaigne P. (1985) Cerebral venous thrombosis — a review of 38 cases. *Stroke*, **16**, 199–213.

Donnan G. A. (1992) Investigation of patients with stroke and transient ischaemic attacks. *Lancet*, **339**, 473–477.

Kopitnick T. A. and Samson D. S. (1993) Management of subarachnoid haemorrhage. *Journal of Neurology, Neurosurgery and Psychiatry*, **56**, 947–959.

Marshall R. S. and Mohr J. P. (1993) Current management of ischaemic strokes. *Journal of Neurology, Neurosurgery and Psychiatry*, **56**, 6–16.

Humphrey P. (1994) Stroke and transient ischaemic attacks. *Journal of Neurology, Neurosurgery and Psychiatry*, **57**, 534–543.

14 | Coma and other disturbances of consciousness

CONSCIOUSNESS

There is no entirely satisfactory definition of consciousness but clinically it means the state of awareness of self and environment. Coma is a state in which a patient is unaware of self and environment and cannot be aroused into a state of awareness.

The structures which are most important in maintaining the state of consciousness are the cerebral cortex and the reticular formation. The reticular formation (from the Latin reticulum, meaning 'a net') consists of large and small cells with their connections which are scattered throughout the brain-stem from the medulla to the thalamus. It is divided anatomically into the brain-stem and thalamic reticular formation. All the major sensory pathways project to the reticular formation which is influenced by, and in turn can modify, the sensory input to the brain. One of the most important functions of the reticular formation is in arousal and in maintaining wakefulness. The part of the reticular formation most concerned with this function is the ascending reticular formation (reticular activating system) in the mid-brain and thalamus which projects diffusely to the cerebral cortex. Destruction of the ascending reticular activating system causes coma and stimulation of it will produce wakefulness in an experimental animal (Fig. 14.1).

Definition of altered states of consciousness

In a state of *alert wakefulness*, when the subjects are fully conscious, they are fully orientated in time and place and respond immediately and appropriately to stimuli. Various grades of impaired or clouded consciousness are recognized and are loosely defined as follows:

Confusional states   Acute confusional states can be produced by intoxication with drugs or toxins, by acute metabolic disturbances such as hypoglycaemia, hypoxia or hypercapnia, by fluid and electrolyte disturbances associated with surgery or shock, by sleep deprivation, pain, alcohol withdrawal or as a transient phenomenon after seizures.

The patient has difficulty in concentrating and thinking. There is lack of attentiveness, some degree of disorientation in time and place, distractability and impairment of memory.

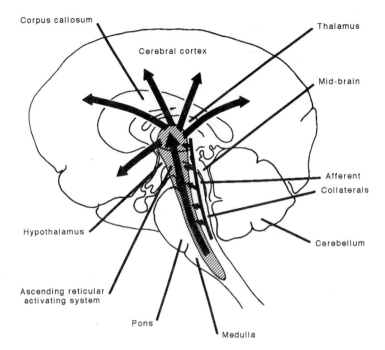

Fig. 14.1 Ascending reticular activating system. (Modified from Lindsay, 1958, *Reticular Formation of the Brain*. Little Brown, New York).

Delirium is a confusional state in which the patient is anxious, excited, agitated and often hallucinating. *Delirium tremens* is a condition seen in heavy drinkers who suddenly cease drinking alcohol, often because of admission to hospital. It is characterized by agitation, mental confusion, hallucinations, tremor, sweating and tachycardia. It may be fatal if not recognized and treated. Other neurological complications of alcoholism include withdrawal seizures (p. 189), peripheral neuropathy (p. 150), cerebellar degeneration (pp. 129–130), Wernicke's encephalopathy (pp. 220–221) and Korsakoff's psychosis (p. 267).

Confusional states and delirium are common and may be caused by a variety of aetiological factors which include drugs, fevers, infections, metabolic disorders, cerebral anoxia, head injuries, cerebrovascular disease and post-epileptic states.

Lethargy The subject is drowsy and indifferent to his surroundings but responds to verbal stimuli. Obtundation is a term also used to describe such a state of dull indifference.

Stupor The patient is unconscious but can be aroused by pain and can give some sort of voluntary response.

Coma The patient is unrousable and primitive reflexes only are present.

These are all terms to describe different states of unconsciousness, but in examining a patient it is most important to make a detailed record of the patient's clinical state and reactions rather than to use one of these labels, which are capable of different interpretations by different observers. The Glasgow coma scale is widely used in the assessment of level of consciousness particularly in patients with head injury; scores are assigned for: (i) eye opening; (ii) verbal response; (iii) motor response (Table 14.1).

There are certain conditions that should be recognized clinically in which there is a chronic state of alteration in consciousness.

Table 14.1   Glasgow coma scale

	Score
Eyes open	
Never	1
To pain	2
To verbal stimuli	3
Spontaneously	4
Best verbal response	
No response	1
Incomprehensible sounds	2
Inappropriate words	3
Disorientated and converses	4
Orientated and converses	5
Best motor response	
No response	1
Extension (decerebrate rigidity)	2
Abnormal flexion of upper limbs (decorticate rigidity)	3
Flexion — withdrawal of pain	4
Localizes pain	5
Obeys commands	6
Total	15

Persistent vegetative state

This is the term given by Jennett and Plum to a syndrome that follows severe brain damage. Following head injury patients are in a deep coma, not opening their eyes for a week or more. They then begin to open their eyes, at first in response to painful stimuli and then spontaneously. They have roving eye movements and the eyes blink to menacing gestures. They appear to be inattentive and have no awareness of their surroundings. They may be in a decorticate or decerebrate posture, they have primitive reflexes including pouting and sucking reflexes, grasp reflex, and withdrawal reflexes on painful stimulation. Plantar responses are extensor. Chewing and teeth grinding are common, they can swallow and may groan or grunt. The condition is due to extensive brain damage of cortical, subcortical and brain-stem structures. *Akinetic mutism* is a term used to describe a state of apparent wakefulness with lack of verbal or motor response.

Locked-in syndrome

This is a condition that may be confused with coma, or the persistent vegetative state and which is important to recognize since the patient is aware. The limbs and lower cranial nerves are paralysed, the patient is unable to speak, but is conscious and can indicate understanding by blinking the eyes and by vertical eye movements. The lesion is most commonly an infarct of the ventral aspect of the pons; it interrupts the motor pathways but spares the tegmentum, including the reticular formation and the supranuclear pathways for eye-movement control.

MECHANISMS OF COMA

Coma is caused by either or both: (i) widespread lesions affecting the whole of the cerebral cortex, e.g. metabolic processes, head injury; (ii) lesions involving directly or indirectly the ascending reticular formation in the thalamus, mid-brain or pons. Small focal cerebral and medullary lesions are not sufficient in themselves to cause coma; it is necessary for the reticular formation to be involved before consciousness is impaired.

Anatomically, the site of lesions causing coma can be subdivided as follows: supratentorial (15%); infratentorial (15%); diffuse disorders affecting the brain, e.g. drug intoxication, metabolic disturbances (70%). Placing the disorder into one of these three categories can usually be effected by careful clinical examination.

Supratentorial lesions

Supratentorial lesions causing coma are those which involve the reticular formation directly or indirectly, such as cerebral haemorrhages, tumours, abscesses, large infarcts, subdural haematomas and head injury.

The reticular formation may be involved by bilateral deep structural lesions in the region of the thalamus, or by unilateral hemisphere lesions that have resulted in displacement of the brain, impairing secondarily the deep-lying structures. The cerebral hemispheres are confined in a rigid compartment bounded by the skull and tentorium cerebelli. When a mass lesion expands, the brain tissue shifts across the mid-line or downwards in the following ways (Fig. 14.2).

Cingulate herniation

The cingulate gyrus is displaced medially under the falx, causing compression of blood vessels; cerebral ischaemia, venous congestion and oedema result.

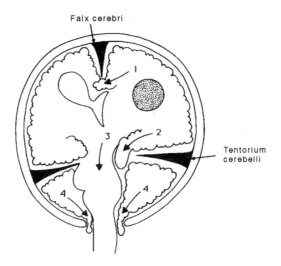

Fig. 14.2   Effect of supratentorial expanding lesions on cerebral structures. The cingulate gyrus may be herniated beneath the falx cerebri (cingulate herniation; 1), a portion of temporal lobe may be compressed between brain-stem and margin of tentorial notch (2), or the brain-stem may be displaced downwards through the tentorial opening (central herniation; 3). In expanding infratentorial lesions, or after injudicious lumbar puncture in the presence of raised intracranial pressure, the cerebellar tonsils may herniate through the foramen magnum (4). (From Lance and McLeod, 1981, with permission of Butterworths, London; modified from Plum and Posner, 1980.)

Central or transtentorial herniation

The brain-stem is forced downwards through the tentorial notch, compressing the diencephalon and mid-brain, and interfering with the blood supply to the brain-stem.

Uncal herniation

The uncus and hippocampal gyrus of the medial temporal lobe are forced through the tentorial notch, compressing the mid-brain and stretching the third nerve on the same side. The *uncal syndrome* consists of a third nerve palsy and signs of mid-brain compression. It is most commonly seen after head injuries and intra-cranial haemorrhage which is rapidly expanding. The presence of a unilateral dilating pupil in a patient after a head injury should prompt immediate neurosurgical intervention.

Subtentorial lesions

The posterior fossa is a tight inelastic compartment, so that expanding lesions such as tumours or abscesses may cause pressure on brain-stem structures with upward herniation of the brain through the tentorial notch and downward herniation of the cerebellar tonsils giving rise to medullary compression and death. Lumbar puncture is highly dangerous and should be avoided when there is raised intra-cranial pressure from any cause and in the presence of space-occupying lesions, particularly those in the subtentorial region, because it may precipitate herniation through the foramen magnum.

Metabolic and other diffuse cerebral disorders causing disturbances of consciousness

Metabolic disturbances, hypoxia, meningitis, drugs and toxins may affect the whole of the cerebral cortex or the reticular formation or both areas. There are usually no focal neurological signs on examination.

Drugs

Drug overdosage is the most frequent cause of coma in a general hospital. The drugs most commonly implicated are barbiturates, benzodiazepines, pheno-thiazines, tricyclic antidepressants, alcohol and opiates (in which case pin-point pupils are characteristic). Chemical screening tests on blood and urine will usually identify the poison.

Disorders of carbohydrate metabolism

This may be due to:

Diabetic coma When caused by diabetic ketoacidosis, the patients are dehy-drated and have deep sighing respirations (Kussmaul breathing). Hyperosmolality usually accompanies diabetic ketoacidosis. However, hyperosmolar coma, in which dehydration is a prominent feature, may occur without the presence of keto-acidosis, it is usually seen in older patients receiving oral hypoglycaemic agents or only small doses of insulin. It should be noted that there are many causes of elevated blood sugar in coma other than diabetes mellitus, e.g. cerebral infarction, head injury, meningitis.

Lactic acidosis This usually occurs in patients receiving metphormin or other oral hypoglycaemic agents. The patients have Kussmaul breathing but no ketosis. Blood glucose may or may not be elevated.

Hypoglycaemia This is often accompanied by signs of sympathetic overactivity i.e. sweating, tachycardia, dilated pupils and tremor. If untreated it will cause irreversible brain damage since brain cells require both glucose and oxygen for their metabolism. The brain contains a reserve of only about 10 g of glucose and when this supply is depleted it metabolizes its own tissues. Hypoglycaemic coma most commonly results from overdose of insulin, sulphonylureas or phenformin in diabetics but can also be caused in non-diabetics by alcohol, fasting, pancreatic islet cell tumours, hypothyroidism and hypopituitarism.

Hypoxia

The brain consumes about 15–50% of the total body oxygen requirements. Brain cells are permanently damaged after 4 min of anoxia; the hippocampus and cerebellum are particularly susceptible. The most common causes of cerebral hypoxia are cardiorespiratory arrest, chronic obstructive airways disease, pneumonia and prolonged hypotension.

Uraemia

Encephalopathy in chronic renal failure is due to multiple causes which include metabolic acidosis, electrolyte disturbances and dehydration. The acidosis is aggravated by hypotension, infection, fluid depletion and sodium restriction.

Calcium disorders

Hypocalcaemia may occur in association with uraemia or in hypoparathyroidism; tetany and fits are common. Hypercalcaemia may be seen in primary hyperparathyroidism, cancer and prolonged immobilization; dehydration, weakness, anorexia, nausea and vomiting are common features.

Hepatic coma

Patients with hepatic encephalopathy usually develop mental confusion or delirium first and then gradually lapse into coma. A characteristic feature is *asterixis*, a periodic inhibition of muscle contraction causing lapses in posture of the hands at the wrists when the arms are outstretched and the hands held dorsiflexed with fingers extended againt the examiner's hand (hepatic flap). The most important factors responsible for the development of hepatic coma are the effects of ammonia and other nitrogenous products or toxic substances such as short chain fatty acids, indoles and drugs normally detoxified in the liver. Hypoglycaemia may also contribute.

Hypothyroidism

Primary or secondary hypothyroidism may cause coma associated with hypothermia. Coma may be precipitated by cold, infection or withdrawal of thyroid drugs. Clinical features include the generalized facial characteristic of myxoedema, low body temperature and delayed relaxation of the ankle jerks. *Hypothermia* in the absence of hypothyroidism can produce almost identical clinical signs.

Water intoxication

Water intoxication may be caused by excess water ingestion, decreased water excretion (e.g. nephrotic syndrome), inappropriate antidiuretic hormone (ADH) secretion due to central cerebral lesions or carbamazepine administration, or occur as a paraendocrine phenomenon associated with carcinoma. The resulting hyponatraemia should be treated cautiously since the rapid correction may lead to a condition known as *central pontine myelinolysis*, in which there is demyelination of the central part of the base of the pons, in severe cases resulting in quadriplegia and pseudobulbar palsy.

Thiamine deficiency

Wernicke's encephalopathy is caused by thiamine deficiency and is most commonly seen in alcoholics. It may be precipitated by increased glucose intake in malnourished alcoholics who have recently been admitted to hospital. The clinical features are mental confusion, nystagmus, bilateral sixth nerve palsies and ataxia; about 80% of patients also have a peripheral neuropathy. Pathological changes are found in the mamillary bodies, the thalamus and hypothalamus, around the third ventricle, around the aqueduct in the mid-brain and the floor of the fourth ventricle. Treatment is 100 mg of thiamine intravenously daily for several days and then regular oral vitamin supplements. It should be remembered that patients with Wernicke's encephalopathy can present in coma as well as with mental confusion.

Infection

Meningitis and encephalitis may cause coma and other disturbances of consciousness. Neck stiffness is a characteristic sign of meningitis in the early stages of the illness but may be absent in a deeply comatose patient.

Epilepsy

Complex partial seizures cause mental confusion and disturbances of consciousness. Postictal state and status epilepticus should be considered in the differential diagnosis of coma.

Subarachnoid haemorrhage

Subarachnoid haemorrhage may cause loss of consciousness with or without focal neurological signs. Neck stiffness is usually present, although it may be absent in a deeply comatose patient.

Psychiatric causes of coma

It is important to remember that apparent coma may be due to hysteria or malingering. In these conditions, the respirations are usually normal in rate and depth, and the pupils react normally unless mydriatic drugs have been administered. The patient usually resists any attempt to open the eyes. Tone and deep tendon reflexes are normal and plantar responses are flexor. Abdominal reflexes are present. Slow, roving eye movements do not occur and on caloric irrigation of the ears with ice cold water, there is no tonic deviation of the eyes to the ipsilateral side, but instead the quick-phase nystagmus to the contralateral side that is characteristic of a conscious patient.

EVALUATION OF THE COMATOSE PATIENT

The questions that must be answered when examining a comatose patient are:
- Where is the lesion? Is the disease focal due to a structural lesion, or is it diffuse, due to a metabolic or toxic process? If it is focal, is it supratentorial or infratentorial?
- Is the condition progressing, improving or remaining static?
- What is the specific pathological process?

While history taking, physical examination and investigations are proceeding to answer these questions, it is essential first to protect the brain by maintaining adequate oxygenation, blood pressure, circulation and metabolism with intravenous glucose and fluids.

History

If possible, obtain from observers a description of the onset of the coma, when the patient was last seen, his behaviour at the time and his habits. Is he diabetic or epileptic? Is he alcoholic or an abuser of drugs? Has he had psychiatric treatment or emotional disturbances? Has he been treated for renal, cardiac, thyroid or respiratory disease?

Physical examination

All details should be carefully recorded.

General

Pay attention to breath, colour, skin, pulse, blood pressure, scalp wounds, temperature, urine and examination of heart, lungs and abdomen. A slowing pulse and rising blood pressure may indicate increasing intracranial pressure. A stiff neck indicates meningeal irritation due to meningitis or subarachnoid haemorrhage.

Neurological

State of consciousness Pay particular attention to, and record carefully the details of, the patient's level of consciousness. Can he be aroused? Does he respond to pain? Is he confused, agitated or delirious? Assess his level of consciousness using the Glasgow coma scale (p. 216). These details will be important in gauging progress.

Respiration Record the rate and rhythm of respiration. Different types of respiration are recognized in comatose patients. These are:

(1) *Cheyne-Stokes* This is a periodic waxing and waning of the amplitude of respiration and usually implies either a metabolic disturbance or bilateral deep hemisphere lesions, e.g. in the thalamus or internal capsule, but sometimes as low as the level of the pons.

(2) *Central neurogenic hyperventilation* Automatic overbreathing which indicates a lesion of the reticular formation in the low mid-brain or pons, or a metabolic disturbance such as diabetic ketosis or salicylate poisoning.

(3) *Apneustic respiration* There are prolonged pauses in the respiratory cycle at full inspiration. The condition is seen in pontine lesions, usually infarction.

(4) *Ataxic respiration* There is a completely irregular respiratory pattern; the condition, which is seen in medullary lesions, has a very poor prognosis.

The pupils Note the size, shape, equality and reaction to light of the pupils. Specific abnormalities to observe are the fixed dilated pupil of a third nerve palsy; Horner's syndrome which may be seen in hypothalamic and brain-stem lesions; the pupils fixed in mid-position and unreactive to light in mid-brain lesions; the pin-point pupils of pontine lesions or narcotic overdosage.

Ocular movements Remember that in unconscious patients with supratentorial hemisphere lesions the eyes are deviated towards the side of the lesion, whereas in pontine lesions the eyes are deviated away from the side of the lesion. It follows that if the patient is hemiplegic the eyes are deviated away from the hemiplegic side in supratentorial lesions, and towards the hemiplegic side in pontine lesions.

In an unconscious patient eye movements can and always should be tested reflexly in order to assist in the localization of the level of the lesion. There are two main reflexes:

(1) *The oculocephalic reflex* This is elicited by brisk head movements (doll's eye phenomenon). Rotation of the head to one side causes the eyes to turn to the opposite side. Flexion of the neck makes the eyes roll upwards and extension of the neck causes the eyes to look downwards.

(2) *The oculovestibular reflex* This is elicited by caloric irrigation. Ice cold water syringed into one ear causes the eyes to deviate to the side of the irrigation; it is a more potent stimulus of eye movements than head movement.

The oculovestibular and oculocephalic reflexes, in general, are present in supratentorial lesions or in metabolic causes of coma. The reflex eye movements are impaired when brain-stem structures are involved.

Lateral pontine lesions result in impaired conjugate eye movements towards the side of the lesion. When the medial longitudinal fasciculus is involved in the pons or mid-brain, an internuclear ophthalmoplegia will be evident. When the third nerve or its nucleus is involved, the features of a third nerve palsy will be evident on reflex stimulation. Damage to the pretectal region of the mid-brain will give rise to impaired upward gaze (Chapter 4).

Motor function Posture of the limbs, spontaneous movements, responsiveness to painful stimuli and reflexes should be observed as these may indicate the presence and site of a focal cerebral lesion. Does the patient spontaneously or reflexly move the limbs more on one side of the body than the other? Decerebrate rigidity (extension of the neck, extension, adduction and pronation of the arms, and extension of the legs with plantar flexion of the feet) is a sign that the mid-brain is involved either primarily or secondarily.

It is important to pay particular attention in comatose patients to *changes* in the patient's condition and in the observations, e.g. slowing pulse, rising blood pressure, dilating pupils.

Clinical features of metabolic disorders and other diffuse conditions causing coma

Since metabolic disorders and diffuse disease of the brain are the most common causes of coma in a general hospital it is important to recognize the clinical manifestations. In general there are no focal neurological signs.

Levels of consciousness

Changes in alertness, orientation and concentration, impairment of memory, and changes in affect and perception are common early signs of metabolic disturbances.

Respiration

Cheyne-Stokes respiration is common in metabolic disorders. Hyperventilation may result from metabolic acidosis (uraemia, diabetes, lactic acidosis or salicylates) and hypoventilation may result from metabolic alkalosis.

Pupils

The pupils usually remain responsive to light in metabolic disorders unless the patient is hypoxic or specific drugs have affected their reactions, such as atropine (causing dilated pupils), morphine, physostigmine, timolol (all causing constricted pupils) or glutethemide (pupils in mid-position).

Ocular movements

Doll's eyes manoeuvre and caloric stimulation produce conjugate movements of the eyes, unless the patient is in deep coma.

Motor activity

Focal neurological signs are not present except in some metabolic disturbances, particularly hypoglycaemia, uraemia and hepatic coma. Tremor, asterixis and myoclonus are common in metabolic disturbances.

MANAGEMENT OF COMA

The immediate management of the comatose patient is to maintain *basic life support* by:
- Clearing the airway of foreign material
- Tilting the head backwards and supporting the jaw
- Applying mouth-to-mouth resuscitation if necessary
- Nursing in the lateral position to allow adequate drainage of saliva and vomitus

After these emergency measures have been undertaken the patient may require *advanced life support* with:
- Oxygen therapy
- Monitoring and maintenance of blood pressure
- Intravenous fluids and restoration of acid-base balance

- Intravenous glucose and thiamine
- Careful nursing care with attention to skin, bowels, and bladder
- Artificial respiration

INVESTIGATIONS IN COMA

General

Full blood count, blood glucose, serum electrolytes (note patterns of abnormality in diabetic hyperosmolar states, inappropriate ADH secretion, lactic acidosis), liver function tests, drug screen, urine examination, chest X-ray.

After blood has been taken inject 50 mL of 50% glucose intravenously as a routine if there is any possibility of hypoglycaemia. Similarly, 100 mg thiamine should be given parenterally if Wernicke's encephalopathy or nutritional deficiency is suspected.

Neurological

A computed tomography (CT) scan or magnetic resonance imaging (MRI) is essential if a mass lesion is suspected. Lumbar puncture is indicated only if infection or subarachnoid haemorrhage is suspected and if a space-occupying lesion has already been excluded.

BRAIN DEATH

Brain death is the state in which brain tissue is damaged to such an extent that vital cerebral functions are irreversibly damaged, regardless of whether or not the heart is beating. It is now widely accepted legally as a criterion of death.

In order to make the diagnosis of brain death the patient must be deeply comatose and there should be no possibility of the coma being due to drugs, hypothermia, or reversible metabolic and endocrine causes. The diagnosis of the cause of brain death must be fully established.

The diagnostic tests for confirmation of brain death are those which establish that all brain-stem reflexes are absent, namely:
- The pupils are fixed in diameter and do not respond to light
- Corneal reflexes are absent
- There are no eye movements in response to caloric irrigation of the ears (absent vestibulo-ocular reflexes)
- There are no reflex responses to noxious stimulation of the face
- Gag reflexes are absent and there is no response to tugging an intratracheal tube.
- There is no spontaneous respiration when the patient is disconnected from a ventilator for a time sufficient to ensure that the carbon dioxide tension has risen above the threshold for stimulation of respiration.

- Brain-stem reflexes remain absent despite repeated testing at intervals of up to 24 hours.

REFERENCES

Bates D. (1993) The management of medical coma. *Journal of Neurology, Neurosurgery and Psychiatry*, **56**, 589–598.

Multisociety Task Force on PVS (1994) Medical aspects of the persistent vegetative state. *New England Journal of Medicine*, **330**, 1499–1508; 1572–1579.

Plum F. and Posner J. B. (1980) *The Diagnosis of Stupor and Coma*, 3rd edn. F. A. Davis, Philadelphia.

15 | Extrapyramidal disorders

THE EXTRAPYRAMIDAL SYSTEM

By definition, the extrapyramidal system consists of all descending motor pathways that do not run through the pyramids of the medulla. Extrapyramidal fibres arise from almost all areas of the neocortex, particularly the sensorimotor area, and project from the cortex to subcortical nuclei, the basal ganglia and then to the brain-stem and spinal cord. Extrapyramidal activity is finally expressed through reticulospinal, rubrospinal and vestibulospinal pathways in the medulla which are influenced by the basal ganglia and cerebral cortex (Fig. 15.1).

The extrapyramidal system complements the function of the pyramidal tract in controlling *tone, posture* and *movement*. It is responsible for maintenance of the upright posture and for movements involving axial (neck and trunk) and proximal muscles, while the pyramidal tract promotes abduction of the upper limbs, flexion of the lower limbs and movement of distal muscles, especially fine skilled finger movements. When normal subjects stand upright with upper limbs flexed and lower limbs extended to resist the force of gravity they are in a posture of reflex standing, determined primarily by vestibulospinal and associated pathways. When this posture is assumed voluntarily, it can be interrupted by pyramidal activity so that the limbs are then placed in a position appropriate for a planned movement, which requires active extension of the upper limbs and flexion of the lower limbs (as in walking). When the posture of reflex standing is assumed involuntarily as the result of damage to the cortex or basal ganglia it cannot be altered voluntarily and is then called the *decorticate posture* or *dystonia-in-extension* (extension here referring to the lower limbs). This posture may be seen as the end result of damage to the caudate nucleus and putamen as in Huntington's chorea and dystonia musculorum deformans. When this posture involves one side only as a result of contralateral cerebral damage it is known as the *hemiplegic posture*. In Parkinson's disease, on the other hand, selective damage to the nigrostriatal system may lead finally to a posture in which both upper and lower limbs are flexed (*dystonia-in-flexion*).

When one pyramidal tract is destroyed in primates (including man), the extrapyramidal system remaining intact, movements may recover 85% of their power and dexterity, leaving slight weakness of upper limb abductors and lower limb flexors and loss of discrete movements of the digits.

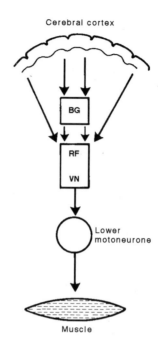

Cerebral cortex

BG

RF

VN

Lower motoneurone

Muscle

Fig. 15.1 Extrapyramidal system. Fibres of cortical origin project to basal ganglia (BG), reticular formation (RF), vestibular nuclei (VN) and other subcortical structures. Extrapyramidal projections to the lower motor neurone are mainly through the reticulospinal and vestibulospinal tracts.

The basal ganglia

The basal ganglia include the *caudate nucleus* and *putamen* (neostriatum) which receive input from the cerebral cortex, mid-line thalamic nuclei and reticular formation, and project to the *globus pallidus* (palaeostriatum) and *substantia nigra*. Output from the neostriatum passes through the globus pallidus to make the following connections: (i) to the ventrolateral (VL) nucleus of the thalamus (Fig. 15.2) either directly by the ansa lenticularis and fasciculus lenticularis which loop across the internal capsule, or indirectly via part of the substantia nigra (zona reticulata) which is homologous to the pallidum and, like the pallidum, projects to the VL nucleus; (ii) to the medial nuclei of the thalamus, which are a rostral extension of the reticular formation (Fig. 15.3); (iii) to the subthalamic nucleus (Fig. 15.4).

Since the VL nucleus of the thalamus projects back to the sensorimotor cortex a circuit is formed (cortex → striatum → thalamus → cortex) which can play a part in the programming of movement or in feedback control of a movement in progress. The connections with the reticular formation on the other hand form a loop concerned with the control of muscle tone through the reticulospinal and vestibulospinal pathways.

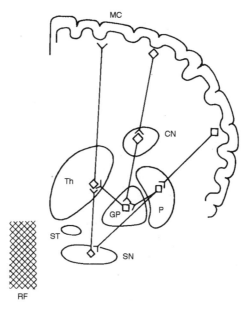

Fig. 15.2 Cortico-strio-thalamo-cortical loop. Corticofugal fibres concerned with the programming and feedback of movement pass to the caudate nucleus (CN) and putamen (P). The caudate nucleus and putamen project to the ventrolateral nucleus of the thalamus (Th) via the globus pallidus (GP) and substantia nigra (SN), and thence to the motor cortex (MC).

There are two other regulatory circuits of clinical significance (Fig. 15.4): (i) part of the substantia nigra (zona compacta) gives origin to the nigrostriatal pathway which regulates activity in the caudate and putamen through a dopaminergic pathway. Degeneration of this pathway is one of the main causes of symptoms in Parkinson's disease. There is a reciprocal pathway from the striatum to substantia nigra using GABA as a transmitter; (ii) the *subthalamic nucleus* projects to globus pallidus by an inhibitory pathway which presumably regulates the control of axial and proximal movements by the striatum, because damage to this pathway releases flinging and rotary movements (ballistic movements) of the limbs which are seen unilaterally in the clinical condition of *hemiballismus*. This condition is usually short lived and settles in a few days.

PARKINSON'S DISEASE

In 1884, Professor Charcot wrote to a Dr Nunn, saying 'I have seen your patient suffering from paralysis agitans, Parkinson's disease as I call it'. This is the first time that the name of James Parkinson was applied to 'shaking palsy' although his monograph was published 67 years before, in 1817. Parkinson's description of the disease reads 'involuntary tremulous motion, with lessened muscular

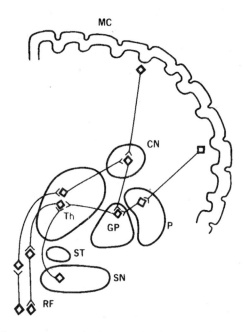

Fig. 15.3 Reciprocal connection with the reticular formation. Fibres from the caudate nucleus (CN) and putamen (P) project through the globus pallidus (GP) to medial thalamic nuclei and thence to the reticular formation (RF) of the mid-brain. Fibres from substantia nigra (SN) also feed into the same pathway. The reticular formation projects back through medial thalamic nuclei to the caudate nucleus. This circuit appears to be concerned with the control of muscle tone.

power, in parts not in action and even when supported, with a propensity to bend the trunk forwards, and to pass from a walking to a running pace: the senses and intellects being uninjured'. The description remains valid except the last phrase, since there is now known to be intellectual failure in some patients.

Aetiology

This condition is a degenerative disorder of the central nervous system affecting primarily the substantia nigra. The most common form of Parkinson's disease (affecting about 1/1000 of the population) is *idiopathic* (*paralysis agitans*); it usually appears after the age of 50 and a family history may be obtained in 4–16% of cases. The *postencephalitic* form which followed a worldwide epidemic of encephalitis lethargica after World War I is now very rare. Parkinson's disease may also be secondary to drugs (especially dopamine antagonists such as pheno-thiazines, alpha methyl dopa and reserpine), carbon monoxide, methyl bromide, manganese poisoning and 1-methyl-4-phenyl-1,2,3,6,-tetrahydropyridine (MPTP), a contaminant of synthetic opiates. A similar extrapyramidal syndrome may follow head injury and vertebrobasilar ischaemia.

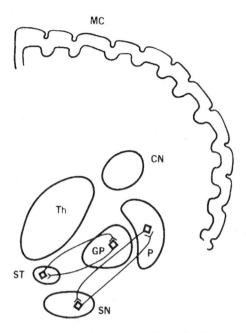

Fig. 15.4 Reciprocal connections modulating basal ganglia function. (i) With the sub-thalamic nucleus (ST). Interruption of this pathway causes hemiballismus; (ii) with the substantia nigra (SN). Striatonigral neurones inhibit SN cells by the release of GABA. The nigrostriatal pathway, which uses dopamine as a transmitter and degenerates in Parkinson's disease, inhibits cells in the putamen (P) and caudate nucleus (CN). GP = globus pallidus; Th = thalamus.

Pathophysiology

The most constant pathophysiological feature of idiopathic Parkinson's disease is the loss of melanin-containing cells in the substantia nigra and locus coeruleus as well as the dorsal motor nucleus of the vagus nerve. Degenerative changes may also be found in the cortex and cortico-striatal fibres. Ehringer and Hornykiewicz reported in 1960 that the concentration of dopamine in the neostriatum was reduced in Parkinsonian patients. There is a relative hyperactivity of striatal cholinergic mechanisms.

The failure of dopaminergic control of basal ganglia mechanisms permits the generation of rhythmic, synchronous bursts of impulses that traverse the pathway from cortex to basal ganglia to thalamus to cortex and propagate down the pyramidal tract as a tremor rhythm. The tremor of Parkinson's disease can thus be controlled by stereotactic lesions in the globus pallidus or ventrolateral nucleus of the thalamus which interrupt this circuit. The same lesions reduce rigidity in 70% of cases because of the reciprocal connections with the reticular formation that promote hyperactivity of alpha and gamma motor neurones in Parkinson's disease. Factors being investigated in the pathogenesis of Parkinson's disease include iron metabolism, increased oxidative stress from free radicals, depletion of reduced glutathion and mitochondrial complex 1 deficiency.

Clinical features

The onset is insidious with symptoms and signs comprising slowness in initiating and performing movement (*bradykinesia*), tremor, cog-wheel rigidity, loss of righting reflexes and autonomic disturbances.

Bradykinesia

There is failure to swing one or both arms on walking and difficulty in moving the feet, leading to a shuffling gait. 'Freezing' (shuffling of the feet on one spot) on attempting to walk is common. The handwriting becomes slower and smaller (*micrographia*) and there is loss of expression from face and voice (*hypomimia*).

Tremors

There are two main types of tremor in Parkinson's Disease — action tremor and resting (alternating) tremor. The characteristic resting tremor of Parkinson's disease begins in one hand although, as the disease progresses, it usually appears in the other hand, in the lower limbs and in the head. It has a median frequency of 4–5 Hz. This tremor is usually most noticeable when the patient maintains a fixed posture. An alternating movement of the thumb over the first finger gives rise to the classic 'pill-rolling' appearance. On movement, resting tremor will suppress briefly to reappear again when a posture is maintained for a few seconds. During muscle contraction, an action tremor at 6–8 Hz with synchronous beats in antagonistic muscles, becomes apparent and may often be detected in patients before resting tremor develops. The frequency of cogwheel beats is determined by the type of tremor dominant at the time of examining muscle tone.

Cog-wheel rigidity

The increased resistance to stretch on passive movement at a joint in Parkinson's disease is uniform throughout the range of movement and has a plastic or 'lead-pipe' quality. It shows little of the dynamic (velocity-sensitive) quality that characterizes the spasticity of upper motor neurone lesions. Flexor spasms and the clasp-knife phenomenon are never observed in Parkinson's disease since they depend on the release of the effects of flexor reflex afferent fibres which, in contrast to spasticity, remain under brain-stem control in Parkinson's disease. The rigidity is interrupted by a superimposed tremor mechanism that imparts a ratchet or cog-wheel sensation to the examiner as the limb is moved.

Glabella tap sign

Glabella tap sign may be present (failure to inhibit eye-blinking when the forehead is tapped repeatedly). It is of little clinical utility.

Tendon jerks

These are usually within the normal range and plantar responses remain flexor.

Posture

Body posture becomes progressively more flexed as the condition advances.

Loss of righting reflexes

Patients tend to fall and are unable to make normal corrective movements to retain balance. They may tend to totter forwards with increasing speed (*festination of gait*) or fall backwards (*retropulsion*). This becomes the most disabling feature of Parkinson's disease in its late stages.

Autonomic disturbances

Postural hypotension, excessive salivation and urgency of micturition occurs in 25% of patients. The postural hypotension is often worsened by the introduction of levodopa.

Change in intellect and mood

Depression is common in Parkinson's disease and dementia may occur later in the disease as a result of the associated cerebral atrophy.

Treatment

Principles

It is important to keep the patient as active as possible and avoid unnecessary bed-rest, to treat the mental depression that is commonly associated, and to start any form of drug therapy in low dosage because of the risk of mental confusion in the elderly.

The aim of medical treatment is to increase dopaminergic activity. This is accomplished by giving levodopa, the precursor of dopamine, since dopamine does not cross the blood-brain barrier. Levodopa is administered with a decarboxylase inhibitor to prevent the transformation of levodopa to dopamine in the gastrointestinal tract or elsewhere in the body and thus to permit higher blood levels of levodopa and greater entry through the blood-brain barrier. There is some controversy as to whether levodopa therapy is best started early in the disorder or deferred until essential to preserve freedom of movement. There is no data from clinical trials to suggest that the early introduction of levodopa is detrimental and most neurologists introduce it as soon as the patient becomes symptomatic. It is advisable for the initiation and maintenance of treatment to be supervised by a neurologist. Early in the course of Parkinson's disease the response to levodopa is gratifying and virtually complete. As the disease progresses and the number of dopaminergic neurones in the substantia nigra decreases treatment becomes more difficult. Patients tend to alternate between dyskinetic side effects of levodopa therapy and severe bradykinesia ('on–off' phenonemon). Sudden failure of dopaminergic transmission may result in 'freezing' episodes. At this point the patients frequently require smaller but more frequent doses of levodopa and the addition of a dopamine agonist such as bromocriptine may be useful. As larger doses of levodopa are used, the risk of mental confusion increases.

Pharmaceutical agents used in the management of Parkinson's disease

Dopaminergic agents

Levodopa   Levodopa is now given in combination with a decarboxylase inhibitor (Chapter 24). Dosage is usually increased slowly from 50–100 mg three times daily to a maximum of 1–1.5 g daily which may be divided into 4–8 doses if necessary to smooth fluctuations in blood levels. Side effects include postural hypotension and involuntary movements usually of the mouth, tongue and extremities (peak dose dyskinesia).

Bromocriptine   Bromocriptine is a dopamine agonist with a long half-life which may be given in low dosage (2.5–40 mg daily) alone or in conjunction with a levodopa preparation. It has also been used in larger doses of 40–60 mg daily. Its long half-life permits fewer daily doses and helps reduce the 'on–off' phenomenon. It often causes mental confusion in larger doses.

Selegiline   This inhibitor of monoamine oxidase B reduces the breakdown of dopamine and is a useful addition to levodopa therapy in resistant cases. There is some evidence to suggest that selegiline may slow the progression of Parkinson's disease by mopping up free radicals and it is used as the initial treatment in many countries for this reason.

Amantadine   Amantadine releases dopamine from body stores and may be helpful in the early stages of the disease.

Anticholinergic (atropine-like) drugs

An example is benzhexol (Artane), available as 2 mg and 5 mg tablets. Dosage is best started at 1 mg three times daily which, if it is well tolerated, can be increased slowly up to 5 mg three times daily. Side effects include mental confusion, dry mouth, blurred vision and difficulty in starting micturition. Anticholinergic drugs are usually contra-indicated in glaucoma and should be used with great caution in the elderly. In recent years, with the availability of a range of dopamine agonists, the anticholinergics have been much less used in the treatment of Parkinson's disease, but are still occasionally useful for the control of resting tremor.

CORTICOBASAL DEGENERATION

Corticobasal degeneration is a rare progressive degenerative disease that affects the extrapyramidal system. It presents with an asymmetrical akinetic rigid syndrome and is often mistaken for Parkinson's disease. There is however no response to levodopa and no resting tremor. There may be flurries of fine myoclonus in the flexor muscles of the forearm on attempted movement and this is often mistaken for an action tremor. The condition usually starts in the hand and is associated with a characteristic dystonic posture with the hand flexed and the thumb flexed across the palm. There is usually a marked apraxia such that the hand becomes useless to the patient although it is not actually weak. The disease progresses to involve the foot on the same side and then spreads to the other side of the body. Late in the disease there may be prominent dysarthria. Intellect is preserved until late in the disease. The disease is associated with neuropathological evidence of degeneration in the basal ganglia and in the motor and premotor cortex. Characteristic large pale ballooned neurones are seen in these areas. These cells are indistinguishable from Pick's cells. The disease is sporadic and of unknown aetiology.

CHOREOATHETOSIS

Two major types of movement disorder, chorea and athetosis are distinguishable but frequently they occur together and are described as choreoathetosis.

Chorea   This consists of involuntary, continuous, rapid, irregular, jerky movements which affect the face, tongue, lips, trunk and limbs, chiefly in their distal parts. Voluntary actions may be severely interrupted and impaired by choreiform movements. The precise site of the lesions causing chorea is not certain, although there is evidence that the caudate nucleus is involved.

Athetosis   An instability or fluctuation of posture which commonly affects the hands, arms and face, and less commonly the lower limbs. The movements are slow and writhing ('mobile spasm') and an alternation between two basic postures is usually recognizable; namely pronated forearm, flexed wrist, flexed metacarpophalangeal joints and extended fingers, and supinated forearm, extended wrist and abducted fingers. The characteristic posture of the foot is inversion and plantar flexion. Athetosis is often associated with lesions of the putamen.

Both types of involuntary movement are often seen together even in conditions labelled as chorea. Choreoathetotic movements are a feature of the following disorders.

Sydenham's (rheumatic) chorea

This is an immune disorder most commonly affecting young women, which follows weeks after a streptococcal sore throat in a manner similar to rheumatic fever. Since the course is benign, autopsy studies are few but cellular infiltration has been reported in cortex, basal ganglia and cerebellum. It usually resolves spontaneously over a period varying from 1 week to several years. Pure choreiform movements are often seen in this condition. Chorea may also be seen in young women with either frank *systemic lupus erythematosus* or circulating anti-phospholipid antibodies (*lupus anti-coagulant*).

Huntington's disease

Huntington's disease is an hereditary progressive dementia, preceded by or associated with choreoathetotic movements, which is inherited as an autosomal dominant characteristic. The age of onset is usually 30–50 years. The caudate nucleus atrophies and neuronal degeneration can also be demonstrated in frontal cortex and putamen. Gamma-aminobutyric acid (GABA), glutamic acid decarboxylase (GAD), and the synthesizing enzyme for acetylcholine, choline acetyltransferase (CAT) are depleted in Huntington's disease. There is no evidence that dopaminergic neurones are released from inhibitory influence but nevertheless there seems to be undue sensitivity of neurones to dopamine. Involuntary movements are made worse by levodopa and are reduced by dopamine-blocking agents such as phenothiazines and butyrophenones (e.g. haloperidol) or by catecholamine-depleting agents such as reserpine or tetrabenazine. Medication does not alter the progressive dementia. Huntington's disease has been shown to be associated with a repeat series of trinucleotides on the short arm of chromosome 4. Subsequent generations may show an increase in the number of repeats and in the clinical severity of the disease. Accurate genetic and pre-natal diagnosis is now available.

Senile chorea

A similar clinical picture to Huntington's disease may be observed in some ageing patients without a family history. The relationship of this condition to Huntington's disease is now being examined with genetic studies.

Cerebral palsy

Infants subjected to hypoxia or other causes of diffuse brain damage *in utero*, at birth, or in early childhood may have choreoathetosis, upper motor neurone signs and intellectual impairment in varying combinations. The main pathological changes are periventricular lesions in the white matter, although signs of old cortical infarction may also be seen. Since mental ability may be normal, every attempt should be made to assess these children accurately so that they can be given appropriate educational opportunity.

Rhesus blood group incompatibility with resulting haemolytic jaundice can cause damage to the basal ganglia (*kernicterus*) because unconjugated bilirubin passes through the blood-brain barrier. The clinical picture resembles cerebral palsy with the addition in some cases of bilateral nerve deafness. Better control of bilirubin levels in neonatal intensive care units has led to a dramatic reduction in the incidence of kernicterus.

Encephalitis in early childhood may also produce a similar syndrome.

Metabolic disorders

Wilson's disease (hepatolenticular degeneration) is a rare deficiency of the copper-binding protein coeruloplasmin in the plasma, with an autosomal recessive inheritance. Copper is deposited in the putamen, thalamus and basal nuclei of the cerebellum and in the outer margin of the cornea where it can be seen as a brown band at the corneo-scleral junction (*Kayser-Fleischer ring*), and is excreted in excess in the urine. The cerebral deposition of copper occurs during episodes of acute hepatic necrosis related to excess copper storage in hepatocytes.

The neurological signs produced include choreoathetotic movements, cerebellar disturbance, a coarse slow postural tremor of the abducted arms ('wing-beating' or 'red nucleus' tremor) and development of dystonia-in-extension. The patients also have progressive cirrhosis of the liver and often aminoaciduria. Progress of the disease may be halted by chelation therapy to help rid the body of excess copper.

Choreoathetosis may also be seen as a sequel to hypoxia or as a symptom of uraemic, hepatic or hypercapnic encephalopathy.

DRUG-INDUCED DYSKINESIAS

Some phenothiazines such as fluphenazine (Stelazine), triethylperazine (Torecan), prochlorperazine (Stemetil) and metoclopramide (Maxolon), and some butyrophenones, such as haloperidol (Serenace), can cause acute dystonic reactions shortly after they are injected or taken orally. The reactions may consist of *akathisia* (motor restlessness), the assumption of a dystonic posture, or choreoathetotic movements. The reaction is rapidly reversed by the injection of an anticholinergic agent such as benztropine (Cogentin), 2 mg, i.v.

The prolonged use of such drugs may cause the gradual development of a persistent choreoathetotic syndrome (*tardive dyskinesia* — 'tardive' because it is slow in developing) which responds poorly to withdrawal of the offending drug and to drug treatment.

DYSTONIA

Dystonia is a disorder in which attempted voluntary movement leads to tonic contraction of antagonistic muscle groups causing part or whole of the body to assume an abnormal posture. At first such postures are transient but may become permanent as 'dystonia-in-flexion' or 'dystonia-in-extension'. Dystonic features may become superimposed on other basal ganglia disorders and may progress until the patient remains in a permanent dystonic posture.

The idiopathic dystonias may be generalized (dystonia musculorum deformans) or focal. Dystonias may be secondary to a known cause (drugs, strokes, kernicterus).

Dystonia musculorum deformans

Dystonia musculorum deformans (torsion dystonia) is a rare disorder which may be familial (autosomal dominant or recessive) or sporadic. An autosomal dominant form in people of Ashkenazi Jewish descent has been localized to chromosome 9

(9q34). The disorder starts in childhood with 'freezing' of gait similar to that seen in Parkinson's disease or with twisting movements of the head and trunk. Speech becomes slow and the mouth may be held open by excessive muscular contraction. The limbs become rigid so that writing and other hand movements are impaired and the patient has to swing the pelvis to place the lower limbs for walking. A form which fluctuates in severity during the day has been reported to respond to levodopa, but generally treatment with dopamine-blocking agents such as tetrabenazine gives greater, although modest, benefit. Anticholinergic drugs, phenothiazines and butyrophenones are also used. Stereotactic thalamotomy is helpful in some cases.

Focal dystonias

These are much more common than dystonia musculorum deformans and are frequently mistaken for manifestations of hysteria, particularly as the symptoms of all basal ganglia disorders become worse with emotional stress. No neuro-pathological changes have been described at autopsy and the focal dystonias are considered most likely to be disorders of neurotransmitters localized to various parts of the basal ganglia. They are made worse by levodopa (indeed they may appear as side effects when levodopa is given to patients with Parkinson's disease) and benefit to some extent from dopamine-blocking agents. Some patients improve with biofeedback training and psychological management. Recognized focal dystonias include:

Occupational dystonias Focal dystonias may appear in the muscles involved in repetitive skilled movements. One of the original descriptions of this was in Morse code operators but its most common manifestation today is writer's cramp. In this condition writing is distorted by co-contraction of antagonistic muscles in the hand and forearm. Undue muscle contraction extends proximally to the shoulder girdle. Occupational dystonias may also be seen in musicians, typists and sportsmen.

Torticollis The head and neck turn involuntarily to one side. The condition is at first spasmodic but may become permanent. *Retrocollis* (extension of the neck) and *anterocollis* (flexion of the neck) are related disorders.

Blepharospasm and orofacial dyskinesia Involuntary closure of the eyelids (blepharospasm) and grimacing movements of the mouth and face (orofacial dyskinesia) may occur as separate entities or in association, in which case the combination is known as *Meige's syndrome*. The onset is usually in late middle age or in the elderly. Blepharospasm has been reported to respond to clonazepam therapy but this has not been our experience. Phenothiazines such as thioridazine (Melleril) are helpful in some cases. Injection of minute quantities of botulinum toxin into the periocular muscles relieves the condition for some months and may be repeated as necessary. Similar injections into neck muscles are useful in the management of torticollis.

Laryngeal dystonia Spasm of the larynx on attempting to speak gives a forced grating quality to the voice resembling that of chronic laryngitis. This also reponds well to treatment with botulinum toxin.

GILLES DE LA TOURETTE SYNDROME

Tics are stereotyped movements usually of the face but less commonly of the upper limbs that are produced as a habit, usually in response to stress. They are very common in childhood and most children will have one or more tics between the ages of 2 and 6.

The syndrome of Gilles de la Tourette is a disorder in which multiple tics develop in children or adolescents. They are frequently accompanied by vocal tics in which grunting or coughing noises interrupt the normal conversation. In some cases expletives may be uttered during the compulsive expiration (*coprolalia*). Tourette's syndrome is commonly familial and is inherited as an autosomal dominant. In some families a linkage has been found to chromosome 18. Severe cases usually respond to therapy with dopamine-blocking agents such as haloperidol.

HEMIBALLISMUS

Destruction of the subthalamic nucleus or its connections by infarction or haemorrhage causes the sudden onset of wild involuntary movements involving the proximal muscles of the limbs on the opposite side of the body. The disorder usually subsides with time but can be controlled with dopamine-blocking agents and abolished by stereotactic thalamotomy on the side contralateral to the ballistic movements.

PAROXYSMAL CHOREOATHETOSIS

This is an unusual and intriguing syndrome in which the assumption of a dystonic posture or involuntary choreoathetotic movements appear transiently and intermittently. There are two main forms:

Paroxysmal kinesigenic choreoathetosis Attacks are induced by startle or movement, hence the term 'kinesigenic', and last for a few seconds to several minutes at a time. The condition may be familial or sporadic.

Paroxysmal dystonic choreoathetosis A rare familial condition, in which the attacks persist much longer, for hours rather than minutes, and are precipitated by excitement or the taking of alcohol or coffee. The cause is unknown but appears to be a periodic disinhibition of basal ganglia mechanisms.

The kinesigenic form responds to anticonvulsants such as carbamazepine (Tegretol) and phenytoin (Dilantin). The dystonic form does not improve with these agents but does appear to be prevented by clonazepam (Rivotril).

TREMOR

Not all tremors are caused by diseases of the basal ganglia but the problem is logically reviewed at the conclusion of a chapter on these disorders. The following tremors are commonly encountered:

Physiological tremor

Maintenance of posture or voluntary movements is accompanied by a fine tremor in normal subjects. This tremor is a reflection of the resonant mechanical properties of an outstretched limb and is provoked by unfused motor unit contractions. The frequency of the tremor is related to the resonant frequency of the body part involved. Thus, for instance, the fingers will have a fast tremor of 12–15 Hz, the wrist a slower tremor of about 8 Hz and the arm at the shoulder a much slower tremor at 3 or 4 Hz. Agents which increase the force of muscle twitch contractions will exacerbate this tremor which is then called *enhanced physiological tremor*. Such situations include increased levels of circulating adrenergic compounds or adrenergic drugs (anxiety, fatigue, hunger, thyrotoxicosis, coffee, beta agonist drugs and theophylline).

Senile tremor

As age advances, many subjects develop an increase in their physiological tremor which may become symptomatic, particularly during slow movements such as drinking a glass of water.

Familial or 'essential' tremor

This may take different forms but commonly resembles an exaggerated physiological tremor or senile tremor with some accentuation on attempting fine coordinated movements. It is improved temporarily by taking alcohol, or more consistently by taking regular medication with the beta-blocking agent propranolol (Inderal), the barbiturate anticonvulsant primidone (Mysoline), or by taking drugs of the benzodiazepine series such as diazepam (Valium). It is inherited as an autosomal dominant trait.

Parkinson's disease

The tremors of Parkinson's disease are centrally generated and comprise alternating (resting) and synchronous (action) tremors. Resting tremor has a frequency of 4–5 Hz which is preserved in all body parts where the tremor is expressed. Although called a 'rest tremor' the tremor may disappear if the subject is lying down and is completely relaxed. It appears on maintenance of any posture including sitting. The tremor is increased in amplitude by walking or by performing mental arithmetic. The movement of the thumb rhythmically over the pulp of the index finger produces the characteristic 'pill-rolling' tremor.

Mid-brain tremor ('red nucleus' or 'wing-beating' tremor)

This is a coarse alternating movement seen in the outstretched or abducted upper limb with lesions of the mid-brain or of the superior cerebellar peduncle. It may be seen in metabolic disorders such as Wilson's disease, or more commonly, in multiple sclerosis or vascular disease.

Intention tremor

Damage to the cerebellar hemispheres or their dentatothalamic projections gives rise to a tremor at 3–8 Hz which increases in amplitude as the limb approaches its target in coordinated movement. Intention tremor (and the mid-brain tremor which occasionally accompanies it) can be diminished by medication with clonazepam and abolished by stereotactic thalamotomy.

Asterixis

This is the so-called 'flapping tremor' of the outstretched hands seen in hepatic encephalopathy and other metabolic disorders. It is not strictly a tremor but is the result of episodic inhibition of muscles sustaining posture against gravity.

Hysteria

Coarse tremors may be observed in hysterical cases, sometimes with jactitations of the limbs resembling an epileptic fit to the unseasoned eye, and sometimes with a calculated and precise misplacement of the finger on approaching a target which could suggest intention tremor to an unwary observer.

REFERENCES

Fahn S. (1992) Parkinson's disease and other basal ganglion disorders. In: *Diseases of the Nervous System*, 2nd edn. Eds A. K. Asbury, G. M. McKhann and W. I. McDonald. W. B. Saunders, Philadelphia. 1144–1158.

Marsden C. D. and Fahn S. (1994) *Movement Disorders*. Butterworth-Heinemann, London.

Marsden C. D. (1994) Parkinson's disease. *Journal of Neurology, Neurosurgery and Psychiatry*, **57**, 672–681.

16 Infections of the central nervous system

The chief infections of the nervous system are meningitis, encephalitis and abscess.

Meningitis is inflammation of the meninges. It may be classified as purulent or pyogenic (i.e. meningitis due to bacterial infections), fungal, or aseptic (most commonly due to viral infections but sometimes caused by chemicals, physical agents, parasites and malignant infiltration).

Encephalitis is inflammation of the brain substance itself. It is often accompanied by inflammation of the meninges (meningo-encephalitis). Acute disseminated encephalomyelitis is a diffuse demyelination of the brain and spinal cord which is usually an immune reaction following infections such as mumps, influenza, chicken pox, rubella, vaccinations or other injections.

MENINGITIS

Acute bacterial meningitis

Infections may reach the meninges through the bloodstream or by direct spread from the middle ear and paranasal sinuses or through skull fractures. The most common organisms causing meningitis are *Neisseria meningitidis* (meningococcus), *Streptococcus pneumoniae* (pneumococcus), and *Haemophilus influenzae*. In the neonatal period Gram-negative organisms (e.g. *E. coli, Proteus, Pseudomonas*) and Group B streptococci are common causative organisms. *Haemophilus influenzae* meningitis occurs in infants predominantly, whereas infection by pneumococcus and meningococcus may occur at all ages. In immunosuppressed patients, less common organisms such as *Listeria monocytogenes* may be responsible.

Pathology

The fundamental process is an inflammation of the leptomeninges with hyperaemia of the meningeal vessels, followed by migration of neutrophils into the subarachnoid space. The exudate rapidly extends into the walls of blood vessels and along cranial and spinal nerves. Foci of necrosis develop in walls of veins and arteries, sometimes leading to thrombosis which may be manifested clinically by convulsions and focal neurological signs. Accumulation of fibrino-purulent exudate at the base of the brain may block the flow of cerebrospinal fluid (CSF) causing hydrocephalus. Loculation of infection to form abscesses may be a further complication.

Clinical features

In adults the signs and symptoms are fever, headache, neck stiffness, nausea, vomiting, drowsiness, confusion and sometimes convulsions. Neck stiffness is a cardinal sign in adults and older children, but it may be absent in infants and neonates in whom the main clinical features are irritability, lethargy, feeding difficulties, vomiting, respiratory distress and fever. Focal neurological signs are usually absent unless complications develop.

Complications include: acute hydrocephalus, with herniation of the brain-stem and temporal lobes through the tentorial notch, or of the cerebellum and medulla through the foramen magnum (Chapter 14); thromboses of venous sinuses or cortical vessels causing seizures, hemiplegia and other focal neuro-logical signs (Chapter 13); cranial nerve palsies and deafness; subdural effusion; communicating hydrocephalus due to adhesions at the base of the brain or non-communicating hydrocephalus from obstruction of the aqueduct of Sylvius or foramina of Luschka and Magendie (Chapter 18).

Management

Lumbar puncture with examination of the CSF is essential for diagnosis and should be carried out without delay when meningitis is suspected. Blood cultures should be performed, and sources of infection should be carefully sought in ears (otitis media), paranasal sinuses, heart (bacterial endocarditis), lungs, and skin.

Treatment consists of:

Antibacterial chemotherapy Initially, therapy should be administered intra-venously. When the organism is unknown treatment in adults is commenced with ampicillin (2 g, i.v. every 4 h) or benzyl penicillin (2.4 g, i.v. every 4 h) usually with cefotaxime (2 g every 8 h) or ceftriaxone (2 g, i.v. once daily). Chloramphenicol (4–6 g/day) is administered only if the patient is allergic to cephalosporins. In children, empirical treatment is commenced with ampicillin (200 mg/kg per day) and cefotaxime (200 mg/kg per day) or ceftriaxone (80 g/kg per day) and chlo-ramphenicol (75–100 mg/kg per day) if there is allergy to cephalosporins. Specific treatment subsequently depends on the results of culturing the causative organism in the CSF.

Supportive measures These include general nursing care, attention to air-ways, reduction of fever, hydration and maintenance of fluid and electrolyte balance.

Treatment of complications Specific treatment is given if they occur, e.g. sei-zures, hydrocephalus, abscess.

Tuberculous meningitis

The onset is usually gradual with non-specific symptoms of lethargy and headaches followed by mental confusion. Later complications include seizures and arteritis causing focal neurological signs. Diagnosis depends on the clinical features and CSF findings; commonly the organism is not cultured but may be detected by polymerase chain reaction (PCR) of the CSF. Treatment is specific chemotherapy, i.e. isoniazid (300 mg/day), rifampicin (600 mg/day), ethambutol (15–25 mg/kg per day) and pyrazinamide (25 mg/kg per day).

Fungal infections

Fungal infections may also cause a chronic meningitis with an insidious onset and clinical features similar to those of tuberculous meningitis. The most common organism is *Cryptococcus neoformans*. Others include *Candida, Aspergillus* and *Histoplasma*. Most cases of fungal infection of the nervous system occur in immunosuppressed patients (especially HIV positive individuals) and in those with lymphoma, leukaemia and other malignancies, but they may present in otherwise healthy patients. Diagnosis is made on lumbar puncture by the characteristic appearances of the CSF and by culturing the organism, as well as detection of capsular antigen in serum and CSF.

Cryptococcal meningitis is treated with amphotericin B and 5-fluorocytosine or fluconazole.

Parasitic infections

Toxoplasmosis causes meningo-encephalitis and brain abscesses usually in patients with AIDS, malignancies, or in those who are receiving immunosuppressive therapy. Treatment is with pyrimethamine and sulphonamide.

Amoebic meningo-encephalitis is most commonly caused by *Naegleria*, and the infection is usually acquired while swimming in freshwater lakes. The onset is acute with headache, fever and neck stiffness.

The nematode *Angiostrongylus cantonensis* causes an acute eosinophilic meningitis. It is well recognized in Southern Pacific regions and is acquired by eating freshwater snails and raw vegetables that have been contaminated by the parasite.

Carcinomatous meningitis

Metastatic spread of carcinoma to the leptomeninges causes a chronic meningeal reaction or meningitis which must be distinguished from infections of the meninges. The CSF contains increased lymphocytes, elevated protein and frequently a reduced glucose level. Malignant cells may be recognized in the fluid.

Viral (aseptic) meningitis

The clinical features of viral meningitis are similar to those of bacterial meningitis. The CSF contains lymphocytes but few if any, polymorphs. The glucose level is normal whereas it is usually markedly decreased in bacterial and fungal meningitis.

The distinctive features of the CSF in the different types of meningitis are shown in Table 16.1.

Table 16.1 Cerebrospinal fluid in infections of the nervous system

Infection	Cells	Protein	Glucose	Bacteriology
Normal	0–4 mononuclears	0.15–0.40 g/L	2.9–4.6 mmol/L	Negative
Acute bacterial meningitis	Thousands of polymorphs	↑	Markedly ↓	+Bacteria
Partially treated bacterial meningitis	Hundreds to thousands of mononuclears or polymorphs	N or ↑	N or ↓	+ or −
Aseptic meningitis**		N or ↑	N*	Viruses
Meningoencephalitis		N or ↑	N*	Negative or viruses
Tuberculous meningitis	Tens to hundreds of mononuclears	↑	↓	+ Acid-fast bacilli
Fungal meningitis		↑	↓	+ Organism
Carcinomatous meningitis		↑	N or ↓	Malignant cells
Neurosyphilis (meningo vascular, syphilitic meningitis, GPI)		↑ Raised γ-globulins	N*	+ Serological tests
Subacute sclerosing panencephalitis	N	↑ Raised γ-globulins	N	Very high measles antibody titre
Creutzfeldt-Jakob disease	N	N	N	N
Progressive multifocal leucoencephalopathy	N	N	N	N

N = normal; ↑ = increased; ↓ = decreased; GPI = general paralysis of the insane.
 * Glucose may be low in herpes simplex and mumps virus infections and acute syphilitic meningitis.
** Polymorphonuclears may predominate in early illness.

Usually the causative virus is not determined, unless viral cultures of the CSF, throat washings and stools are performed but the most common causes of viral meningitis are ECHO, Coxsackie, mumps, herpes simplex and measles. The polio virus can cause an aseptic meningitis but fortunately poliomyelitis is now rare.

ENCEPHALITIS

Encephalitis is usually caused by a viral infection of the brain and is associated commonly with aseptic meningitis. The main clinical features are headaches, fever, delirium, convulsions and focal neurological signs. Herpes simplex, mumps and arboviruses are the most commonly identified organisms.

Herpes simplex encephalitis

Herpes simplex encephalitis is caused by the herpes simplex virus (HSV), usually type 1, and is one of the most common sporadic viral infections of the central nervous system. The virus enters the nervous system by way of the olfactory bulb, or a latent infection in the trigeminal ganglion may be reactivated and spread to the brain through its branches innervating the meninges. The pathology is that of a focal necrotizing encephalitis localized predominantly in the temporal lobes. Although the onset may be acute, symptoms of headache, fever, mental confusion and epileptic seizures usually evolve over several days. Examination of the CSF reveals an increased number of cells, mainly lymphocytes, and increased protein content. The virus may be detected by CSF culture (low sensitivity) or PCR for HSV in CSF (high sensitivity). Herpes simplex virus antibodies may be detected but are of little diagnostic value since they may be present in anyone who has had a previous HSV infection. Electroencephalogram (EEG) and computed tomography (CT) scans characteristically demonstrate abnormalities in one or both temporal lobes. Mortality is high and can be significantly reduced by early treatment with acyclovir (30 mg/kg per day, i.v.).

Herpes zoster

Herpes zoster is a common infection with an annual incidence of about 4/1000. The herpes zoster-varicella virus invades during primary varicella infection and lies latent in sensory ganglia. When reactivated, the symptoms of herpes zoster (shingles) are manifested by pain, a vesicular eruption and loss of sensation in the distribution of the particular nerve root. Nearby motor nerves may sometimes be involved causing localized muscle weakness and wasting. Thoracic and trigeminal nerve roots are most commonly affected. When the first division of the trigeminal nerve is involved (*herpes ophthalmicus*) corneal ulceration and iritis may result in blindness. High dose acyclovir should be administered early to prevent this complication.

The *Ramsay-Hunt syndrome* (geniculate herpes) consists of a unilateral facial palsy with herpetic eruptions in the external auditory meatus and is thought to be due to viral invasion of the geniculate ganglion although the pathogenesis is controversial. The pain of herpes zoster may persist after the rash has subsided (*post-herpetic neuralgia*) and is very distressing. It is more common after the age of 50. There is some evidence that early treatment with high dose acyclovir can reduce the incidence of post-herpetic neuralgia.

Arbovirus encephalitis

Arboviruses are arthropod-born viruses which are spread by mosquitoes and ticks. The best known are equine encephalitis and St Louis encephalitis in the United States, Japanese B encephalitis and Murray Valley (Australian) encephalitis. Ross River fever is caused by an arbovirus, but encephalitis is not a complication. The clinical features are headache, drowsiness, vomiting, convulsions and frequent focal neurological signs which may be permanent. There is no specific treatment.

Subacute sclerosing panencephalitis (SSPE)

Subacute sclerosing panencephalitis is caused by the measles virus and affects children and adolescents, evolving over some months. Early symptoms are mental and behavioural changes followed by myoclonic jerks. Death usually occurs within 1–2 years. The EEG shows characteristic periodic complexes which may be diagnostic. The CSF cell content is not increased but the protein is elevated with high immunoglobulin levels and high titres of measles virus antibodies. There is no specific treatment.

Progressive multifocal leucoencephalopathy (PML)

This is caused by the SV40 or JC papova viruses and occurs mainly in patients with HIV infection, lymphoproliferative diseases and other disorders associated with disturbed immunity. There are progressive multifocal lesions in the cerebral white matter.

Acquired immunodeficiency syndrome (AIDS)

The neurological manifestations of human immunodeficiency virus type 1 (HIV-1) infection result from opportunistic infections or from direct invasion of the brain by the retrovirus or cerebral lymphoma. Opportunistic infections of the nervous system occur in about 20% of AIDS patients and account for about 40% of the neurological manifestations. The most common are cytomegalovirus, toxoplasma and cryptococcal infections.

Cytomegalovirus (CMV)

This causes acute encephalitis or meningoencephalitis with confusion, headache, seizures and focal neurological signs; dementia, stupor and coma may supervene.

Lumbosacral polyradiculoneuropathy, retinal and optic nerve involvement, and peripheral neuropathy are other complications. Treatment is usually with ganciclovir.

Cerebral toxoplasmosis

This can present with a sudden onset of seizures and focal neurological signs, or there may be more gradual onset with fever, headache, confusion and hemiparesis or other focal signs. Computed tomography scans with contrast characteristically show ring enhancing lesions. Pyrimethamine, sulphadiazine and folinic acid are used in treatment.

Cryptococcal meningitis

Cryptococcal meningitis usually presents with fever, headache, mental confusion and seizures (see above).

Other opportunistic infections include papova viruses causing progressive multifocal leucoencephalopathy, herpes simplex and zoster, syphilis and Listeria.

AIDS-dementia complex

This is an important complication resulting from direct invasion of the brain which occurs in over 30% of AIDS patients. There is progressive mental confusion, intellectual deterioration, slowing of motor function and hyper-reflexia. Other manifestations of direct viral invasion include vacuolar myelopathy, the symptoms of which are leg weakness and paraesthesiae, ataxia and incontinence, acute or chronic inflammatory polyneuropathy and aseptic meningitis. Treatment is with high-dose zidovudine (AZT).

Prion diseases

Prions are small proteinaceous infectious particles that differ from viruses and cause transmissible degenerative diseases of the nervous system. Prion diseases are also known as slow virus infections or subacute transmissible spongiform encephalopathies. The human prion diseases include *kuru* (a disease of the cannibal New Guinea Fore Tribe, characterized by rapid, progressive cerebellar ataxia and dementia which is transmitted by eating human brains), *Creutzfeldt-Jakob* disease and *Gerstler-Sträussler-Scheinker* disease (an autosomal dominant condition linked to chromosome 20 and also characterized by ataxia and dementia). Prion diseases in animals include scrapie in sheep and bovine spongiform encephalopathy ('mad cow disease').

Creutzfeldt-Jakob disease

Creutzfeldt-Jakob disease usually presents in middle age as a rapidly progressive dementia associated with ataxia and myoclonus. Some cases are familial. Like SSPE, there is a characteristic EEG abnormality consisting of periodic complexes.

The CSF is normal. Death usually occurs within 1–2 years and there is no specific treatment.

NEUROSYPHILIS

The central nervous system is usually invaded within 2 years after the primary infection, if at all. The principal types of neurosyphilis are acute syphilitic meningitis, meningovascular syphilis, general paralysis of the insane (GPI), and tabes dorsalis. Atypical presentations may occur with HIV infection.

Acute syphilitic meningitis
Meningeal involvement usually takes place within the first 2 years of disease. Most cases are asymptomatic but others present with the typical symptoms of acute meningitis, i.e. headache, mental confusion and neck stiffness. The CSF contains an increased number of lymphocytes (100–1000 cells/mm³), elevated protein, reduced glucose and positive serological tests for syphilis.

Meningovascular syphilis
This develops about 6–7 years after the primary infection. As well as meningeal inflammation there is vasculitis with thrombotic occlusions of blood vessels. The clinical manifestations are those of cerebrovascular disease; neurosyphilis should be considered in the differential diagnosis of young people with strokes. The CSF shows increased lymphocytes, raised protein and immunoglobulin and positive serology. Spinal syphilis and syphilitic optic atrophy are specific complications of chronic syphilitic meningitis.

General paralysis of the insane
This complication usually develops about 15–20 years after the primary infection and is characterized by dementia, dysarthria, tremor, epileptic seizures, pyramidal tract signs and sometimes Argyll Robertson pupils. The CSF is abnormal with increased lymphocytes (50–200 cells/x10⁶ per L), increased protein and immunoglobulin and positive serological tests.

Tabes dorsalis
This is covered in more detail in Chapter 7.

Treatment
Benzylpenicillin 12–20 million units, i.v. daily for at least 10 days followed by either further benzylpenicillin, i.v. or daily procaine penicillin, i.m. or weekly benzathine penicillin 2.4 million units, i.m. for a total of 4 weeks. In the case of minor penicillin allergy, cefotaxime or ceftriaxone are given; in more severe penicillin sensitivity, oral tetracycline (0.5 g six-hourly for 30 days) should be prescribed.

BRAIN ABSCESS

Brain abscesses occur: (i) as complications of penetrating head wounds; (ii) following extension of infections from the middle ear or paranasal sinuses; (iii) following bloodstream infection, frequently in association with cyanotic congenital heart disease, bacterial endocarditis and pulmonary infections.

Initially, the infection commences as an inflammation of the brain parenchyma (cerebritis) with oedema, and is followed by necrosis in the centre of the lesion with pus formation. Headache, fever, lethargy, seizures and focal neurological signs are the usual presenting symptoms. The brain abscess acts as an expanding lesion causing raised intracranial pressure and papilloedema. Lumbar puncture should never be performed when an abscess is suspected. Most abscesses are visible on CT or radionuclide scans.

Treatment is antibiotic therapy; neurosurgery may be required later. Abscess has a high mortality rate and epilepsy is a complication in over 50% of survivors. Abscesses, as well as forming within the brain substance, may collect in the subdural space (subdural empyema) or in the spinal epidural space (spinal epidural abscess).

REFERENCES

Anderson M. (1993) Management of cerebral infections. *Journal of Neurology, Neurosurgery and Psychiatry*, **56**, 1243–1256.

Asbury A. K., McKhann G. M. and McDonald W. I. (Eds). (1993) Infections. In: *Diseases of the Nervous System*, 2nd edn. W. B. Saunders, Philadelphia. 1288–1379.

Department of Health and Community Services, Victoria (1994) *Antibiotic guidelines*, 8th edn.

Prusiner S. B. (1994) Prion diseases of humans and animals. *Journal of the Royal College of Physicians of London*, **28** (suppl), 1–30.

Rudge P. (Ed.) (1992) Neurological aspects of human retroviruses. *Baillière's Clinical Neurology 1:1*. Baillière Tindall, London.

Sanford J. P. (1994) *Guide to Antimicrobial Therapy*. Antimicrobial Therapy Inc., Dallas, Texas.

17 | Neoplasms

CEREBRAL TUMOURS

Next to stroke, tumour is the most common cause of intracranial disease. Primary tumours may be benign or malignant. Since the prognosis is good in many cases if treated early, it is important to recognize early symptoms and provide appropriate treatment.

Tumour types

There are many different forms of brain tumours and they are classified according to the types of cell from which they arise. The incidence of different types of tumour depends on the age groups studied and the method of selection of patients in different series. Approximate frequencies of tumours for all ages are: glioma 45%; meningioma 15%; metastases 15%; pituitary tumours and cranio-pharyngioma 10%; acoustic neuroma 7%; others 8%. Some tumours are more frequent in children (e.g. medulloblastoma, pinealoma) and some are more frequent in adults (glioma, meningioma, metastases). Some of the more common tumours will be briefly described.

Malignant tumours

Gliomas   These arise from glial cells and include astrocytomas which arise from astrocytes, oligodendrogliomas arising from oligodendrocytes and ependymomas from ependymal cells.

Astrocytomas are classified in different ways according to their grade of malignancy, but a widely accepted classification is low grade astrocytoma (grade 1), malignant astrocytoma (grade 2) and glioblastoma multiforme (grade 3). Glioblastoma multiforme represents about 50% of all gliomas.

Medulloblastomas   Medulloblastomas arise from primitive neuronal cells and represent about 20% of childhood brain tumours. They usually arise in the midline cerebellum.

Cerebral metastases   These occur in about 30% of patients with cancer and in half of these metastatic disease is confined to the central nervous system. Tumours which commonly metastasize to the brain are melanomas and carcinomas of the lung, breast and kidney.

Primary cerebral lymphoma This is not common but is being seen with increasing frequency in patients who have been on long-term treatment with immunosuppressive drugs (e.g. azathioprine) and in patients with the acquired immunodeficiency syndrome (AIDS). The lymphoma is usually of the non-Hodgkin's large cell type.

Benign tumours

Meningiomas These are the most common form of benign cerebral tumour. They originate from cells in the arachnoid layer of the meninges. They are classified according to their anatomical site of origin e.g. falx, sphenoidal ridge or olfactory groove meningiomas. Clinical features result from compression of surrounding structures and, as with other cerebral tumours, these vary according to their site of origin.

Pituitary adenomas Pituitary adenomas arise from the anterior lobe of the pituitary gland and are classified according to cell type using immunocytochemical analysis of hormones (prolactin, growth hormone and corticotrophin).

Craniopharyngiomas These present mainly in children and young adults. They are suprasellar tumours that arise from pharyngeal epithelium in Rathke's pouch.

Acoustic neuromas Acoustic neuromas arise from Schwann cells of the vestibular nerve. They may arise sporadically as solitary tumours, or they may be a manifestation of neurofibromatosis 2 (an autosomal dominant disorder linked to chromosome 22) in which case they are often bilateral.

Clinical features of cerebral tumours

The cranial cavity is a closed inexpansible box and tumours produce symptoms because they grow and expand inside the space, compressing and displacing the brain and other structures. They may present as focal cerebral lesions, or with signs of generalized disturbance of cerebral function. The clinical features depend upon their site in the brain, the type of tumour, its rate of expansion and the presence of cerebral oedema.

Non-focal signs

Change in mental function Dullness, apathy, lack of initiative, abnormal social behaviour, forgetfulness, personality change, weakness, tiredness and dizziness are common symptoms. These features are seen especially in frontal and temporal lobe and corpus callosum tumours.

Headaches These are usually dull, non-pulsatile, worse in the morning and aggravated by sneezing, coughing or head movement. They are caused by displacement of blood vessels and other pain-sensitive structures or by raised intracranial pressure (Chapter 11). About 30% of patients with cerebral tumour experience headaches as a presenting symptom.

Vomiting This is usually associated with a headache and may be projectile in type, without associated nausea.

Epilepsy　About 20–50% of patients with cerebral tumour are subject to seizures that may be either focal or generalized in type.

Raised intracranial pressure　The symptoms of raised intracranial pressure are headache, vomiting, mental changes, unsteadiness of gait and incontinence. Obscurations of vision (transient loss of vision or blindness) are usually precipitated by movements such as bending, coughing or straining that further increase the intracranial pressure; they are an ominous sign of impaired circulation to the optic nerve and retina. Papilloedema is the major clinical sign of raised intracranial pressure. Raised intracranial pressure may give rise to false localizing signs (Chapter 18).

Cerebral oedema　This is usually associated with brain tumours. The most common type is *vasogenic oedema* which is confined to the cerebral white matter and results in an increase in permeability of capillary endothelial cells so that plasma enters into the extracellular space. Since there is no lymphatic drainage in the brain the fluid accumulates and adds to the mass effect of the tumour on surrounding structures. *Cytotoxic oedema* refers to the swelling of brain cells due to increased intracellular fluid content and characteristically occurs after hypoxia but is also seen in brain tumours.

Focal signs

Tumours, regardless of type, may give rise to focal signs appropriate to their anatomical site in the cerebral hemispheres (frontal, temporal, parietal or occipital; Chapter 3), corpus callosum, cerebellum, optic chiasm or brain-stem.

Specific signs

Some tumours have specific signs, for example:

Acoustic neuromas　Acoustic neuromas arise from the VIII nerve in the cerebellopontine angle. They initially cause deafness and in more advanced cases lower motor neurone facial weakness, sensory loss on the face, absent corneal reflex, and incoordination on the side of the lesion (due to compression of nerves V and VII and the cerebellum).

Pituitary tumours　These may be non-secreting causing only pressure effects on surrounding structures or hormone-secreting causing acromegaly, Cushing's disease, or hyperprolactinaemia in addition to pressure effects. They often extend superiorly from the pituitary fossa, compressing the optic chiasm and causing bitemporal hemianopia (Figs 4.2, 4.3, 4.6). Sometimes they invade the cavernous sinus laterally involving the third, fourth, fifth (first and second division) and sixth nerves (Fig. 4.12).

Sphenoidal wing meningioma　If the tumour is near the superior orbital fissure, it causes unilateral exophthalmos and involves nerves III, IV, V (first division) and VI. A more medially placed tumour may compress the optic nerve as it passes through the optic foramen causing unilateral loss of vision and optic atrophy.

Olfactory groove meningiomas　These rise from the floor of the anterior cranial fossa and compress the olfactory bulb causing anosmia. As they expand they may cause a frontal lobe syndrome.

Pinealoma These arise from the pineal gland and compress the tectal region of the mid-brain causing Parinaud's syndrome (dilated pupils which do not react to light; impairment of upward gaze and vergence; p. 58) and raised intracranial pressure.

Investigations

Computed tomography (CT) scanning with contrast and enhancement will demonstrate most brain tumours. Magnetic resonance imaging (MRI) is more sensitive and may detect low grade astrocytomas and some tumours in the posterior fossa at the base of the skull that are not so easily visible on CT scanning. Positron emission tomography (PET) demonstrates hypermetabolism in actively growing tumours and is a useful technique for differentiating between tumour recurrence and post-radiation necrosis. In the case of cerebral metastases, investigations of other parts of the body may be necessary to detect the primary tumour.

Management

Medical

Epileptic seizures will require treatment with appropriate anticonvulsants (Chapter 12). Cerebral oedema may be reduced by dexamethasone (4 mg every 4–6 hours); this treatment temporarily relieves symptoms and lowers intracranial pressure.

Surgery

A pre-operative diagnosis of tumour type can frequently be made from knowledge of the clinical features and anatomical site of the tumour and its appearance on neuro-imaging. Histological diagnosis is essential in the management of brain tumours. This can be done by open operation or stereotactic surgery under CT or MRI control and an intra-operative diagnosis can be given by smear or frozen section methods. A definite diagnosis is made on paraffin sections. Benign tumours, such as meningiomas, acoustic neuromas and pituitary tumours can frequently be completely removed. Malignant tumours cannot usually be completely excised but are often partially removed or de-bulked to reduce their mass effect and to remove necrotic tissue. Laser technology has improved the results of neurosurgery.

Radiotherapy

Malignant gliomas are usually treated post-operatively with radiotherapy (5000–6000 rads or cGy) over 5–6 weeks. Craniopharyngiomas, pituitary adenomas and some metastases are also radio-sensitive. Focal irradiation (e.g. proton beam, gamma knife) is preferable to general brain irradiation which may cause: (i) cerebral oedema during treatment causing an increase in the neurological deficit, which can be treated with corticosteroids; (ii) late radio-necrosis (due to progressive occlusion of blood vessels) which commences months to years after irradiation. It presents as a progressive neurological deficit that is very difficult to distinguish clinically from tumour recurrence but may be differentiated by PET scanning.

Chemotherapy

Different types of chemotherapy have been tried but none has so far been found to influence the outcome significantly.

SPINAL CORD TUMOURS

Primary tumours of the spinal cord represent only about 15% of primary tumours of the central nervous system; they tend to be benign. The most common tumours are meningiomas and neurofibromas which are extramedullary, and ependymomas and gliomas which are intramedullary.

Metastases to the spine are far more common than primary spinal neoplasms and they are most commonly epidural; intramedullary metastases are rare and leptomeningeal metastases cause carcinomatous meningitis with CSF pleocytosis (Chapter 16). Epidural spinal cord compression in most cases (85%) arises from spread from bony metastases in the vertebral column; about 50% of cases of metastatic epidural compression in adults arise from breast, lung or prostate carcinoma but other frequent primary tumour sources include lymphoma, melanoma, renal cancer and multiple myeloma.

The clinical features of spinal cord compression are described in Chapter 7. In about 95% of adults the initial symptom of metastatic epidural compression is pain.

PARANEOPLASTIC SYNDROMES

A number of disorders of the central and peripheral nervous systems are manifestations of the remote effects of neoplasms, many of which have an autoimmune mechanism.

Peripheral neuropathy

Predominantly sensory neuropathy may be a remote manifestation of small cell carcinoma of the lung, rarely other tumours, and is associated with the presence of anti-neuronal nuclear antibodies. Inflammatory neuropathies, when secondary to malignancy, are usually complications of lymphoma. A sensorimotor neuropathy, the pathogenesis of which is uncertain, may be associated with many other malignancies (carcinoma, lymphoma, multiple myeloma).

Myasthenic syndrome (Lambert-Eaton syndrome)

This is an autoimmune syndrome usually associated with a small cell carcinoma of the lung (Chapter 10).

Polymyositis

This may present as a remote manifestation of an underlying malignancy.

Paraneoplastic cerebellar degeneration

This may be the presenting feature of an underlying malignancy, usually carcinoma of the lung, breast or ovaries. Anti-neuronal antibodies are present in most cases, especially when the condition is secondary to ovarian or other gynaecological cancers.

Limbic encephalomyelitis

This presents with confusion and dementia and is a paraneoplastic manifestation of some cancers, particularly small cell carcinoma of the lung.

Myelopathy

Myelopathy is rarely seen as a paraneoplastic syndrome.

REFERENCES

Adams R. D. and Victor M. (1993) *Principles of Neurology*, 5th edn. McGraw-Hill, New York.

Black P. M. (1991) Brain tumours. *New England Journal of Medicine*, **324**, 1471–1476, 1555–1564.

Shapiro W. R. and Shapiro J. R. (1992) Primary brain tumours. In: *Diseases of the Nervous System*, 2nd edn. Eds A. K Asbury, E. M. McKhann and W. I. McDonald. W. B. Saunders, Philadelphia. 1074–1092.

Byrne T. E. (1992) Spinal cord compression from epidural metastases. *New England Journal of Medicine*, **327**, 614–619.

18 | Raised intracranial pressure

The brain and spinal cord are bathed in cerebrospinal fluid (CSF), the pressure of which reflects that within these structures.

CEREBROSPINAL FLUID

The chief functions of the CSF are to:
- Provide physical support for the brain and spinal cord
- Act as a vehicle for the excretion of waste products of brain metabolism
- Control the chemical environment of the central nervous system
- Enable intracerebral transport of chemicals and hormones, e.g. hypothalamic releasing factors

Anatomy and physiology

The total volume of the CSF is approximately 150 mL, of which 75 mL are in the intracranial cavities. The ventricular volume of the CSF is only about 16 mL of which 7 mL are in each lateral ventricle, 1 mL in the third ventricle and 1 mL in the fourth ventricle.

Formation

The CSF is mainly formed and secreted by the choroid plexus of the cerebral ventricles, but there is also evidence for extrachoroidal formation in the brain and spinal cord with transependymal secretion. The CSF formed in the lateral ventricles flows into the third ventricle through the interventricular foramina and then through the aqueduct into the fourth ventricle to reach the subarachnoid space by way of the foramen of Magendie and the foramina of Luschka. In this space it fills the cerebral cisterns, flows down and back up again in the spinal subarachnoid space, and passes upwards over the convexity of the cerebral hemispheres (Fig. 18.1). The rate of CSF formation is relatively constant at 500 mL/day (0.35 mL/min).

Absorption

Most of the reabsorption of CSF is through the arachnoid villi in the intracranial venous sinuses but there is also some absorption in the spinal canal adjacent to the spinal roots. The rate of absorption, within broad limits, is directly related to the CSF pressure. The blood-brain barrier is maintained by tight junctions of capillary endothelial cells, choroidal epithelium and arachnoid membranes. In some regions such as the area postrema, parts of the hypothalamus and sub-fornical and subcommisural organs, the barrier does not exist.

The blood-brain barrier can be altered by pathological states including anoxia, ischaemia, toxins, infections and some endocrine disorders.

Characteristics

Adults and older children

Glucose: 2.9–4.6 mmol/L
Protein: Ventricular 0.05–0.15 g/L
          Cisternal   0.15–0.25 g/L
          Lumbar   0.15–0.40 g/L (0.15–0.30 g/L) in children
          Ig G   0.07–0.38 g/L (5–12% of total protein) in adults
                       0.07–0.17 g/L (3.5–8.7% of total protein) in children
Cells: 0–4 × 10^6 cells/L (normally lymphocytes/monocytes)
Pressure: 65–195 mm CSF (5–15 mmHg)

Newborns

The CSF protein is high at first (up to 1.2 g/L) and gradually drops to childhood levels by about 3 months of age. The white cell count is also elevated in the newborn; up to about 20 × 10^6 cells/L being common, often with a predominance of polymorphs. Xanthochromia is also common in the neonate.

Lumbar puncture

The CSF pressure may be measured at lumbar puncture or through a catheter inserted into a lateral ventricle. Lumbar puncture is described in Chapter 23.

CAUSES OF RAISED INTRACRANIAL PRESSURE

The brain and CSF are in a rigid compartment and any increase in the volume of one or other will result in an increase in the intracranial pressure. The major causes of this are:
- Increased brain volume, due to cerebral tumour, cerebral haemorrhage or infarction, abscess or other space-occupying lesions, or to cerebral oedema
- Extracranial masses, such as subdural or extradural haemorrhage

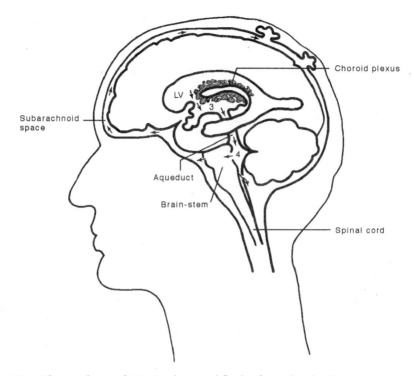

Fig. 18.1 The circulation of CSF. Cerebrospinal fluid is formed in the choroid plexuses in the lateral ventricles (LV), third ventricle (3) and fourth ventricle (4), passing out from the ventricular system through the foramina of Magendie and Luschka to pass over the hemisphere in the subarachnoid space and to be absorbed in the arachnoid villi. (From Lance, 1975, Headache, by permission of Charles Scribner's Sons, New York.)

- Increased venous pressure due to heart failure or superior mediastinal obstruction
- Hydrocephalus
- Benign intracranial hypotension

Hydrocephalus

Hydrocephalus is an increase in the volume of CSF associated with dilatation of the cerebral ventricles.

Causes

Obstruction   This can be intraventricular or extraventricular in origin

(1) *Intraventricular (non-communicating hydrocephalus)*   The obstruction is within the ventricular system and may be at the foramen of Monro, third ventricle, aqueduct, fourth ventricle, or foramina of Luschka and Magendie.

The causes of the obstruction include congenital neoplasms, congenital defects and inflammatory lesions such as meningitis. Mumps and possibly other intra-uterine infections may cause aqueduct stenosis.

(2) *Extraventricular (communicating hydrocephalus)* There is a free communication of the ventricular system with the subarachnoid space. This type of hydrocephalus may result from adhesions of the subarachnoid space at the base of the brain following infections or haemorrhage. Other causes include congenital defects such as the *Arnold-Chiari malformation* (a tongue of cerebellar tissue with an elongated medulla protruding into the spinal canal) or developmental absorptive defects of the arachnoid villi.

Defective absorption Impaired venous sinus drainage may be caused by lateral or sagittal sinus thrombosis, or congenital or acquired (e.g. inflammation, high CSF protein) defects of the arachnoid villi. The lateral sinus may thrombose as a complication of mastoiditis (otitic hydrocephalus).

Overproduction This is known to occur only in the very rare condition of choroid plexus papilloma.

Aetiology and pathology

The most common type of congenital hydrocephalus is that associated with the other major congenital abnormalities of meningomyelocoele and encephalocoele. Hydrocephalus is associated with 80% of cases of myelomeningocoele. It is due either to aqueduct obstruction or to associated Arnold-Chiari malformation. In occasional cases, intra-uterine infection (toxoplasmosis, cytomegalovirus infection and syphilis) is the aetiological factor. Rare cases have a genetic basis (X-linked recessive).

The aqueduct is the most common site of obstruction in congenital hydrocephalus; it may be congenitally abnormal (e.g forked) or simply of very small calibre (aqueduct stenosis). There is ventricular enlargement, proximal to the site of block. The cerebral white matter is greatly thinned whereas the grey matter of the cerebral cortex is preserved until late in the course of the disease.

Clinical features

In congenital hydrocephalus developing in infancy the most common symptoms and signs are head enlargement, delayed motor skills, pyramidal tract signs in the lower limbs due to stretching of corticospinal fibres (those destined for the lower limbs have a long course around the lateral ventricles from their origin on the medial side of the hemisphere and are thus most liable to damage), and optic atrophy, which is a late complication of chronic papilloedema due to increased intracranial pressure.

In older children and adults with acquired lesions there are symptoms of raised intracranial pressure such as headaches, nausea, vomiting and diplopia.

Diagnosis

Head measurement The circumference of the head should be compared with normal values on a standard head-size chart (Figs 2.1, 2.2). Serial measurements showing a crossing of percentiles are very important. Increased head size may also be caused by megalencephaly (brain of excessive size and weight), bone abnormalities (e.g. achondroplasia and rickets), chronic subdural haematoma in infancy and some other rare conditions.

Transillumination of the head A torch is held against the baby's head in a dark room. Abnormal redness around the torch indicates an excessive amount of fluid beneath the torch, i.e. hydrocephalus, subdural effusion or localized cerebral cysts.

Skull X-ray A large head and widened sutures may be seen in a child with hydrocephalus. The sutures can widen with raised intracranial pressure until around the age of 10 years. In older children and adults, after the cranial sutures have fused, the signs of raised intracranial pressure are erosion of the dorsum sellae and clinoid processes.

Neuroradiology Computed tomography (CT) and magnetic resonance imaging (MRI) scans will demonstrate enlarged ventricles and possibly the site of obstruction.

Echo-encephalography This is a useful non-traumatic investigation for diagnosing and following the size of the lateral ventricles in children under the age of about 4 years.

Treatment

Treatment is removal of the primary lesion neurosurgically if possible (e.g. posterior fossa tumour) or insertion of a shunt.

A variety of methods for diverting CSF flow have been devised. The current popular methods are the ventriculo-atrial and ventriculo-peritoneal shunts using non-reactive tubing and pressure valves.

Unfortunately complications do occur with the shunts including blockage causing raised intracranial pressure, infection, pulmonary emboli with ventriculo-atrial shunts, and shunt nephritis, an immunologically determined disorder due to secondary *Staphylococcus albus* infection.

Normal pressure hydrocephalus

Normal pressure hydrocephalus is a syndrome of adults characterized by insidious onset of memory and intellect impairment, which progresses to a severe dementia with apraxia of gait and urinary incontinence. Headache is not a feature and there are no signs of raised intracranial pressure; there is no papilloedema and CSF pressure is normal.

There is marked ventricular dilatation present on the CT scan without evidence of cortical atrophy. These findings are in contrast to those in cerebral atrophy where the sulci are very prominent and secondary ventricular enlargement occurs (*hydrocephalus ex vacuo*). Normal pressure hydrocephalus is, in fact, a communicating hydrocephalus with obliteration of the subarachnoid space over the surface of the cerebral hemispheres. It may be secondary to subarachnoid haemorrhage, meningitis or trauma or may occur spontaneously. The CSF pressure is said to be normal or low (hence the term normal pressure hydro-cephalus); however, continuous monitoring of intracranial pressure through an intraventricular catheter shows that rises of pressure to abnormally high levels occur at times, particularly during sleep. Isotope cisternography is helpful in the diagnosis. This investigation consists of introducing a radio-isotope into the CSF and then performing radionuclide scanning to observe its flow. In normal pressure hydrocephalus the radio-isotope remains in the ventricular system and does not appear in the subarachnoid space over the surface of the brain.

About 50% of patients with normal pressure hydrocephalus respond well to surgical shunting procedures.

Benign intracranial hypertension (pseudotumour cerebri)

Benign intracranial hypertension is a condition in which increased intracranial pressure occurs in the absence of a space-occupying lesion or obstruction to CSF flow. The ventricles can be of normal size or small.

Aetiology and pathology

In most adults the cause is unknown. It is however most commonly seen in obese young females and thus presumably has an endocrine basis. It may be secondary to a thrombosis of one or more of the dural sinuses, particularly the lateral sinus as a sequel to otitis media or mastoiditis (otitic hydrocephalus). Benign intracranial hypertension may follow withdrawal of corticosteroids, Vitamin A intoxication, tetracycline and nalidixic acid administration.

Clinical features

The symptoms are those of raised intracranial pressure: headache, vomiting, blurred vision and diplopia due to an abducens nerve palsy (a false localizing sign). Papilloedema is almost invariably present. In contrast to raised intracranial pressure secondary to an expanding lesion, the patient looks well and has a normal level of consciousness and normal intellectual function. Apart from the signs due to raised intracranial pressure, there are no other abnormal neurological findings.

Diagnosis

Investigations to exclude a space-occupying lesion must be undertaken and a diagnosis of benign intracranial hypertension cannot be made until these are all demonstrated to be normal. On CT or MRI scans there are no space-occupying lesions visible and the ventricles are normal or small in size.

Prognosis

Although the disease is often self-limiting, treatment of the intracranial hyper-tension is necessary in order to prevent blindness occurring as a result of chronic papilloedema which, in turn, may lead to secondary optic atrophy.

Treatment

The raised intracranial pressure may be reduced with corticosteroid therapy. Other forms of treatment such as acetazolamide and other diuretics and repeated lumbar puncture are also employed. Ventricular shunting procedures may be necessary, particularly the insertion of a shunt from the spinal subarachnoid space to the peritoneum (lumbar–peritoneal shunt).

REFERENCE

Fishman R. A. (1992) *Cerebrospinal Fluid in Diseases of the Nervous System*, 2nd edn. W. B. Saunders, Philadelphia.

19 | Dementia

Dementia is a progressive loss of global intellectual function, including memory, caused by organic disease of the brain. It may be the result of primary degenerative brain disease (e.g. Alzheimer's disease, Huntington's disease) or secondary to other, potentially treatable, conditions (e.g. cerebral tumour, subdural haematoma, hydrocephalus, vascular disease and infection; Table 19.1). It is important to distinguish circumscribed intellectual failure resulting from a single cerebral lesion from multiple focal lesions and from a global impairment of all cortical function. Severe depressive or psychotic states may mimic dementia.

CLINICAL FEATURES

Dementia may present in many ways but early features include changes in personality, apathy, faulty judgement, forgetfulness, difficulty in concentrating, irritability, disorientation, and slowness in speech and movement. These symptoms and signs, which are initially subtle, gradually become more obvious; memory becomes grossly impaired, there is loss of interest in other people and the surroundings, and there is deterioration in personal cleanliness and hygiene. In the early stages the only abnormality on neurological examination may be impairment of memory and poor performance on neuropsychological tests of intellectual function. In the later stages there is a shuffling gait, akinesia and appearance of primitive reflexes such as the grasp, snout and sucking reflexes (Chapter 3). The presence of focal neurological signs should always alert the clinician to the likelihood of space-occupying or other focal lesions that may be treatable.

CAUSES OF DEMENTIA

Although there are many causes of dementia numerically the most important are Alzheimer's disease (50%) and vascular dementia (25%). Combined vascular and Alzheimer pathology account for 13% and the remaining 12% are due to other causes (Table 19.1) which are nevertheless important because many of them are potentially treatable.

Table 19.1   Causes of dementia

Cerebrovascular disease
   Multi-infarct dementia
   Lacunar infarcts

Head injuries

Intracranial space-occupying lesions
   Tumours
   Abscesses
   Subdural haematomas

Normal pressure hydrocephalus

Nutritional
   Wernicke-Korsakoff syndrome
   Vitamin B_{12} deficiency
   Folate deficiency
   Pellagra

Metabolic
   Myxoedema
   Cushing's syndrome, Addison's disease
   Hypocalcaemia
   Renal, hepatic failure
   Inappropriate anti-diuretic hormone secretion
   Intoxications

Infections
   Creutzfeldt-Jakob disease
   AIDS-dementia complex
   Neurosyphilis (general paralysis of the insane; GPI)
   Chronic meningitis e.g. cryptococcal, tuberculous
   Abscess

Degenerative diseases
   Huntington's disease
   Pick's disease
   Parkinson's disease
   Parkinson's-dementia complex
   Spinocerebellar degenerations
   Progressive supranuclear palsy
   Corticobasal degeneration

Senile dementia of the Alzheimer type

The association of dementia with old age has been recognized for centuries. The most common form of dementia and the usual cause of senile dementia is Alzheimer's disease, originally described by Alois Alzheimer in 1907. As Alzheimer's disease is a pathological diagnosis, it is usual to refer to clinical cases of dementia where Alzheimer's disease is suspected as senile dementia of the Alzheimer's type (SDAT). The prevalence is about 1% of the population aged 65 but rises steeply to about 20% of the population over the age of 80. About 50% of the nursing home population has Alzheimer's disease. As well as age, genetic factors play a part in the aetiology since there is a familial incidence of the disease; linkages have been demonstrated on chromosomes 14 and 21. It may be significant that adults with Down's syndrome have similar neuropathological changes to those with Alzheimer's disease.

The characteristic pathological features consist of:
- Cortical atrophy and loss of cells, particularly the large neurones
- Neurofibrillary tangles in cortical neurones, consisting of paired helical filaments that are argyrophilic (take up silver stains)
- Neuritic or senile plaques which are degenerating nerve terminals with a central core of amyloid. The major protein component of the amyloid (A4 protein) is coded on chromosome 21. The number of neuritic plaques correlates with the severity of the dementia. Senile plaques and neurofibrillary tangles are found in the brains of many individuals who are not clinically demented during life. The incidence of these pathological findings rises from about 5% among people in their sixties to over 70% in people in their eighties. Whether or not all people with plaques and tangles will eventually develop dementia is not yet certain.

Depletion of chemical transmitters, particularly acetylcholine, due to the death of cholinergic neurones may play an important part in the mental changes of Alzheimer's disease. There is a reduction in cholinergic activity in the brain and a loss of neurones in the major cholinergic projections to the cerebral cortex from the basal nucleus of Meynert in the substantia innominata. Some other neurotransmitters are also depleted but not to the same extent nor as consistently as the cholinergic markers. Treatment of patients with cholinergic drugs, such as oral tetrahydroaminoacridine, has not produced any lasting benefit.

Vascular dementias

Multi-infarct dementia

Focal loss of cerebral tissue due to damage by ischaemic stroke leads to the loss of the cerebral function associated with the area destroyed. In general, such focal loss does not constitute dementia. However, in some patients who have had infarctions that involve several areas of cerebral cortex, their overall function may be so impaired as to render them demented.

Ischaemic white matter disease

Otto Binswanger, a German neuropathologist, described in 1894 a condition of progressive dementia accompanied by focal neurological signs which post-mortem proved to be accompanied by macroscopic loss of white matter and ventricular enlargement. Later pathologists noted that such cases had marked narrowing and hyalinization of arterioles entering the white matter of the brain. In some areas of the white matter, small (lacunar) infarctions are seen while in other areas there is ischaemic demyelination without frank tissue death. Patients with this pathology are frequently male and hypertensive. They present with a dementing illness, often characterized by early difficulty in walking, which is in contrast to Alzheimer's disease. They tend to have a stepwise clinical progression and pseudobulbar palsy may be a feature.

Although the fully developed entity of *Binswanger's disease* or subcortical arteriosclerotic encephalopathy is rare, the picture is complicated by modern imaging techniques. On computed tomography (CT) scanning and, in particular, on magnetic resonance imaging of the cerebral white matter, many asymptomatic elderly people are seen to have areas of oedema in the deep white matter of the cerebral hemispheres. This radiological appearance has been given the descriptive term of *leukoariosis*. This finding may be seen in up to 30% of intellectually normal individuals over the age of 60. The incidence of such findings is however much higher in groups of patients with intellectual decline. There is a correlation between declining intellectual abilities and the extent of leukoariosis.

Pick's disease

This is a rare condition that presents with a clinical picture similar to Alzheimer's disease although typically there is more early evidence of focal cortical dysfunction. Such patients may, for instance, present with a primary progressive aphasia or primary progressive constructional difficulty or signs suggestive of unilateral frontal lobe damage. It is characterized pathologically by very severe cortical atrophy often confined to the frontal and temporal lobes. On microscopy there are characteristic silver staining intracellular inclusions (Pick bodies) in pale, swollen cortical neurones.

Wernicke-Korsakoff syndrome

Wernicke's encephalopathy (pp. 220–221) is frequently associated with Korsakoff's psychosis. They are both most commonly caused by thiamine deficiency in chronic alcoholics and are together known as the Wernicke-Korsakoff syndrome. Korsakoff's psychosis is characterized by severe impairment of memory and inability to acquire new information. Frequently the memory defects are disguised by *confabulation* (fanciful invention or fabrication of information to take the place of that which has been forgotten). There is also accumulating evidence that alcoholics may develop cognitive impairment due to frontal lobe degeneration in addition to the Wernicke-Korsakoff syndrome. This damage may be partly reversible whereas Korsakoff's psychosis is permanent.

AIDS-dementia complex

This is discussed further on p. 248.

INVESTIGATION AND MANAGEMENT

A careful history from the patient, relatives and friends is essential. A progressive dementia must be distinguished from acute confusional states due to metabolic and other diffuse cerebral disorders (Chapter 14). Careful enquiry should be made about a history suggestive of stroke (multi-infarct dementia), head injuries, headaches and fits (space-occupying lesions), and drug or alcohol abuse. Careful testing of the mental state should be performed and supplemented by more detailed neuropsychological tests. Physical examination should be directed towards a search for focal lesions and evidence of systemic disease. Laboratory investigations should include a CT scan, chest X-ray, EEG, full blood count and erythrocyte sedimentation rate, serum folate and Vitamin B_{12} levels, thyroid and liver function tests, serum calcium, blood sugar, HIV antibodies, a screening test for syphilis and cerebrospinal fluid examination.

Treatment will depend on the underlying cause, the most common being Alzheimer's disease for which there is no specific therapy. Supportive treatment of the patient and their carers plays a major part in management.

REFERENCES

Rossor M. N. (1992) Unusual dementias. *Baillière's Clinical Neurology.* Baillière Tindall, London.

Whitehouse P. J. (1993) *Dementia.* F. A. Davis, Philadelphia.

20 | Multiple sclerosis

Demyelinating diseases of the central nervous system are characterized by foci of degeneration of the myelin sheath around nerve fibres in the white matter of the central nervous system. The axon may also be damaged but the primary pathological process involves destruction of myelin. Multiple sclerosis is the most common and important of these conditions but there are other demyelinating diseases which include acute disseminated encephalomyelitis, neuromyelitis optica (Devic's disease) Balo's concentric sclerosis and diffuse sclerosis (Schilder's disease).

MULTIPLE SCLEROSIS

Multiple sclerosis is an autoimmune disease that affects mainly people in the younger age groups and, in its most common form, is characterized by relapses and remissions. The lesions are disseminated in both space (different parts of the central nervous system white matter) and time (new foci of demyelination occur at intervals over a period of many years).

Aetiology

Although the cause of multiple sclerosis remains unknown, it is clear that both environmental and genetic factors are involved. The environmental factor may be a virus infection that triggers immune-mediated demyelination in people with a genetically determined susceptibility.

Environmental factors

The chief evidence for an environmental agent is epidemiological. The frequency of multiple sclerosis is related to latitude in both Northern and Southern hemispheres; there is a higher prevalence in temperate climates than in tropical and subtropical climates. In Australia the prevalence increases from 11.8/100 000 population in tropical Queensland to 75.6/100 000 in Hobart, Tasmania (Fig. 20.1). Migration studies indicate that a subject moving from a high risk to a low risk zone in adult life has a greater chance of later developing multiple sclerosis than someone migrating as a child. This observation suggests that critical exposure to environmental factors occurs in early years of life.

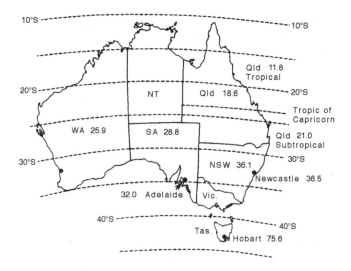

Fig. 20.1 Prevalence of multiple sclerosis in Australia. Standardized prevalence expressed as number of cases per 100 000 population at 30 June 1981. (From McLeod J. G., Hammond S. R. and Hallpike J. F. (1994). Epidemiology of Multiple Sclerosis in Australia. *Medical Journal of Australia*, **1**, 117–122.)

Genetic factors

There is familial incidence of multiple sclerosis; approximately 10% of patients have an affected relative. The concordance rate in monozygotic twins is 25%, whereas in dizygotic twins it is 2.5%. There is a strong association of the disease with the human leucocyte antigen (HLA) system. In Caucasian races, there is an association with HLA-A3, HLA-D7 and HLA-DR2. Over 60% of patients are HLA-DR2 positive compared with only 15–20% of controls. In Arab populations, there is an association with HLA-DR4.

Pathology

The acute lesion is a perivenular infiltration of lymphocytes, macrophages and plasma cells associated with demyelination. In the later stages glial cells proliferate; some axons are lost and only a very limited degree of remyelination occurs. The gliotic areas form discrete grey coloured areas within the white matter and are termed plaques. Plaques of demyelination occur predominantly in the white matter of the periventricular regions of the cerebral hemispheres, brain-stem and cerebellum, subpial regions of the spinal cord and the optic nerves.

Immunology

The earliest change in multiple sclerosis is a breakdown of the blood-brain barrier, mediated by T cells that allow lymphocytes, macrophages and humoral factors to enter the central nervous system. There is presumed to be an antigen-specific immune response against an unidentified antigen that results in this breakdown. Sensitized T cells produce cytokines which may participate in causing damage to oligodendrocytes and myelin. Oligoclonal immunoglobulin G (IgG) found in the cerebrospinal fluid (CSF) is produced by clones of B cells, but the antigen against which it is produced has not been identified.

Clinical features

The age of onset is most commonly between 20 and 50 years. Approximately 20% of cases arise before the age of 20 but only about 20–30% have an onset after the age of 50 years. Females are affected more commonly than males in the ratio of about 2:1. Symptoms usually develop rapidly within hours but may develop more slowly over several days. The most common initial symptoms are as follows:

Weakness

There may be abrupt onset of weakness in one or more limbs causing mono-plegia, hemiplegia or paraplegia. The patient may complain of heaviness or stiff-ness of a limb or tiredness, weakness or a tendency to fall. Fatiguability is common and weakness and other symptoms may be more pronounced in hot weather or after hot baths because a rise in temperature causes a block in conduction across the demyelinated zone in affected nerve fibres.

Optic neuritis

This is also discussed on p. 49. Acute optic neuritis is a common early symptom. The vision becomes blurred and sight may be lost completely in one eye. There may be associated pain on eye movement and on pressure applied to the eye. The vision usually improves over a few days to weeks, and normal vision may return although there is commonly some residual impairment of colour vision. If the lesion lies near the optic disc, swelling of the disc may be observed on ophthalmoscopic examination but, if the lesion is more posteriorly placed in the optic nerve, no abnormality will be seen. On plotting the central fields of vision, a central or paracentral scotoma is usually present and this can be more readily detected with a red target. Optic atrophy with pallor of the disc, especially in the temporal part, may be a sequel to optic neuritis. Permanent blindness is rare. Visual evoked potentials, which enable the conduction of the visual pathways to be assessed neurophysiologically, are abnormal in about 90% of patients with clinically definite multiple sclerosis even though they may give no history of optic neuritis. Patients who have had optic neuritis in the past may experience temporary blurring of vision following exercise, or after hot baths (*Uhthoff's phenomenon*). The physiological explanation of this symptom is that conduction across demyelinated fibres is reduced by slight rises in temperature.

Sensory symptoms

Numbness of one or more limbs or of the face is common in multiple sclerosis. A lesion in the dorsal columns may cause sensations of apparent swelling of the limbs or feelings similar to tight bandages or strings being wrapped around the limb. A band-like sensation around the waist may develop. A plaque in the cervical cord may cause a sensation resembling an electric shock down the back on flexing the spine (Lhermitte's sign). A clumsy or useless hand may result from a lesion that involves a dorsal root entry zone and dorsal columns by impairing proprioception. Trigeminal neuralgia may sometimes be caused by demyelination.

Unsteadiness of gait

Ataxia of gait due to weakness, proprioceptive disturbance or cerebellar dysfunction is common.

Double vision

Brain-stem lesions may cause double vision by involvement of the ocular motor pathways. Internuclear ophthalmoplegia, due to a lesion in the medial longitudinal fasciculus, is a common cause of diplopia in multiple sclerosis (p. 58).

Vertigo

Vertigo may be an early symptom of multiple sclerosis and results from a brain-stem lesion involving the vestibular pathways and the pons.

Sphincter disturbances

Frequency, urgency and precipitancy of micturition or retention of urine may be initial symptoms of multiple sclerosis and sphincter disturbances are very common in later stages of the disease. Impotence frequently occurs.

Mental changes

Mental changes are rarely initial symptoms of multiple sclerosis but are found later in the disease. Emotional instability, depression, impaired cognitive function and euphoria are common, and dementia may occur in the later stages of the disease.

Fatigue

Fatigue is one of the commonest complaints in patients with established multiple sclerosis.

Precipitating and aggravating factors

There are a number of factors which are considered, but not proven, to precipitate attacks of multiple sclerosis. They include viral infections, trauma, surgical operations, pregnancy, emotional stress, exertion and fatigue, and vaccinations and inoculations. There is a slightly increased risk of exacerbation occurring during pregnancy or after delivery but there is no evidence that this makes any difference to the long-term course or prognosis of the disease. Immunization may precipitate relapse and should be avoided if possible. Emotional stress is difficult to evaluate objectively but there is no firm scientific evidence that it influences the course of multiple sclerosis.

Clinical course and prognosis

About 80% of patients have a relapsing and remitting course and in a proportion of these the disease may subsequently become progressive. The remaining 20% have a progressive course from the outset. The chronic progressive form tends to have a later age of onset and a worse prognosis. About 10% of patients die within 15 years but the mean survival is 30 years and many patients live longer. Guides to a poor prognosis are a late onset, a short interval between the first two relapses and the onset of a progressive phase of the disease.

Diagnosis

The clinical diagnosis of multiple sclerosis depends upon evidence from the history and examination of lesions in the central nervous system at more than one site and various episodes of involvement separated by an interval of time. According to the degree of certainty of the diagnosis, it may be classified as clinically 'definite', 'probable' or 'possible'. Investigations such as evoked potentials and magnetic resonance imaging may be used to establish the presence of lesions which are not apparent clinically, and the presence of oligoclonal bands in the CSF increases the likelihood of a diagnosis of multiple sclerosis. In taking the history it is important to ask about any previous neurological symptoms, such as blurring or loss of vision, numbness, tingling, weakness, double vision and sphincter disturbances. Occasionally symptoms are paroxysmal in nature, e.g. episodes of ataxia, or dysarthria of short duration. Tic douloureux and Bell's palsy may also be manifestations of multiple sclerosis. On physical examination it is important to look carefully for more than one site of involvement, e.g. if the patient has spastic paraparesis explicable by a single spinal cord lesion, examine carefully for evidence of cranial nerve involvement, such as optic atrophy and nystagmus. If all the symptoms and signs can be explained by a lesion at one site in the nervous system, multiple sclerosis should not be diagnosed and every effort should be made to exclude by appropriate investigations other causes, such as a tumour. Other diseases that can produce multiple lesions in the central nervous system which are disseminated in space and time should be considered in the differential diagnosis. These include systemic lupus erythematosus (SLE) and other connective tissue diseases, sarcoidosis, HIV infections and metastases.

Certain diagnostic tests may be of value in confirming the diagnosis:

Cerebrospinal fluid

Cells   The cell count is normal (less than 3–4 lymphocytes/mm³) in 60–70% of patients in remission. However, during relapse about 60% of patients have an increased cell count. The cell count rarely exceeds 50 cells/mm³.

Protein   The total CSF protein is raised in about 30% of patients with multiple sclerosis and it is exceptional for the value to be greater than 1.0 g/L.

Gamma globulin   The gamma globulin tends to be elevated in patients with multiple sclerosis. The IgG/albumin ratio in the CSF is normally less than about

25% and it is increased in approximately 60% of patients with clinically definite multiple sclerosis. Immunoglobulin G index compares the IgG/albumin ratio in the CSF and blood and is abnormal in about 90% of patients with clinically definite multiple sclerosis.

Oligoclonal bands   Oligoclonal IgG may be detected by agarose gel electrophoresis of the CSF or by isoelectric focusing. The latter technique is more sensitive but has a higher incidence of false positive results. Blood and CSF must be studied simultaneously to be certain that the IgG is synthesised intrathecally. Abnormalities are detected in about 90% of patients with clinically definite multiple sclerosis.

Electrophysiological studies

Also refer to pp. 305–306.

Visual evoked responses   These are a means of testing conduction in the visual pathways. The stimulus to the retina is usually that of a moving chequerboard pattern and the potential from the visual cortex is recorded through scalp electrodes. The potential is delayed or reduced in amplitude in the presence of demyelinating lesions in the optic pathway and is abnormal in about 90% of patients with clinically definite multiple sclerosis. ·

Somatosensory evoked potentials   These may be recorded through scalp electrodes over the sensory cortex or from over the cervical spine on stimulating sensory nerves in the arms or legs. They are abnormal in about 70% of patients with clinically definite multiple sclerosis.

Auditory or brain-stem evoked potentials   These can be recorded through surface electrodes after click stimuli are applied to the ears. They are abnormal in less than 50% of patients with clinically definite multiple sclerosis, the abnormalities indicating a lesion in the brain-stem.

One or more evoked potentials are abnormal in over 90% of patients with clinically definite multiple sclerosis. The techniques are valuable in detecting clinically silent lesions and they therefore enable lesions in unsuspected sites to be diagnosed. The electrophysiological abnormalities persist; rarely do they return to normal.

Computed tomography scan

The CT scan may sometimes reveal plaques of demyelination but the yield of abnormalities is relatively low. Its main value is to exclude other diagnoses such as tumours and vascular disease.

Magnetic resonance imaging (MRI)

Demyelinating lesions in the brain are readily demonstrated as areas of high signal intensity on T2-weighted images in over 90% of patients with clinically definite multiple sclerosis (Fig. 23.3). They are more difficult to demonstrate in the spinal cord, but the yield is increased by the use of the contrast agent gadolinium that demonstrates regions where there has been breakdown of the blood-brain barrier.

Treatment

Acute attacks

Adrenocorticotropic hormone and corticosteroids in short courses reduce the duration of an acute attack, but have no influence on the long-term course of the disease. The treatment of choice is methylprednisolone 500 mg daily by intravenous infusion for 5 days, or 1000 mg daily for 3 days. Oral prednisone, 60 mg daily for one week, 40 mg daily in the second week, 20 mg daily in the third week, 10 mg daily in the fourth week and 5 mg daily in the final week may be given instead of intravenous therapy but is not as effective. Adrenocorticotropic hormone injections given in reducing doses over four weeks are also effective but are now rarely given.

Complications

Spasticity Possibly improved by baclofen, 10–25 mg three times daily or by diazepam 5–10 mg three times daily.

Bladder disturbances These may be treated by anticholinergic and other drugs (Chapter 24).

Depression Depression may require treatment with tricyclic antidepressants or other drugs.

Trigeminal neuralgia and other paroxysmal disturbances Such disturbances can be helped by carbamazepine 200–400 mg three times daily.

Fatigue One of the most common and troublesome symptoms and is usually treated with antidepressants, counselling and occasionally amantadine.

Long-term therapy

Beta-interferon has been shown to reduce the frequency of relapses and the number of demyelinating lesions seen on cranial MRI. It is being extensively trialled. Alpha-interferon has not proved beneficial and gamma-interferon makes the disease worse. Immunosuppressive agents including azathioprine, cyclophosphamide, cyclosporin and corticosteroids have significant side effects and do little to alter the course of the disease.

OTHER DEMYELINATING DISEASES

Acute disseminated encephalomyelitis

Acute disseminated encephalomyelitis is acute demyelination of the white matter of the brain and spinal cord, characterized pathologically by perivascular cellular infiltration and perivenous demyelination. It usually follows exanthematous viral infections such as measles, chicken pox, rubella and smallpox (post-infectious encephalomyelitis), but may also follow vaccinations (post-vaccinial encephalomyelitis).

The onset is commonly about 5–20 days after the exanthem or vaccination and the condition has an immune basis. The onset is usually abrupt with headache, drowsiness, fever and sometimes convulsions. There is a combination of pyramidal tract, cerebellar and brain-stem signs. The mortality rate may be as high as 30%; in the remainder of cases, recovery occurs with a variable degree of neurological deficit.

Neuromyelitis optica (Devic's disease)

Neuromyelitis optica is probably a specific form of multiple sclerosis. It is characterized by the rapid onset of bilateral optic neuritis and transverse myelitis occurring within days or weeks of each other. Either the spinal or optic nerve lesion may appear first.

Balo's concentric sclerosis

This is a variant of multiple sclerosis characterized pathologically by concentric rings of demyelination mainly in the frontal white matter. Dementia is a prominent clinical feature and the disease has an inexorably progressive course.

Diffuse cerebral sclerosis

This is a condition first described by Schilder in which there is massive demyelination of the cerebral white matter characterized clinically by progressive visual failure, spasticity and dementia. It is very rare and it probably represents a heterogeneous group of metabolic and inflammatory disorders.

REFERENCES

Ebers G. C. (1994) Treatment of multiple sclerosis. *Lancet,* **343**, 275–279.
Ffrench-Constant C. (1994) Pathogenesis of multiple sclerosis. *Lancet,* **343**, 271–275.
Matthews W. B. (Ed) (1991) *McAlpine's Multiple Sclerosis*, 2nd edn. Churchill Livingstone, Edinburgh.

21 | Degenerative diseases

MOTOR NEURONE DISEASES

Amyotrophic lateral sclerosis

This is also discussed in Chapter 7. Amyotrophic lateral sclerosis is a degenerative disorder of upper and lower motor neurones that presents most commonly in later life. In about 10–20% of cases there is autosomal dominant inheritance. In some families there is linkage to chromosome 21 (21q22.1– q22.2). Progressive weakness leads to death, on average, about 4 years from the time of diagnosis. There are characteristic pathological changes of degeneration in the anterior horn cells of the spinal cord, the motor nuclei of the medulla and the corticospinal tracts (Fig. 7.7).

The presenting clinical features vary depending upon the extent of involvement of lower and upper motor neurones and may consist predominantly of muscle wasting or spasticity, or a combination of the two. There are three recognized modes of presentation:

Progressive muscular atrophy

Muscular wasting and fasciculation are usually noticed first in the small muscles of the hand or in the lower limbs, accompanied by foot-drop, and spread slowly to involve all muscles except those concerned with eye movements and bladder control. Painful muscle cramps are a common complaint.

Progressive lateral sclerosis

This is a less common variant of motor neurone disease in which signs of upper motor neurone degeneration, spasticity and hyper-reflexia precede those of lower motor neurone involvement. This is in contrast to the usual situation in amyotrophic lateral sclerosis where upper and lower motor neurone signs occur together giving a characteristic combination of wasted muscles with increased reflexes in the affected limbs.

Progressive bulbar palsy

Impairment of bulbar function (swallowing, coughing and articulation of speech) may be the presenting symptom, but in any event it always develops at a later stage of the disease with atrophy and fasciculation of the tongue. The upper motor neurone (corticobulbar tract) is often involved as well, so that voluntary elevation of the palate is less than that provoked by the gag reflex and the jaw jerk is increased (*pseudobulbar palsy*). Pseudobulbar palsy is also characterized by loss of control over emotional reactions so that patients may laugh and cry inappropriately. Dysphagia may be aggravated by spasm of the cricopharyngeus muscle and partially relieved by its division (myotomy).

The cause is unknown and there is no specific treatment. Management involves helping patients cope with the various symptoms as they arise and providing assistance in the home when they become disabled. Many patients derive comfort from membership of the Amyotrophic Lateral Sclerosis (ALS) Society. Death is usually caused by bulbar and respiratory weakness with inhalational pneumonia. By mutual agreement between patient, relatives and medical staff, resuscitation measures are usually avoided in the terminal phase when relief of pain and distress becomes more important than the prolongation of life.

Chronic proximal spinal muscular atrophy (Kugelberg-Welander syndrome)

This is a mild, slowly progressive disorder with a benign prognosis; it is compatible with a normal life-span. Inheritance is usually autosomal recessive, but dominant and X-linked forms have also been described. The recessive types of spinal muscular atrophy are linked to chromosome 5 (5q12.2–q.13.3). The onset is in childhood or adolescence with difficulty in walking because of hip-girdle weakness. Proximal muscles in the upper and lower limbs are mainly affected and the distribution of muscle weakness may cause the condition to be mistaken for muscular dystrophy. However fasciculations are often seen and the neurogenic nature of the disorder is confirmed by electromyography and muscle biopsy. Bulbar musculature is spared and upper motor neurone signs are rarely present. There is no specific therapy.

Acute infantile spinal muscular atrophy (Werdnig-Hoffman disease)

This is a rapidly progressive anterior horn cell degeneration with an autosomal recessive inheritance and the same genetic linkage as Kugelberg-Welander syndrome. It may be apparent at birth (floppy baby syndrome) or develop during the first 6 months of life. The mean survival is 6 months and most children are dead by 18 months of age. A more slowly progressive variant is recognized.

HEREDITARY SPASTIC PARAPLEGIA

The pure form of hereditary spastic paraplegia is a degeneration of the cortico-spinal pathways, usually inherited as an autosomal dominant characteristic, causing progressive spasticity with hyper-reflexia and extensor plantar responses. The legs are primarily affected and the arms are rarely involved. The age of onset and degree of disability vary in different families.

There are complicated forms of hereditary spastic paraplegia in which the features of spasticity may be combined with muscle wasting (amyotrophy), mental retardation, ataxia, optic atrophy, extrapyramidal features or sensory neuropathy.

EXTRAPYRAMIDAL DISEASE

Parkinson's disease, Huntington's disease, dystonia musculorum deformans and Wilson's disease are described in Chapter 15.

A mixed pyramidal and extrapyramidal degeneration of late onset, characterized by impairment of voluntary vertical eye movements, especially downgaze, axial rigidity and gait disturbance, is known as progressive supranuclear palsy (Steele-Richardson syndrome).

A rare autosomal recessive disorder is associated with deposition of iron in the basal ganglia (Hallevorden-Spatz disease). It runs a slowly progressive course over 10–20 years with extrapyramidal and pyramidal features.

HEREDITARY ATAXIAS

The hereditary ataxias are a group of disorders that are classified according to their clinical, genetic and pathological features.

Friedreich's ataxia

This is a disease with an autosomal recessive inheritance (chromosome 9–9q12.13) with onset under the age of 25 years (mean 12 years), the first symptom usually being ataxia of gait. Other clinical features are dysarthria, incoordination, absent reflexes in the lower limbs, impaired position and vibration sense, extensor plantar responses, pes cavus, scoliosis and cardiomyopathy. Diabetes may be a complication. Pathologically it is characterized by degeneration of the spinocerebellar tracts, posterior columns, corticospinal tracts, and of the cell bodies in the dorsal root ganglia with their large afferent fibres mediating proprioception and tendon reflexes (Fig. 7.7). Optic atrophy and deafness may also be associated. The condition is progressive and the mean age of death is 37 years, usually due to heart failure, pneumonia or diabetes. Treatment is limited to supportive measures and the management of cardiac dysrhythmias or failure and diabetes in some patients. Friedreich's Ataxia Associations and other support groups exist in most large cities.

Other early onset cerebellar ataxias

In some types of early onset cerebellar ataxia the tendon jerks are retained (in contrast to Friedreich's ataxia) and scoliosis, impaired proprioception, cardiac abnormalities and diabetes are less common than in Friedreich's ataxia.

Another form of cerebellar ataxia in which the pathological changes are those of cerebello-olivary atrophy was first described by Holmes. Since the degenerative changes are confined to the cerebellum and its connections and the spinal cord and peripheral nerves are unaffected, there are no associated pyramidal tract or peripheral nerve signs and the reflexes remain intact. Inheritance is usually autosomal recessive.

Progressive cerebellar ataxia of early onset may be associated with myoclonus. This autosomal recessive disorder is known as the Ramsay-Hunt syndrome. The age of onset is usually between the ages of 5 and 15 years. This syndrome, and related system degenerations with myoclonus, are prevalent in countries surrounding the Baltic Sea and are included in the term 'Baltic myoclonus'. Myoclonus may also be associated with cerebellar degeneration in storage diseases (Lafora body disease, cerebral lipidosis), and mitochondrial myopathy.

Late onset cerebellar ataxia

Olivopontocerebellar atrophy is a form of progressive cerebellar ataxia of middle life which usually has an autosomal dominant mode of inheritance. Pontine and mid-brain structures degenerate in addition to the cerebellum, and clinical features include ataxia, dysarthria, nystagmus, pyramidal tract signs, optic atrophy and ophthalmoplegia.

Other forms of late onset cerebellar ataxia exist in which there is no family history.

MULTIPLE SYSTEM ATROPHY

Multiple system atrophy (MSA) is a group of disorders characterized by progressive autonomic failure, cerebellar ataxia, pyramidal tract signs and Parkinsonism. They have in common the pathological finding of oligodendroglial and neuronal intracytoplasmic and intranuclear inclusions. Multiple system atrophy includes the conditions: Shy-Drager syndrome, adult onset striato-nigral degeneration and sporadic olivopontocerebellar degeneration.

OPTIC ATROPHY

Optic atrophy may be found in combination with many of the disorders described above.

Leber's optic atrophy

This is a hereditary disorder transmitted exclusively through the maternal line to males. In the second or third decade of life, central vision deteriorates, first in one eye then the other, sometimes occurring suddenly but usually occurring in a period of time ranging over days to months. It is caused by a point mutation on mitochondrial DNA.

Retinitis pigmentosa

This is also more common in males and may be of recessive or dominant inheritance. It starts with night blindness, followed by peripheral constriction of the visual fields. A network of pigment can be seen extending throughout the retina, sparing the macula. It may be associated with other hereditary disorders such as hereditary ataxias, familial spastic paraplegia, ocular myopathy, polyneuropathy and deafness (Refsum's disease), and a syndrome of obesity, hypogonadism, mental retardation and syndactyly (Laurence-Moon-Biedl syndrome).

DEAFNESS

Hereditary perceptive (nerve) deafness may be associated with many neurological disorders, such as optic atrophy, polyneuropathy, familial myoclonic epilepsy and hereditary ataxias.

PERIPHERAL NEUROPATHY

Peripheral neuropathy is covered in more detail in Chapter 10.

Peroneal muscular atrophy (Charcot-Marie-Tooth Disease)

This is a heterogeneous group of disorders manifested by predominantly motor neuropathy, usually with autosomal dominant inheritance. It has been separated on electrophysiological, genetic and histological grounds into hereditary sensorimotor neuropathy (HMSN) types Ia and Ib with demyelination and hypertrophic changes, and HMSN type II with axonal degeneration. Another form of Charcot-Marie-Tooth disease, known as the Roussy-Levy syndrome, is associated with tremor.

Hypertrophic polyneuropathy (Déjèrine-Sottas disease HMSN III)

This is a recessively inherited demyelinating neuropathy with hypertrophic changes that becomes clinically apparent in the first decade. Sensory disability is greater and the condition progresses more rapidly than Charcot-Marie-Tooth disease. It may be a heterogeneous group of conditions.

Hereditary sensory neuropathy

There are several different types of this disorder. The most common is a dominantly inherited neuropathy in which sensory symptoms and signs are predominant, although some members of affected families may develop distal wasting resembling that of Charcot-Marie-Tooth disease. Lightning (stabbing) pains may be a distressing symptom. Loss of pain sensation may be so profound that joints are destroyed

(Charcot joints), and trophic ulcers develop on the feet for want of protective reflexes.

Familial dysautonomia is a rare congenital, recessively inherited poly-neuropathy with defective autonomic function (Riley-Day syndrome).

Congenital insensitivity to pain

These are rare syndromes of universal analgesia; pain pathways may be abnormal in either the peripheral or the central nervous system. Congenital indifference to pain is a condition in which pain can be perceived but is disregarded.

Rare metabolic neuropathies

Refsum's disease is an autosomal recessive polyneuropathy associated with cerebellar ataxia, retinitis pigmentosa and nerve deafness and an increase in blood phytanic acid. Other metabolic neuropathies are caused by disorders of lipoprotein metabolism and include *a-beta-lipoproteinaemia, (Bassen-Kornzweig syndrome)* which is associated with acanthocytosis, and *an-alpha-lipoprotein-aemia (Tangier disease)*. Metachromatic leucodystrophy is characterized by accumulation of sulfatide and symptoms of mental retardation, leucodystrophy and peripheral neuropathy (see below). There are several different types of *familial amyloid neuropathy*.

MUSCULAR DYSTROPHY

This is discussed in more detail in Chapter 10.

NEUROCUTANEOUS SYNDROMES (THE PHAKOMATOSES)

Tuberous sclerosis

This is a congenital disorder, occurring sporadically or as an autosomal dominant condition, characterized by areas of ectodermal or mesodermal hyperplasia in the skin, nervous and other systems. The abnormal gene has been assigned to the long arm of chromosome 9 (9q32). It usually presents as epilepsy in a child with some degree of mental retardation and is recognized initially by the nature of the skin lesions. The following anomalies may be present:

Skin

Reddish papules are found over the nasolabial folds, cheek and chin ('adenoma sebaceum'). There are fibrotic areas in the skin, usually on the back, known as shagreen (sharkskin) patches and leaf-shaped areas of hypo-pigmentation on the trunk or limbs called 'ash leaf patches'. Tumours of the nail-bed (subungual fibromas) may exist.

Nervous system

Tubers of astrocytes and giant cells are scattered throughout the brain and in the walls of the lateral ventricles and are the cause of epilepsy in this condition. They commonly calcify and may be seen readily on a computed tomography (CT) scan and sometimes on a plain radiograph of the skull.

Retina and other organs

Gliomatous nodules (phakomas) may be seen in the vicinity of the optic disc.

Rhabdomyomas of the heart, lung cysts ('honeycomb lungs'), and benign tumours or cysts of the kidney, liver and other organs are not uncommon.

Neurofibromatosis

There are two forms of this disorder, NF1 and NF2.

NF1: Von Recklingbausen's disease

This is autosomal dominant with variable penetrance and affects about 15/100 000 of the population. The gene is located on 17q11.2. The clinical manifestations are:

Skin Areas of skin the colour of milk coffee (*café au lait* patches) are found of larger size and in greater number than in the general population. Some 80% of patients have six or more large patches. Multiple freckles may be seen in the axilla or over the lower abdomen, buttocks and upper thighs. Spots of depigmentation may be found in the skin elsewhere.

Cutaneous tumours may feel hard or soft to palpation. Firm subcutaneous nodules may be felt attached to nerves and overgrowth of subcutaneous fibrous tissue may produce deformities.

Iris A small hamartoma may be seen as a pale spot in the iris in most instances.

Peripheral nerves Peripheral nerves may be palpable in the posterior triangle of the neck, elbow or popliteal fossa. Nerve palsies may develop as a 'mononeuritis multiplex'.

Brain Neuromas on the acoustic, trigeminal or other cranial nerves. Gliomas and meningiomas are also more common in this condition.

Spinal cord Tumours of spinal nerves may compress the spinal cord, enlarge the appropriate intervertebral foramen and form a paravertebral mass ('buttonhole neurofibromas'). Spinal root or cauda equina tumours may simulate root compression by a cervical or lumbar disc lesion but radicular pain is usually the first and most persistent symptom of radicular neurofibromas.

Other organs A phaeochromocytoma develops in about 0.5% of patients with neurofibromatosis. From the other aspect, neurofibromatosis is present in 5–20% of patients with phaeochromocytoma.

NF2: Central neurofibromatosis

This is an autosomal dominant disorder that is rarer than NF1 (2/100 000). Clinical manifestations are bilateral acoustic Schwannomas, multiple meningiomas and spinal root Schwannomas. Linkage is to chromosome 22q12.2.

Sturge-Weber syndrome

In this condition, there is an association of a capillary haemangioma (port-wine stain) in the distribution of the first division of the trigeminal nerve with a meningeal naevus and calcification in the gyri of the underlying cortex. The calcification, which shows up as parallel lines in plain X-rays (tramline calcification), is readily seen in CT scans and is usually more prominent over the posterior half of the affected hemisphere. The facial naevus may involve the eye, causing glaucoma. The intracranial anomaly is usually accompanied by a mild contralateral hemiparesis and focal (partial) motor seizures. The condition is not associated with intracerebral arteriovenous malformations, nor is there any tendency to subarachnoid haemorrhage. It is not usually familial.

Familial telangiectasia (Osler-Weber-Rendu disease)

Telangiecteses are seen as small red spots, blanching on pressure, on the skin and on the lips in this autosomal dominant disorder. Mucosal telangiecteses often give rise to epistaxis or intestinal bleeding. Telangiectasia is an uncommon cause of intracerebral or intraspinal haemorrhage but should be kept in mind when a young patient suffers a catastrophe of this sort without demonstrable cause.

Ataxia telangiectasia

This is an autosomal recessive disorder beginning with ataxia and choreoathetotic movements in the first decade of life, associated with telangiecteses on the conjunctiva and other areas of the face or neck. There is a deficiency of immunoglobulin A and an immune deficiency state that renders the patient prone to repeated infection or the development of lymphoma. Death usually occurs in the second or third decade of life.

Von Hippel-Lindau disease

This association of retinal angioma with cerebellar haemangioblastoma is an autosomal recessive disorder, the gene being located on chromosome 3p25. The tumour secretes erythropoietin which can cause polycythaemia. The retinal and cerebellar lesions are treated independently by laser and surgical excision, respectively.

STORAGE DISEASES AND OTHER INHERITED METABOLIC ABNORMALITIES

Lysosomal storage diseases result from specific enzyme deficiencies that permit the accumulation of a metabolite which would normally be degraded. Some examples of cerebral lipidosis are given in the following sections.

Tay-Sachs disease

A disease of infancy, characterized by mental regression, pyramidal tract degeneration, myoclonus and the development of a cherry-red spot at the macula. Death occurs by the age of 5 years. The deficient enzyme is hexosaminidase A and the accumulated metabolite is GM_2 ganglioside. The condition is restricted to the Jewish race, and the gene is located on chromosome 15 (15q23–q24).

Juvenile cerebroretinal degeneration

Infantile, juvenile and adult forms of cerebral lipidosis are recognized in which macular degeneration, myoclonus, generalized seizures and mental retardation are salient features.

Metachromatic leucodystrophy

A sphingolipid storage disease caused by the absence of aryl sulfatase A, leading to the accumulation of sulfatide. There are infantile, juvenile and adult forms, with autosomal recessive inheritance. There are mutations in the gene encoding aryl sulfatase A (22q 13–13qter). It is characterized by mental regression, pyramidal and cerebellar signs and peripheral neuropathy. The diagnosis may be confirmed by the presence of metachromatic granules in a nerve biopsy. The condition runs a progressively downhill course over a period of 5 years.

REFERENCES

Baraitser M. (1990) *The Genetics of Neurological Disorders*, 2nd edn. Oxford University Press, Oxford.

Harding A. E. (1992) The Hereditary Ataxias and Related Disorders. In: *Diseases of the Nervous System*, 2nd edn. Eds A. K. Asbury, G. M. McKhann and W. I. McDonald. W. B. Saunders, Philadelphia. 1169–1178.

Marsden C. D. (1993) The motor disorder of multisystem atrophy. *Journal of Neurology, Neurosurgery and Psychiatry*, **56**, 1239–1242.

Martin J. P. (1993) Molecular genetics in neurology. *Annals of Neurology*, **34**, 757–773.

22 | Trauma

HEAD TRAUMA

In Australia there are about 26 deaths per 100 000 population from head injury each year, about two-thirds of which are due to motor vehicle accidents. Head injuries may be *closed*, where there is no communication between the cranial cavity and the external environment, in contrast to *open* head injuries.

Closed head injury

Most civilian head injuries are closed and, if severe enough to cause brain damage, almost always result in loss of consciousness. Any impairment of consciousness following a head injury is commonly referred to as *concussion*.

Pathophysiology of closed head injury

Damage to the brain in closed head injury is due to the rapid acceleration and deceleration of the deformable brain within the rigid cranial cavity. It has been shown in experimental animals that even very severe blows will not cause brain injury if the head is restrained so that it is unable to move, and conversely that rapid acceleration without any physical blow can produce closed brain injury. Rotational forces during head injury may lead to the brain moving past rough internal surfaces of the skull causing cortical contusions or lacerations that tend to be mainly frontal, presumably because this portion of the skull has more internal protuberances. Shearing forces within the deep white matter may lead to axonal injury or disruption with subsequent distal degeneration of the axons. Pathologically this is marked by the appearance of axonal retraction balls, myelin loss and gliosis. If this process is widespread it is referred to as *diffuse axonal injury.* As CNS axons are unable to restore their appropriate connections, even if axonal regrowth occurs, such injuries result in permanent structural changes to the brain.

Although fractures are frequently seen in association with closed head injury severe diffuse axonal injury may occur without skull fracture or significant cortical lacerations. Secondary changes may occur in the brain as a consequence of the intracerebral oedema associated with diffuse axonal injury. These changes include herniation of one frontal lobe underneath the falx cerebri or of one temporal lobe through the tentorium cerebelli. In severe head injury intracranial pressure may rise enough to cause regions of secondary infarction. These changes result in further swelling with subsequent progression and usually lead to the death of the patient.

Management

Unfortunately the management of closed head injury is largely expectant. There is no specific therapy since the neural damage has all taken place at the time of the initial insult. If large extradural, subdural or intra-cerebral haematomas (Chapter 13) occur these may require surgical drainage. In order to reduce the secondary changes due to raised intra-cerebral pressure, intracranial pressure (ICP) is monitored and the patient's fluid balance is manipulated with fluid restriction or osmotic diuretics (mannitol) to try and keep the ICP below set limits. Since raised intracranial pressure is a manifestation of severe diffuse axonal injury, such patients usually have a poor outcome even if they survive.

Outcome of closed head injury

There is a correlation between the outcome of closed head injury and the depth of the coma, which can be assessed with the Glasgow Coma Scale (Table 14.1) that scores from 3 to 15. Scores of less than 8 indicate a severe head injury with a poor prognosis, scores between 9 and 12 a moderate injury with an intermediate prognosis and scores of more than 13 a mild injury with a good long-term prognosis. These indicators relate specifically to closed head injury and a Glasgow Coma Scale score should not be used to prognosticate in coma due to other causes. *Post-traumatic amnesia* is the interval from the onset of injury to recovery of memory of events, and this also correlates with the degree of diffuse brain damage and with long-term outcome.

Mild injury   Patients may suffer persistent symptoms after even mild head injury. These may take the form of headaches, impaired concentration, tiredness, vertigo and depression. Patients who undergo a series of mild head injuries may develop more serious impairment of intellectual functions; e.g. prize fighters who are knocked unconscious on several occasions may develop a progressive syndrome, *dementia pugilistica*, characterized by forgetfulness, slow thought processes, slurring dysarthria, slowed movements and a wide-based shambling gait that appears Parkinsonian. The existence of this condition suggests that there may be a degree of axonal injury that occurs with even very short-lived periods of unconsciousness following closed head injury and, for this reason, patients who have had one concussive injury should be advised to avoid situations that might produce further such injuries.

Moderate injury   Patients with more severe injuries may have persistent focal signs such as hemiparesis, hemianopia, dysarthria or cranial nerve palsies. In addition, however, many patients have disturbances of higher intellectual function that are more disabling. They are often impulsive, show poor organizing abilities, have poor memory and display hypersexuality or other signs of release or disinhibition. Their families frequently complain that their personalities have changed from the pre-morbid state.

Severe injury   About 5% of patients admitted to hospital with closed head injury will develop a *persistent vegetative state* (p. 216). They may survive for many years and present serious moral, emotional and financial difficulties to society and to their families. They do not meet brain death criteria and cannot therefore have medical support withdrawn under most existing legal codes.

Post-traumatic epilepsy

About 5–10% of patients admitted to hospital with head injury will develop persistent post-traumatic epilepsy. A number of patients will have early seizures while still in hospital and of these, about 30% will go on to have late seizures together with a proportion who did not have immediate post-traumatic seizures. The latent interval between the injury and the first seizure may be 5 years or longer. Most people who have a seizure after a long latent interval will go on to have persistent epilepsy. Patients with intracranial haematomas and depressed skull fractures have an especially high risk of post-traumatic epilepsy.

Open head injury

A head injury is defined as open when the skin is breached in association with a depressed skull fracture (compound fracture) or when there is dural rupture in association with a fracture at the skull base allowing cerebrospinal fluid (CSF) to leak into the middle ear or paranasal sinuses. In the latter case the open nature of the fracture may not be clinically obvious. Sometimes air may be seen on a skull film or computed tomography (CT) and such a finding always implies an open head injury. Minor CSF leaks, particularly from the external auditory meatus, may occasionally heal spontaneously. Persistent leaks require surgical repair. The major risk in cases of open head injury is infection. The occurrence of bacterial meningitis, particularly if an unusual organism is involved in a patient who has a history of serious head injury, should always prompt a search for a CSF leak. Such an event may be delayed for years after the original injury.

SPINAL TRAUMA

Although motor vehicle accidents are the single largest cause of spinal injury a significant percentage occur during sporting and recreational activities. Damage to the spinal cord is almost invariably accompanied by damage to the vertebral column and frequently by head injury.

Cervical spine injury

Mechanism

Cervical spine injuries usually result from force applied to the head causing hyperextension or hyperflexion of the neck. Hyperflexion usually results in a crush fracture of the anterior portion of the vertebral body at the level of greatest force. The vertebral body beneath may be fractured and driven backwards into the spinal canal (fracture dislocation). Lesser degrees of force may produce fracture without dislocation. Hyperextension of the neck causes collision of the spinous and articular processes of the midcervical vertebrae with subsequent separation of the vertebral bodies at the intervertebral disc. The resultant dislocation traps the cord between the body of the superior vertebra and the processes of the inferior vertebra. If the movement is very violent there may be complete rupture of the anterior spinal ligament. Both flexion and extension injuries most commonly occur at the C6/7 vertebral junction. If the vertebral column has reduced flexibility due to cervical spondylosis, ankylosing spondylitis or congenital spinal canal stenosis the risk of spinal cord injury for a given degree of force is increased. The combination of ankylosis and ligamentous disruption seen in rheumatoid arthritis may lead to dislocation at the atlanto-odontoid joint. Damage to the spinal cord usually occurs at the time of the injury. The exception to this is fractures and dislocations in those with relatively fixed spines where the amount of force required to produce bony injury is much less. In all spinal cord injuries the detection of any voluntary movement below the level of the lesion on the first day after the injury is a good prognostic sign.

Pathology

The cord is squeezed by the vertebral bodies with destruction of grey and white matter. There is often some haemorrhage within the area of damage, which is usually confined to the level of the injury or one or two segments above and below.

The cord is almost never completely transected except by gross, usually fatal, injuries. There may be subsequent development of post-traumatic syringomyelia with progression of disability many years later.

Management

Cervical spine injury produces quadriparesis or quadriplegia (Chapter 7). Surgical stabilization of the spine may be undertaken in some cases. Abrupt loss of spinal cord function leads to loss of temperature and blood pressure control as well as to loss of all bowel and bladder function during the stage of spinal shock. Complete loss of sensation below the level of the lesion puts the patient at risk of decubitus ulceration and immobility leads to hypercalcaemia and hypercalcuria. The usual mechanism of death in quadriplegic patients who survive the acute episode is urinary tract infection. Because of these complications acute spinal cord injuries are best managed in dedicated spinal injury units with a multidisciplinary approach. Life for quadriplegic patients is difficult and most such patients remain dependent on care from family members or paid help. As many such patients are young, risk-taking males, whose body image was central to their ego integrity the late management of spinal cord injury involves complex social and psychological issues as well as medical care. Most spinal injury units undertake long-term support of such patients.

Lumbar spine injury

The second most common anatomical site for spinal injury is the junction of the thoracic and lumbar spine. As the spinal cord ends at the level of the first lumbar interspace, injuries in this region often involve the cauda equina rather than the cord. This leads to wasting in the muscles whose innervation is lost rather than the upper motor neurone syndrome seen with higher injuries. These injuries are still devastating as they produce paraplegia accompanied by loss of bladder, bowel and sexual function. However, because of the preservation of control of the upper limbs and trunk and of thoracic autonomic outflow, patients are much easier to manage and have a better long-term prognosis than those with cervical cord injuries and most become independent with appropriate aids.

REFERENCES

Byrne T. and Waxman S. G. (1990) *Spinal Cord Compression: Diagnosis and Principles of Management.* F. A. Davis, Philadelphia.

Jennett B. and Teasdale B. (1991) *Management of Head Injuries,* 2nd edn. F. A. Davis, Philadelphia.

Johnson R. A. (1993) The management of acute spinal cord compression. *Journal of Neurology, Neurosurgery and Psychiatry,* **56**, 1046–1054.

Part 3

INVESTIGATION AND TREATMENT OF NEUROLOGICAL DISORDERS

23 | Investigation of neurological disorders

IMAGING TECHNIQUES

Plain X-rays

Simple radiography of the skull and facial bones is indicated when a fracture is suspected or to confirm the diagnosis of sinusitis. Skull X-rays will also demonstrate enlargement, or a double floor, of the pituitary fossa when it is expanded by a tumour, and displacement of the calcified pineal gland from the mid-line with a unilateral space-occupying lesion. Computed tomography (CT) or magnetic resonance imaging (MRI) gives more information in these cases. A chest X-ray should be taken if an intracranial lesion is suspected since it may show primary or secondary tumours, tuberculosis, sarcoidosis, bronchiectasis or other conditions of relevance.

Plain X-ray of the cervical spine demonstrates cranio-spinal anomalies such as platybasia, abnormalities of the vertebrae, narrowing of disc spaces and osteophytic projection from neurocentral and facet joints which may narrow the intervertebral foramina in cervical spondylosis and cause root compression. Radiography of the lumbar spine is less informative but will show disc degeneration or spondylolisthesis.

Computerized axial tomography (CT)

A thin beam of X-rays scans the head or spine in a series of planes and the differential absorption of each area is calculated by computer and displayed as a pictorial representation of the structures scanned (Fig. 23.1) Computed tomography scanning demonstrates hydrocephalus, cerebral atrophy, haemorrhages and most infarcts, tumours and other intracranial lesions. It is particularly helpful in recent strokes for detecting haemorrhages. An intravenous injection of contrast medium is given to display the vascular system and may demonstrate an aneurysm or arteriovenous malformation. Where the blood-brain barrier is defective, in the vicinity of tumours or infarcts for example, the contrast medium enters cerebral tissue and is seen as an area of enhancement on the scan. Some tumours and subdural haematomas in an isodense phase may escape detection. Computed tomography scanning, especially when it is used in conjunction with myelography,

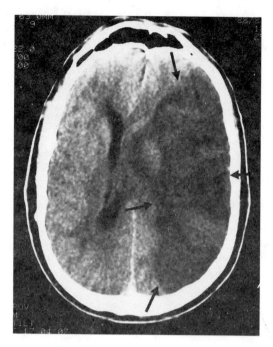

Fig. 23.1 Computed tomography scan of brain. The dark low-density area in left hemisphere (arrowed) represents an infarct in the distribution of the middle cerebral artery.

will demonstrate abnormalities of spinal cord and roots such as syringomyelia, tumours and disc protrusions.

Magnetic resonance imaging (MRI)

Magnetic resonance imaging depends on a strong magnetic field orienting hydrogen ions in the body in a north–south direction, followed by the application of a lateral magnetic pulse to displace these ions. The field generated during this process and the return to the previous orientation is analysed by computer to depict anatomical structures as a function of their water content (Fig. 23.2). The technique is complementary to CT scan and has advantages in showing small lesions in the grey matter (hamartomas, cryptogenic haemangiomas, and hippocampal sclerosis or other areas of gliosis producing epileptogenic foci) and particular white matter diseases, areas of demyelination in multiple sclerosis (Fig 23.3) and some infiltrating tumours such as pontine glioma that may elude the CT scan. Magnetic resonance imaging also provides clear images of the spinal column, cord and roots that may make a definitive diagnosis of spinal cord compression or intrinsic lesions such as tumours, multiple sclerosis, plaques or syringomyelia. Magnetic resonance angiography (MRA) images blood vessels and may be a suitable alternative to invasive techniques of angiography.

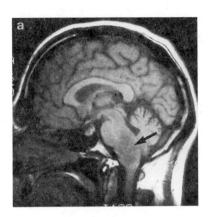
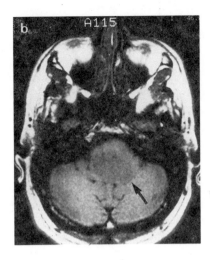

Fig. 23.2 Magnetic resonance imaging (MRI) of brain. (a) Mid-line sagittal MRI scan showing the ventricular system and aqueduct with enlargement of the medulla by a glioma (arrowed); (b) horizontal MRI scan of the same patient, demonstrating the medullary lesion (arrowed).

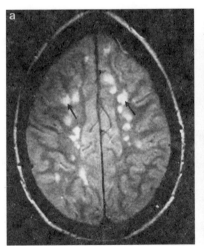
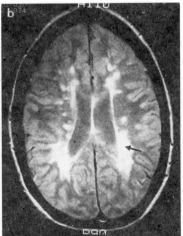

Fig. 23.3 Magnetic resonance imaging of brain in multiple sclerosis. (a) White areas (arrowed) represent plaques in cerebral white matter; (b) periventricular demyelination (arrows).

Angiography

Injection of a contrast medium into the circulation, usually by means of a catheter inserted into the femoral artery and insinuated into the appropriate artery, demonstrates the carotid or vertebrobasilar vessels. Aneurysms, angiomas and the blood supply to tumours can be demonstrated in this way. Smaller doses of the contrast agent can be used intra-arterially if the images are enhanced by computer (digital subtraction angiography or DSA).

Myelography

A water-soluble contrast medium is inserted into the cerebrospinal fluid (CSF) by lumbar puncture to outline the spinal cord and roots radiologically. Myelography is used to determine the site and extent of spinal cord compression if it is not adequately displayed by MRI. It should be followed by CT scanning while the contrast medium is still present to provide more accurate information about structural change at certain segmental levels. The contrast medium may later enter the spinal cord and demonstrate a central lesion such as syringomyelia. It is important to discuss the patient's clinical signs with the radiologist so that the suspected level is thoroughly investigated. A lumbar myelogram is of no help in diagnosing a lesion of the thoracic cord! A CSF sample is usually taken for examination at the time of the insertion of the contrast medium. Sufficient fluid should be taken to allow for immuno-electrophoresis of CSF proteins to determine whether oligoclonal bands are present in the globulin fraction.

Isotope ventriculography

To determine the rate of clearance of CSF from the ventricular system, a radioactive isotope can be injected into the lumbar sac and the ventricular content of isotope monitored for 48 hours thereafter. This technique is sometimes employed in the diagnosis of hydrocephalus and in the detection of leaks of the CSF, e.g. CSF rhinorrhoea after head injuries or CSF leakage from the lumbar sac in prolonged low pressure headaches after lumbar puncture.

Positron emission tomography (PET)

Positron emission tomography is a technique that utilizes positron emitting radiopharmaceuticals to map the physiology, biochemistry and pharmacology of the human brain. The radioisotopes are produced by a medical cyclotron and are incorporated into compounds that are biologically active in the body. The scanner provides cross-sectional images of the distribution of these radiolabelled compounds in the brain and other organs. Glucose metabolism is measured with fluorine-labelled glucose ([18F]-fluoro-2-deoxy-D-glucose or FDG); labelled water is used for measuring cerebral bloodflow, levodopa is employed to study presynaptic dopamine terminals in the brain, and [11C]- and [18F]-labelled compounds have been used to examine post-synaptic dopamine receptors. Other neurochemical receptors can be studied in similar ways.

The major clinical applications of PET scanning are in localizing epileptogenic foci (the focal lesions are hypoactive in between attacks and hyperactive during attacks) and in localizing and determining the degree of malignancy of tumours by measuring their metabolic activity with FDG.

Functional scanning, using ^{15}O-labelled compounds to measure cerebral bloodflow, has provided important information about localization of function such as speech and vision within the brain since bloodflow increases during cerebral activity.

Single-photon emission computed tomography (SPECT)

Single-photon emission computed tomography isotopes emit single photons which can be detected with simpler equipment than is required for PET. The radio-isotopes (e.g. technetium) are produced by a cyclotron but have a longer half-life than those used with PET. Single-photon emission computed tomography is used for measuring cerebral bloodflow and for localizing epileptogenic foci. The resolution is not so precise as that with PET scanning, but the cost is considerably less.

NEUROPHYSIOLOGY

Electromyography (EMG)

Electromyography is the recording through a needle or surface electrode of electrical activity from muscles which is amplified and then displayed on an oscilloscope. The signals are also broadcast through a loudspeaker so that an examiner can hear the auditory equivalent of the electrical potentials. Normally there is no electrical activity from muscle fibres at rest but injury to either muscles or nerves can produce abnormal potentials.

Fibrillation potentials

These arise from denervated muscle fibres. If a nerve fibre is destroyed then all of the muscle fibres connected to it will begin to generate spontaneous biphasic action potentials within 7–14 days from the time of denervation (Fig. 5.7). The same process may also produce positive sharp waves. These denervation potentials may also be recorded in some primary muscle disease, (e.g. polymyositis, Duchenne muscular dystrophy), because the terminal innervation of some muscle fibres is damaged by the disease process.

Fasciculation potentials

These are single motor unit action potentials produced by spontaneous discharges in degenerating nerve fibres. Their occurrence in isolation in a relaxed muscle is characteristic of motor nerve fibre degeneration.

Recruitment patterns

On voluntary activation of muscle the smallest motor neurone in the motor neurone pool will begin to fire slowly. This will produce a stereotyped recurrent individual motor unit action potential discharge on the oscilloscope screen. As the subject's effort increases more motor units will be recruited. Initially these will be identifiable as individual potentials on the oscilloscope screen but as more and more units are recruited they begin to overlap and produce an *interference pattern*. If there is poor drive from the upper motor neurone then a sparse interference pattern with few units is seen. This pattern of recruitment may be seen in upper motor neurone lesions but it is also seen in patients who do not make an adequate voluntary effort.

Chronic partial denervation

After denervation of a muscle, the surviving nerve fibres will sprout and re-innervate some or all of the denervated muscle fibres. This process leads to motor units having more muscle fibres in them than is usual for that particular muscle. On the oscilloscope screen such units will appear as complex (polyphasic) potentials of larger than usual amplitude. Such high amplitude polyphasic potentials are characteristic of partial denervation with subsequent re-innervation (Fig. 5.8).

Myopathic potentials

Primary muscle fibre diseases lead to muscle fibre splitting and smaller motor units than is usual for a given muscle. Electrically this produces a full interference pattern with motor unit action potentials that are polyphasic but of low amplitude (Fig. 5.8).

Needle electromyography is very successful in demonstrating denervation and spontaneous potentials and myopathic potentials in muscular dystrophies. It is also very helpful in structural myopathies where the motor unit architecture is disturbed but in many of the metabolic myopathies motor unit action potentials may be within normal limits.

Nerve conduction studies

Nerve conduction studies are normally carried out on patients with suspected peripheral nerve disease. They are useful in confirming the presence of a generalized peripheral neuropathy and may indicate the nature of the underlying pathology. In mononeuropathies they may indicate the site of entrapment or other focal pathology. Nerve conduction studies also provide a quantitative assessment of nerve function that may be useful in following the course of a disease or in assessing the response to therapy.

Motor nerve conduction studies

Motor nerve conduction studies are usually performed by recording EMG activity with surface electrodes over the belly of a muscle. A compound muscle action potential (CMAP) is recorded after electrical stimulation of the motor nerve through surface electrodes applied to the skin. After the signal has been amplified and displayed on the oscilloscope the delay (latency) between the time the stimulus was delivered and the time at which the onset of the CMAP is observed can be measured. This measurement is the *distal motor latency*. If the same nerve is stimulated again at a more proximal point, the distance between the two stimulus sites can be divided by the difference in latency for the two responses to give a conduction velocity in m/s. This conduction velocity is a measure of conduction in the fastest conducting fibres in the nerve (Fig. 23.4), that are large in diameter and well myelinated. It should be noted that conventional nerve conduction studies do not assess the function of small myelinated and unmyelinated fibres. In normal adults the velocity in the fastest conducting motor fibres of the major upper limb nerves in the forearm is approximately 50–65 m/s and is somewhat less, in the range of 40–50 m/s, in the nerves of the lower limbs.

Because nerve fibres are greater in diameter proximally than distally, conduction velocities are a little greater in proximal than distal nerve segments. In full-term newborn infants the motor conduction velocity is approximately one half that of adult values and increases with age to approach adult values at about 3–5 years. Nerve conduction velocity is also temperature dependent and this again contributes to lower velocities in the distal portions of nerves. Nerve conduction velocity in a nerve increases at about 1.9 m/s per °C over the physiological

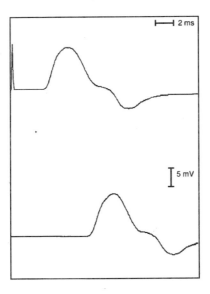

Fig. 23.4 Compound muscle action potentials recorded from abductor pollicis brevis while stimulating the median nerve at the wrist (top) and elbow (bottom). The latency to the onset of the response at the wrist is 3.6 ms and at the elbow 8.2 ms so that the conduction time from wrist to elbow is 8.2 − 3.6 = 4.6 ms. The distance between the stimulating sites is 260 mm. The motor conduction velocity in the forearm is 260/4.6 = 57 m/s.

range. For this reason it is important to maintain careful control of limb temperature during nerve conduction studies.

Areas of localized pressure to nerves produce focal demyelination with
marked delay in conduction at the site of pressure. The resulting focal slowing is
very useful in localizing common entrapment neuropathies such as those of the
median nerve at the wrist (carpal tunnel syndrome) and the ulnar nerve across the
elbow.

Sensory nerve conduction studies

Sensory nerve action potentials (SNAP) may be recorded from surface electrodes
over mixed or sensory nerves following stimulation of distal sensory fibres. The
median and ulnar nerves in the hand are commonly assessed by stimulating
electrically the index or little fingers, respectively, with ring electrodes (Fig. 23.5)
and recording the signals over the nerves at the wrist. The sural nerve action

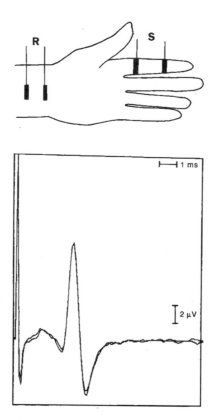

Fig 23.5 Top: Technique for recording the median sensory nerve action potential. The
digital nerves are stimulated with ring electrodes on the fingers (S) while the potential is
recorded with surface electrodes at the wrist (R). Bottom: Median sensory nerve action
potential recorded with the method shown in (A). Note the initial stimulus artefact and
the triphasic waveform typical of sensory nerve action potentials.

potential is usually recorded in the lower limbs. Sensory nerve action potentials are of very small amplitude (10–20 μV) compared with compound muscle action potentials (2–20 mV). For this reason, sensory nerve conduction studies are more technically demanding than motor nerve conduction studies.

Mixed nerve conduction studies

It is also possible to record conduction velocities in mixed nerves such as the median, ulnar and common peroneal nerves stimulating and recording from the nerve trunk directly with surface electrodes. Such potentials may be recorded from nerve trunks. Since the largest diameter fibres in mixed nerves are afferent, the conduction velocity recorded is in afferent rather than motor fibres. Abnormalities of latency, amplitude and conduction velocity of sensory and mixed nerve action potentials are usually a more sensitive index of a presence of the neuropathy than changes in the motor conduction velocities.

Pathological correlates

Wallerian degeneration   Nerve fibres continue to conduct impulses at normal or near normal conduction velocities until conduction ceases altogether at 1–4 days following transection of the nerve when the nerve fibres become totally inexcitable. Conduction may be restored following nerve fibre regeneration but conduction velocities rarely attain their previous values.

Axonal degeneration   Conduction fails over the distal degenerating part of the axon in the same way that it does in Wallerian degeneration but the intact proximal segments conduct with normal conduction velocities. Conduction velocities remain normal in individual fibres until conduction fails completely. Since clinical neurophysiological techniques measure conduction in the fastest conducting fibres, velocities are slightly reduced (usually by less than 20–30%) due to failure of conduction in large fibres. The measured conduction velocity is in the normally conducting, unaffected smaller diameter fibres. The amplitude of the CMAP will be smaller than normal because fewer motor units are activated by the stimulus.

Segmental demyelination   There are two major physiological consequences of demyelination, conduction block and slowing of conduction. Conduction block is the complete failure of nerve fibres to transmit electrical impulses across a demyelinated segment; it may be seen following nerve compression e.g. after prolonged application of a tourniquet or pneumatic cuff and in inflammatory neuropathies (e.g. Guillain-Barré syndrome and chronic inflammatory demyelinating polyneuropathy (CIDP)). It is assessed by attenuation of the compound muscle action potential when the stimulus is moved from a distal to a proximal site. Greater than 30% reduction between two sites is generally regarded as good evidence of failure of conduction in at least some nerve fibres.

Slowing of conduction is usually quite marked across demyelinated or remyelinating segments of nerve and distal latencies may be disproportionately prolonged. In normal myelinated fibres the impulses conduct rapidly from one node of Ranvier to the next by saltatory conduction, but, in demyelinated nerve fibres either conduction becomes continuous across the demyelinated segments as it is in unmyelinated fibres, or conduction time between nodes is delayed. Temporal dispersion of the action potential is a feature of the slowed conduction in demyelination and remyelination. Other abnormalities of conduction that occur in demyelinated fibres are impairment of the ability to transmit faithfully rapid trains of impulses, increased sensitivity to mechanical stimulation, generation of spontaneous impulses from the demyelinated zones and an increased susceptibility to changes in temperature.

Late waves

The *H-reflex* (named after Hoffman who described it) is a monosynaptic reflex recorded from a muscle following low intensity electrical stimulation of its motor nerve supply. It is usually recorded from the calf muscles after stimulation of the medial popliteal (posterior tibial) nerve. This small stimulus selectively activates the largest fibres in the nerve, the Ia fibres originating from the muscle spindles. The H-reflex is the electrical counterpart of a deep tendon reflex, except that the muscle spindle apparatus has been bypassed. The H-reflex provides a means of quantitating reflex changes. It is decreased or absent in most peripheral neuropathies and increased in upper motor neurone disorders.

F-waves are late responses following the initial direct muscle action potential (M-wave) after the application of a supramaximal stimulus to a motor nerve. They are caused by backfiring of some motor neurones in response to antidromic stimulation. The latency of the F-wave is a measure of the time of conduction in motor fibres from the site of stimulation to the motor neurone and then back again to the recording site, and is a useful measure of conduction in the proximal segments of nerves and spinal roots.

Central motor conduction

It is possible to stimulate upper motor neurones in the motor cortex by the application of surface electrodes to the scalp. In order to achieve this, quite high voltages must be used which are painful to the subject. *Cortical magnetic stimulation* is a technique used to stimulate cortical motor neurones by the application of a strong, rapidly changing magnetic field which causes minimal discomfort to the subject. After stimulation of the cortex through the scalp a small CMAP is recorded from the relevant muscle group, usually in the hands or feet. The CMAP produced are always significantly smaller than those produced by stimulation of peripheral nerves, but can be increased considerably by having the subject make a low level voluntary contraction of the muscle at the time of stimulation. The latency from the stimulus to onset of the CMAP represents the conduction time in both the central motor pathways and the peripheral motor nerves. The peripheral conduction time can be calculated either by stimulating the spinal cord with an electric or magnetic stimulus, or by recording F-wave latencies thus enabling calculation of a *central motor conduction time*. This is useful in assessing central motor pathways in central nervous system diseases (e.g. multiple sclerosis, motor neurone disease and cerebrovascular disease). It can be used to demonstrate intact motor pathways in patients suspected of having weakness due to psychiatric disorders such as hysteria, conversion reactions and malingering.

Electroencephalography

The electroencephalogram (EEG) is a recording, through electrodes attached to the scalp, of the electrical field generated by the neuronal activity of the underlying brain. Electrodes are distributed approximately equidistantly over the surface of the scalp according to an international convention (10–20 System). Potential differences between pairs of electrodes or combinations of electrodes can then be displayed either on a paper trace or on an oscilloscope screen.

Normal EEG rhythms, which usually have an amplitude of 50–200 µV, are designated according to their primary frequency. The *alpha* rhythm (8–13 Hz) is recorded over the occipital region when eyes are closed and is attenuated by opening the eyes or by mental activity. The occipital alpha rhythm depends upon synchronous discharge of cells in the visual cortex. *Beta* activity (14–22 Hz) is maximal over the sensorimotor area and is diminished by hand clenching. *Theta* activity (4–7 Hz) is prominent in children, gradually diminishing during adolescence. *Delta* activity (1–3 Hz) is a normal finding only in early childhood. Occasionally other normal variants may be seen: the *mu* rhythm is of alpha frequency but has a characteristic appearance like the top of a picket fence or the Greek letter µ and is distributed asymmetrically in the central regions. *Lambda* waves are generated in the occipital region by saccadic eye movements when the eyes are open.

The most common abnormal EEG patterns are:
- Generalized slow wave activity, encountered in coma and any diffuse cerebral disorder such as a metabolic disturbance
- Localized slow wave activity, recorded over the site of any focal lesion such as an infarct, abscess, herpes simplex encephalitis or tumour
- Localized spike discharges or sharp waves that indicate a potentially epileptogenic focus (Fig. 23.6)
- Generalized spike-wave discharges which are called 'typical' if they are well-formed at 3 Hz and atypical if they are of higher or lower frequency or if their pattern includes multiple spikes (polyspike-wave complexes; Fig. 23.7). Such patterns are commonly associated with epilepsy (Chapter 12)
- Episodic discharges may recur regularly in certain pancortical diseases such as subacute sclerosing panencephalitis (SSPE), Creutzfeldt-Jakob disease and metabolic encephalopathies

The resting pattern of the EEG is recorded for several minutes. Following this, the patient is asked to hyperventilate for 2–3 minutes because the resulting hypocapnia induces vasoconstriction. This brings out slow rhythms and may delineate a focal abnormality that previously escaped notice, or it may induce a paroxysm of spike-wave activity. At the conclusion of the record, the patient is exposed to a stroboscopic light flashing at varying frequencies to provoke seizure patterns in susceptible patients. Other techniques used to identify epileptic foci are *sleep recordings*, which may reveal abnormalities not evident when the subject is

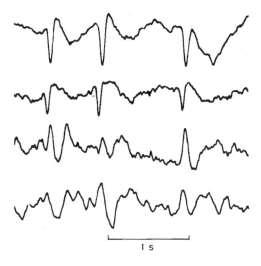

Fig 23.6 Electroencephalogram showing sharp-waves over an epileptogenic focus.

awake, and prolonged (6–8 h) *telemetric recordings.* There is considerable variation in the normal EEG and minor deviations can be erroneously designated as abnormal or, even worse, as indicative of epilepsy or other cerebral disorders.

The EEG is very useful for the accurate diagnosis of epilepsy and, if seizure activity occurs during the recording, it is diagnostic. It is of some assistance in determining the nature of some pancortical disturbances such as SSPE or Creutzfeldt-Jakob disease. It can confirm the clinical localization of some cerebral

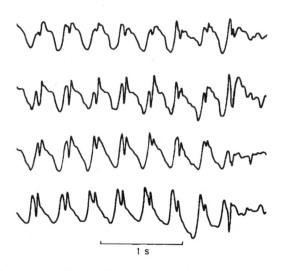

Fig 23.7 Electroencephalogram showing typical 3 Hz spike and wave activity.

lesions but imaging techniques do this much more effectively. An EEG should never be requested without a clear idea of the question it is required to answer.

Cerebral evoked responses

It was noted by early workers performing EEG that in response to stroboscopic stimulation, time-locked waves could be seen in the occipital region. These waves are difficult to detect because they are much smaller in amplitude than the background EEG signal. By averaging the EEG signal recorded after a series of stimuli it is possible to eliminate the background random EEG activity and enhance the time-locked, event-related activity. The resulting signal is called a sensory evoked potential or *event related potential* and is useful in examining central nervous system sensory pathways. Three types of sensory evoked potential are commonly performed.

Visual evoked responses (VER)

Because the original flash-evoked response was found to be rather insensitive, modern VER testing is done with a black and white checker board pattern. This alternates from second to second so that each area of the retina that was previously dark becomes light and vice versa but the overall luminance of the whole retina does not change. This produces a characteristic waveform over the occipital region of the head (Fig. 23.8). This waveform is dependent on synchronous conduction in the optic pathways and is a sensitive test for the presence of demyelinating disease in the optic nerves, tracts or radiations.

Brain-stem auditory evoked response (BAER)

A series of pure tones is applied to the ear while electrical activity is recorded over the mastoid process or earlobe. A characteristic waveform (Fig. 23.9) with five identifiable peaks is produced. The first peak (wave I) is produced in the cochlea and the last (wave V) is produced in the inferior colliculus. Brain-stem auditory evoked responses are much less sensitive in detecting demyelination than VER as they examine a relatively short segment of central pathways. They do, however, provide a useful means of assessing cochlear and auditory nerve function. They are a particularly sensitive method of detecting the presence of acoustic neuromas and are useful in assessing brain-stem function in patients who are suspected of having pontine damage.

Somatosensory evoked response (SSER)

The SSER is measured by applying electrical stimuli to sensory or mixed peripheral nerves while recording from sites over the spinal cord, brain-stem and scalp. Characteristic waveforms are produced from each of these locations (Fig. 23.10). The SSER tests the integrity of large sensory fibres and their central pathways through the dorsal columns, medial lemniscus and thalamus to the cortex. The SSER is almost as sensitive as the VER in detecting central demyelination and is a useful test for examining patients with suspected multiple sclerosis. Somatosensory

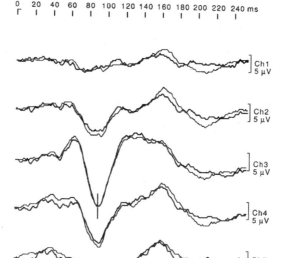

Fig 23.8 Visual evoked potential (VER): The patient is watching an alternating chequerboard pattern. The signals have been recorded from a line of electrodes across the back of the skull overlying the visual cortex. The middle trace is in the mid-line above the inion. Each trace is the average of the response to 1000 consecutive stimuli. The averaged responses are overlaid to show reproducibility. The major downgoing peak P100 (marked with a cursor) occurs 91 ms after the stimulus in this subject.

evoked responses are the most time-consuming and technically difficult of the evoked responses to record and are best ordered from laboratories who perform them frequently. Somatosensory evoked potentials are occasionally used during spinal procedures to demonstrate the continued integrity of spinal cord function during operations to correct kyphoscoliosis. The slow conduction velocity of small fibres leads to temporal dispersion of their afferent volley so that they do not contribute to the SSER, which may thus be normal in spite of a lesion in the spino-thalamic tracts.

LUMBAR PUNCTURE

Because the spinal cord normally ends at about the level of the first lumbar vertebra, a needle can be inserted into the spinal subarachnoid space below this level without fear of cord injury.

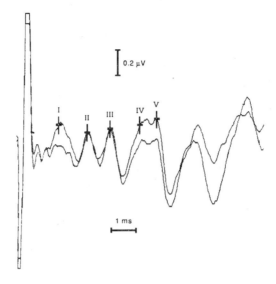

Fig. 23.9 Brain-stem auditory evoked potential (BAEP). The patient is listening to a series of clicks and the signals have been recorded from an electrode over the mastoid process. Wave I is generated by the cochlear nerve (cranial nerve VIII) adjacent to the cochlea. Waves II and III are generated by the cochlear nucleus and the superior olivary nucleus, respectively. The wave IV/V complex is probably generated in the lateral lemniscus.

Indications

Diagnosis of diseases The main value of CSF examination is to diagnose meningeal inflammation (Chapter 16) or bleeding (Chapter 13) into the subarachnoid space. Although changes in the CSF occur in other diseases (e.g. tumours and vascular disease) the changes are often non-specific and a diagnosis can often be reached with more accuracy and safety by other means.

Introducing agents into the subarachnoid space Lumbar puncture is used to introduce therapeutic agents or local anaesthetics into the subarachnoid space. Diagnostic agents can also be introduced in this way, e.g. contrast media such as metrizamide for myelography and CT scanning, radio-isotopes for ventriculo-cisternography, and air for pneumoencephalography.

Measurement of CSF pressure This should rarely be the sole indication for lumbar puncture, except in neurosurgical hands (see contra-indications below). However, the CSF pressure must always be measured whenever a lumbar puncture is performed.

Therapy Regular lumbar puncture has been employed as a means of reducing CSF pressure in benign intracranial hypertension.

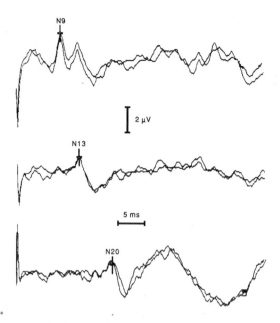

Fig. 23.10 Somatory evoked potential (SER): The stimulus is an electric shock applied to the median nerve at the wrist. The top trace has been recorded from an electrode at Erb's point and the N9 potential represents the nerve action potential traversing the brachial plexus. The middle recording is from an electrode over the cervical spine and the N13 potential arises from the sensory relay in the dorsal column nuclei. The bottom trace has been recorded from a scalp electrode overlying the sensory cortex and the N20 potential probably arises from this region.

Contra-indications

The presence of papilloedema is an absolute contra-indication to lumbar puncture until a CT scan has excluded a space-occupying lesion, and suspicion of raised intracranial pressure is a relative contra-indication to the procedure. Thus, a lumbar puncture should not be done primarily to see if the pressure is raised. The danger of lumbar puncture in the presence of raised intracranial pressure is that withdrawal of fluid may cause herniation of the medulla through the foramen magnum (coning), leading to medullary compression and death. In supratentorial space-occupying lesions, herniation of the medial temporal lobe may occur through the tentorial opening which results in compression of the mid-brain and possible death (uncal herniation; Chapter 14). The mortality of lumbar puncture in cases of cerebral abscess is appreciable.

Infection of the skin in the lumbar region near the site of puncture is also a contra-indication.

Complications

- Headache, caused by reduced pressure. Treatment involves the patient lying flat with the foot of the bed elevated and drinking copious fluids
- Pressure coning as discussed above
- Damage of a spinal root, which is usually caused by placing the needle too far laterally
- Infection. When usual sterile precautions are taken, this is very uncommon.
- Transient back stiffness

Abnormalities of CSF

Naked eye appearance

CSF is normally clear and colourless.

Turbidity This is due to excessive numbers of cells, usually polymorphs, e.g. meningitis.

Blood Presence of blood may be due to either traumatic tap or subarachnoid haemorrhage. In a traumatic tap the CSF is most heavily stained at the beginning and then usually clears gradually. In a subarachnoid bleed it remains evenly blood-stained. If the CSF is collected in three separate tubes in a traumatic tap, the fluid usually appears clearer in the third tube than in the first ('the three tube test').

Xanthochromia The presence or absence of xanthochromia (yellow colouration) after the fluid has been centrifuged is the most valuable method of distinguishing a subarachnoid bleed from a traumatic tap. Xanthochromia appears about 4 hours after a subarachnoid bleed, reaches a maximum after about 36 hours and gradually disappears over 7–10 days. It is due to the presence of oxyhaemoglobin, bilirubin and methaemoglobin.

Cells

The cell count normally does not exceed 4×10^6 cells/L, all mononuclear.

Polymorphs Polymorphs usually indicate an acute inflammation, e.g. acute bacterial or viral meningitis. However, they may also appear after chemical irritation (e.g. myelography, air encephalography) or with trauma, haemorrhage or infarction.

Mononuclear cells Mononuclear cells are increased in chronic inflammations such as tuberculous, fungal, and carcinomatous meningitides and in viral infections, demyelination, cerebral infarction and some other conditions.

Protein

A mild or moderate rise in protein up to about 0.8 g/L is common but non-specific since it occurs in many disease states. High protein levels (over 1.0 g/L) are seen most commonly in spinal cord tumour causing obstruction of the subarachnoid space, meningitis, haemorrhage, demyelinating polyneuritis and some brain tumours.

Immunoglobulins

The CSF immunoglobulin G (IgG) is normally between 5 and 12% of the total CSF protein. It is increased in a number of conditions, but has particular diagnostic value in multiple sclerosis. In clinically definite multiple sclerosis it is raised in about 80–90% of cases. The ratio of IgG to albumin in the CSF can be measured and is usually less than 25%. Discrete oligoclonal bands of IgG may be demonstrated on electrophoresis in about 90% of patients with clinically definite multiple sclerosis.

Glucose

Glucose content is very low or absent in pyogenic meningitis and moderately low in chronic meningitides (e.g. tuberculous, fungal, carcinomatous). The level is high in diabetes mellitus, paralleling the blood glucose. When an abnormality in CSF glucose is suspected it should be compared with a blood glucose level taken simultaneously with the CSF; it is normally 60–80% of the blood glucose level.

Serological tests for syphilis

The most commonly employed screening tests are the Reiter protein reagin (RPR) and treponema pallidum haemagglutination (TPHA) tests. Positive serological tests in the CSF are virtually diagnostic of neurosyphilis, although false positives may occur if there is a 'bloody tap'. The tests may remain positive when disease is inactive.

BIOPSIES

Muscle

Muscle biopsies are necessary for the diagnosis of most forms of muscle disease. Electromyography and nerve conduction studies can usually distinguish between primary muscle disease (myopathies) and neurogenic causes of muscle atrophy (anterior horn cell, spinal root and peripheral nerve disorders); however muscle biopsies are necessary to diagnose many of the specific causes of primary muscle disease (polymyositis, mitochondrial myopathy, muscular dystrophies and congenital myopathies with specific pathology). Needle biopsy can be performed as an outpatient procedure but only a small sample of muscle is obtained. Open biopsy is necessary to obtain larger samples of muscles. The selection of the appropriate muscle to biopsy is important; a weak muscle should be selected but not one so severely affected that all the muscle has been replaced by connective tissue. Histochemical staining with ATPase, succinic dehydrogenase and other stains will differentiate the type 1 (slow contracting, aerobic metabolism) from the type 2 (fast contracting anaerobic metabolism) fibres. Specific patterns of degeneration distinguish primary muscle disease from neurogenic causes. Electron microscopy may provide additional information in some cases.

Nerve biopsy

Nerve biopsy is performed in selected patients with peripheral neuropathy where the cause is uncertain. With appropriate staining and quantitative techniques, specific patterns of nerve fibre degeneration can be distinguished. Nerve biopsy is necessary for diagnosis in most cases of vasculitis, amyloid, leprosy, and many hereditary and inflammatory neuropathies. The sural nerve is usually biopsied at the ankle under local anaesthetic.

Brain and meninges

There are very few indications for brain biopsies except in the case of cerebral tumours. Rarely it is necessary to biopsy the brain or meninges to establish potentially treatable causes of encephalitis or chronic meningitis, respectively. Cerebral arteritis, a rare condition, which may respond to treatment with cortico-steroids and immunosuppressive agents, may require brain biopsy for diagnosis.

Blood vessels

Temporal artery biopsy is usually necessary for the diagnosis of temporal arteritis.

Skin biopsy

Skin biopsy may help establish the diagnosis of some rare hereditary and metabolic disorders.

MOLECULAR GENETIC TECHNIQUES

Molecular genetic techniques, using DNA analysis, have greatly improved the accuracy of diagnosis of many hereditary diseases and the ability to provide informed genetic counselling. In disorders where the gene has been isolated, it may be detected by DNA analysis of blood samples from affected individuals. Diseases which may be diagnosed in this way include Duchenne muscular dystrophy, Charcot-Marie-Tooth disease Type 1 (HMSN Ia), facio-scapulo humeral muscular dystrophy, dystrophia myotonica, neurofibromatosis type I (NF1), and mitochondrial diseases such as Leber's optic atrophy and mitochondrial myopathy.

In conditions where the gene has not been identified but the chromosomal location is known (e.g. Friedreich's ataxia), linkage analysis is necessary which involves testing DNA in blood samples from as many family members as possible, unaffected and affected. Diseases which fall into the category include Huntington's disease and Friedreich's ataxia.

24 | Treatment of neurological disorders

There is much more to treatment than the prescription of medication. Treatment starts from the moment patients recognize that you are taking their problem seriously and doing your best to find the cause. Sometimes a careful history and physical examination, followed by discussion and reassurance, will be all that is necessary. At all times the patient should be regarded as a partner in the therapeutic process.

Neurosurgery plays an important role in the management of neurological disorders but it is unfortunately beyond the scope of the present text to discuss this in any detail. In this Chapter therefore, emphasis will be on the medical rather than the neurosurgical aspects of managing neurological disorders.

MENTAL COMFORT OF THE PATIENT

A medical examination can be an ordeal for some people. They may be afraid of giving silly answers to the doctor's questions, of taking off their clothes, of being prodded in sensitive and vulnerable areas and, when all is done, of being diagnosed as having some unpleasant or incurable disease. Tension is usually eased by a friendly approach and some words of explanation from the doctor as the examination progresses. Any discussion about the nature of the illness or advice about management must be expressed in words that the patient understands. Even intelligent and sophisticated patients may be vague about the location of their internal organs and what they do. Simple sketches may help your patient understand what is going on and what you propose to do about it.

The most important aspect of treatment is often the advice given to the patient; advice about personal relationships, life-style, family affairs, occupation, and personal habits such as diet, exercise, smoking and the consumption of alcohol and drugs. Some conditions such as hyperventilation may be cured completely by explanation alone. Depression is common in neurological disorders, not only as an understandable reaction to disability but often as an integral part of the disorder. Antidepressant medication is then indicated and consultation with a psychiatrist is advisable for those with serious emotional disturbances.

Where should patients be treated? Are they able to continue work, should they rest at home or would they be better off in hospital? In any event, there should be close communication between general practitioner and specialist to ensure continuity of patient care.

In a hospital setting, the patient's well-being depends as much on the nursing and paramedical staff as on medical care. Close and courteous collaboration between doctors and nurses, physiotherapists, occupational therapists, speech pathologists and social workers is essential for the best results.

PHYSICAL COMFORT OF THE PATIENT

As a general rule, the less time anyone with a degenerative neurological disorder spends in bed the better. Prolonged bed-rest will cause a patient with ataxia or Parkinson's disease to become more disabled and will often prolong convalescence. Every person should have the maximum amount of exercise compatible with his or her disability.

Attention to bladder and bowel function and protection of the skin are obvious essentials. Incontinence often results from retention with overflow which requires bladder catheterization or disimpaction of faeces. The doctor should be conversant with the principles of management of respiratory paralysis, coma, and disturbances of fluid balance, electrolytes and nutrition.

Simple physical measures may pay dividends. The elevation of a painful or swollen limb, a cradle to keep the weight of bedclothes off a tender or paralysed limb, a foot-drop support or other measures to prevent overstretching of weakened muscles are simple examples. Extension exercises to strengthen the back muscles are important for the relief and prevention of pain in lumbar disc injuries. Traction, mobilization and some cautious forms of manipulation may be helpful in cervical or lumbar spondylosis. A soft or plastic supportive collar is often used for patients with cervical pain. It is a tautology to say 'cervical collar' since all collars are, by definition, applied to the neck.

Relaxation therapy, with or without biofeedback, is a useful adjuvant to treatment of patients with tension headache and other conditions accompanied by overcontraction of muscles, particularly those of the jaw and face.

Attention should turn to rehabilitation as early as possible. A home visit by a physiotherapist or occupational therapist assists in planning to make the patient's life easier once returned home, by the installation of ramps, railings or other devices to allow disabled persons to function efficiently. All these things seem self-evident but are sometimes neglected. Above all, the aim is to have a happy as well as a healthy person back in the home environment as soon as possible.

MEDICATIONS AND PROCEDURES SHARED WITH OTHER FIELDS OF MEDICINE

The list that follows is a summary, serving to direct attention to the appropriate chapters in this book.

Analgesics, anticoagulants, antibiotics and antiviral agents

Antibiotics and antiviral agents are covered in Chapter 16 while anticoagulants appear in Chapter 13.

Vitamins

Thiamine   Thiamine is used for Wernicke's encephalopathy (Chapter 14) and some cases of peripheral neuropathy (Chapter 10).

Hydroxycobalamin   This forms cyanocobalamin (Vitamin B_{12}) in the body. It is used in tobacco–alcohol amblyopia and Leber's optic atrophy, for mental changes, subacute combined degeneration or peripheral neuropathy caused by defective absorption of Vitamin B_{12}.

Vitamin B_{12}   Cyanocobalamin 1000 µg daily for 5 days, followed by 100 µg weekly then monthly, is the usual regimen for treatment of pernicious anaemia and its associated neurological disorders (Chapters 7, 10).

Vitamin E   Some cases of spinocerebellar degeneration are associated with Vitamin E deficiency.

Folate   Folic acid deficiency may be found in patients on long-term anticonvulsant therapy. A supplement of 0.4–0.8 mg daily is recommended for patients taking anticonvulsants in pregnancy.

Corticosteroids

Cerebral oedema   Extracellular oedema — post-operative or surrounding tumours — responds to high dosage steroids; e.g. dexamethasone, 16–64 mg daily, in divided doses. Intracellular oedema after stroke does not respond to this therapy (Chapter 17).

Temporal arteritis   See Chapter 11.

Brachial radiculitis   Neuralgic amyotrophy.

Acute herpes zoster   Steroids can be given in addition to acyclovir 400–800 mg, five times daily, or by half-hour intravenous infusions of 10 mg/kg solution, at eight hourly intervals (Chapter 16).

Polymyositis   See Chapter 10.

Tuberculous meningitis   When CSF protein is high corticosteroids are sometimes administered in association with antituberculous therapy (Chapter 16).

Myasthenia gravis   In resistant cases (Chapter 10).

Relapse of multiple sclerosis   Pulsed methylprednisolone, 0.5–1.0 g given by intravenous infusion daily for 3–5 days, has been shown to hasten recovery from a relapse. Oral steroids or the intramuscular injection of adrenocorticotropic hormone, are also useful in the management of an acute relapse of multiple sclerosis (Chapter 20).

Bell's palsy   The value of steroids in the acute phase of Bell's palsy remains controversial. The rationale is to reduce oedema of the facial nerve in the styloid canal.

Chronic inflammatory demyelinating polyradiculoneuropathy   See Chapter 10.

Cerebral vasculitis   Vasculitis and other connective tissue diseases (Chapter 10).

Immunosuppressant agents

Used in polyarteritis nodosa, systemic lupus erythematosus and other connective tissue diseases, and in some cases of polymyositis, chronic demyelinating polyradiculoneuropathy, and myasthenia gravis (Chapter 10).

Plasmapheresis (plasma exchange)

Guillain-Barré syndrome   Plasma exchange is useful when used within 10 days of onset if the disease is progressive and severe (Chapter 10).

Myasthenic crisis   See Chapter 10.

Some cases of chronic inflammatory demyelinating polyradiculoneuropathy   See Chapter 10.

Intravenous immunoglobulin infusion

These are effective in conditions that respond to plasmapheresis — Guillain-Barré syndrome, chronic inflammatory demyelinating polyneuropathy, myasthenia gravis (Chapter 10).

MEDICATIONS AND PROCEDURES USED CHIEFLY IN NEUROLOGY

Note that medication should be started with a low dose to minimize the possibility of side effects.

Pain syndromes

Lightning (stabbing) pains   (e.g. trigeminal neuralgia)
- Carbamazepine (Tegretol), 100–400 mg three times daily
- Baclofen (Lioresal), 10–20 mg three times daily

Constant (burning or pressing) pains   (e.g. post-herpetic neuralgia, chronic daily headaches)
- Amitriptyline (Tryptanol), 10–150 mg *nocte*. Note that the blood levels of amitriptyline may vary ten-fold with the same dose per kg bodyweight in

different patients so that dosage must be increased slowly and adjusted for the tolerance of the individual.

Intractable pains

- Psychological management
- Transcutaneous electrical stimulation (TENS)
- Acupuncture
- Analgesics
- Epidural or intrathecal morphine in selected cases
- Surgical procedures in selected cases

Episodic headache

See Chapter 11.

Acute migraine requires the early administration of one or more of the following:
- Metoclopramide (Maxolon), 10 mg i.v., i.m. or orally; aspirin, 600 mg; ergotamine tartrate, 1–2 mg orally, rectally or by inhalation
- Sumatriptan (Imigran) 100 mg orally or 6 mg, s.c.
- Dihydroergotamine, 1.0 mg, i.m., 8-hourly
- Naproxen, 500 mg, ibuprofen 400 mg

Prophylactic (interval) therapy involves:
- Beta-blockers, e.g. non-selective: propranolol (Inderal), 40–120 mg twice a day; timolol (Blocadren), 5 mg two or three times daily; or selective beta$_1$- blockers: atenolol (Tenormin), 50–100 mg daily; metoprolol (Betaloc, Lopresor), 50–100 mg daily
- Pizotifen (Sandomigran), 0.5 mg, 2–6 tablets *nocte*
- Naproxen, 250 mg, one or two tablets twice daily
- Calcium channel-blocking agents (Chapter 11)
- Methysergide (Deseril), 1–2 mg three times daily
- Amitriptyline (Tryptanol) 10–75 mg at night
- For resistant cases, the monoamine oxidase (MAO) inhibitor phenelzine (Nardil) 15 mg two or three times daily, may be used with due precautions

Cluster headache

Episodic
- Ergotamine tartrate, 2 mg *nocte* (for nocturnal cluster pain)
- Methysergide (Deseril), 2 mg three times daily
- Prednisone, 50 mg daily, with reducing dosage (Chapter 11)
- Oxygen inhalation (for acute attack)

Chronic
- Lithium carbonate, 250 mg, two or three times daily with monitoring of blood levels
- Calcium channel-blockers
- Surgical procedures (rarely)

Chronic paroxysmal hemicrania (CPH)

- Indomethacin (Indocid) 25 mg three times daily

Epilepsy

See Chapter 12.

Partial (focal) and generalized (tonic–clonic, grand mal) seizures

- Carbamazepine (Tegretol), 100 mg and 200 mg tablets, syrup (100 mg/5 mL). Usual dose adult: 100–400 mg three times daily; children 15–20 mg/kg per day. Dosage to achieve blood levels 20–50 µmol/L, i.e. 3–8 µg/mL
- Phenytoin (Dilantin) 50 mg tablets, 30 mg/5 mL suspension, capsules of 30 mg or 100 mg. Usual dose 100–200 mg twice daily: 6 mg/kg per day for adults and 5–10 mg/kg per day for children. The required blood levels are 40–80 µmol/L, i.e. 10–20 µg/mL
- Sodium valproate (Epilim) 100 mg, 200 mg and 500 mg (enteric coated tablets); 200 mg/5 mL liquid or syrup. Usual dose 200–500 mg, three times daily. The blood levels are irrelevant.
- Barbiturates: Phenobarbitone, 30 mg tablets. Usual dose: 30–90 mg twice daily. Methylphenobarbitone (Prominal), 30 mg, 60 mg and 200 mg tablets. Usual dose: 60–200 mg twice daily. Primidone (Mysoline), 250 mg tablets. Usual dose: 250–500 mg twice daily. Blood levels are of little help in assessing efficacy
- Benzodiazepines: Clonazepam (Rivotril), 0.5 mg and 2 mg tablets; drops, 2.5 mg in 1 mL. Usual dose is 0.5–2.0 mg two or three times daily. Clobazam (Frisium), 10 mg tablets. Usual dose 10 mg two or three times daily as add-on therapy. Blood levels are unnecessary
- Vigabatrin (Sabril) 500 mg, increasing to 2–4 g daily
- Lamotrigine (Lamictal) 25 mg, 50 mg, 100 mg, increasing to 50–200 mg twice daily
- GABApentin (Neurontin) 300 mg, 400 mg capsules, increasing to 1200–2400 mg/day

Minor generalized seizures (petit mal absences)

- Sodium valproate, as above
- Clonazepam, as above
- Ethosuximide (Zarontin), 250 mg capsules; syrup, 250 mg in 5 mL. Blood levels are unnecessary

Myoclonus

- Sodium valproate, as above
- Clonazepam, as above
- Serotonin precursors may be used for post-hypoxic myoclonus or progressive myoclonic epilepsy

Status epilepticus
- Clonazepam, 1 mg in 2 mL bolus or continuous i.v. infusion
- Diazepam, 10 mg in 2 mL bolus or continuous i.v. infusion
- Phenobarbitone sodium, 200 mg in 1 mL, i.m.
- Phenytoin (Dilantin), 100 mg in 2 mL, or 250 mg in 5 mL, i.v., a loading dose of 15–18 mg/kg infused over 1 hour. Phenytoin should never be given i.m.
- Thiopentone (Pentothal), i.v., in resistant cases

Narcolepsy

Special authority is usually required to prescribe these stimulant drugs:
- Methylphenidate (Ritalin), 10 mg two or three times daily
- Dexamphetamine (Dexedrine), 5 mg, 1–2 tablets two or three times daily
- Amphetamine (Benzedrine), 5 mg, 1–2 tablets two or three times daily

Cataplexy
- Imipramine (Tofranil), 25 mg three times daily

Tremor
See Chapter 15.

Essential tremor, action tremor
Alcohol is helpful in socially acceptable amounts and no treatment is required in most cases. If treatment is required then the following are employed:
- Propranolol, 40–120 mg two or three times daily
- Primidone, 250 mg, 0.5–2 tablets twice daily
- Diazepam, 5 mg, 1–2 tablets three times daily

Resting tremor of Parkinson's disease (see below)
- Stereotactic thalamotomy for unilateral tremor in some cases

Rubral (red nucleus, 'wing-beating') tremor, intention tremor and hemiballismus
- Clonazepam, 0.5–2.0 mg two or three times daily
- Thioridazine (Melleril), 10 mg and 25 mg tablets, dosage 10–50 mg two or three times daily
- Stereotactic thalamotomy in some cases

Parkinson's disease
See Chapter 15.

Anticholinergic agents

May be useful for the control of resting (alternating) tremor. Start with very small doses in the elderly, as these drugs may cause confusional states. Most commonly used is:

- Benzhexol (Artane), tablets of 2 mg and 5 mg. Usual dose, 1–5 mg three times daily

Dopamine-releasing agents

- Amantadine, 100 mg capsules. Usual dose, 100 mg morning and at mid-day

Dopamine precursor

Levodopa with decarboxylase inhibitor in one of the two preparations given below. Whichever preparation is used, start with a small dose containing 50–100 mg levodopa and increase the dose slowly to that required to improve performance without inducing involuntary movements or confusion.

- Levodopa with carbidopa tablets in the ratios 100 mg : 10 mg, 100 mg : 25 mg and 250 mg : 25 mg (Sinemet)
- Levodopa with benserazide, 200 mg : 50 mg tablets or capsules in the ratios 50 mg : 12.5 mg, 100 mg : 25 mg, 200 mg : 50 mg (Madopar)

Dopamine agonists

- Bromocriptine (Parlodel), 2.5 mg tablets, or capsules of 5 mg and 10 mg. Used as adjuvant therapy with levodopa or as the primary agent in some cases. Start with low doses and increase slowly to avoid side effects (Chapter 15)

Monoamine oxidase B (MAO B) inhibitor

Used to prolong the life and action of dopamine.

- Selegiline (Deprenyl) inhibits MAO B. 5 mg tablets. Added to levodopa therapy in resistant cases, 5–10 mg daily.

  Since deprenyl has little effect on MAO A, there is no need for the restriction on diet and drugs essential for patients on MAO A inhibitors. At present, in Australia, selegiline is available for use only in patients not adequately controlled by levodopa preparations.

Choreoathetosis (including tardive dyskinesia)

See Chapter 15.

- Diazepam (Valium), 2 mg, 5 mg and 10 mg tablets. Usual dose 2–10 mg three times daily
- Clonazepam (Rivotril), 0.5 mg and 2 mg tablets. Usual dose 0.5–2.0 mg twice daily
- Thioridazine (Melleril), 10 mg and 25 mg tablets. Usual dose 10–50 mg two or three times daily
- Tetrabenazine (Nitoman), 25 mg tablets. Use is restricted to severe cases, e.g. Huntington's chorea. One tablet two or three times daily

Dystonia

See Chapter 15.

- Benztropine (Cogentin), 2 mg tablets. Usual dose 2–4 mg twice daily. An injectable form (2 mg in 2 mL) is available for i.v. use in acute dystonia, e.g. following the use of phenothiazine drugs
- Benzhexol (Artane), 2 mg and 5 mg tablets. Dosage 5–10 mg three times daily. Higher doses have been used in young patients with success
- Drugs listed above for use in choreoathetosis

Gilles de la Tourette syndrome

See Chapter 15.

- Clonidine (Catapres), tablets of 100 µg and 150 µg. Usual dose one tablet three times daily
- Haloperidol (Serenace, Pacedol, Haldol), tablets of 0.5 mg, 1.5 mg and 5 mg. Usual dose: 1.5–5 mg three times daily
- Pimozide (Orap), 2 mg tablets. Usual dose 2 mg two or three times daily

Spasticity and flexor spasms

- Baclofen (Lioresal), 10 mg and 25 mg tablets. Usual dose:10–25 mg three times daily
- Diazepam (Valium), 2 mg, 5 mg and 10 mg tablets. Usual dose 5–10 mg three times daily

Multiple sclerosis

See Chapter 20.

Acute relapse

- Methylprednisolone, 1000 mg, i.v., infused over 1–2 hours daily for 3 days, or 500 g daily for 5 days
- Adrenocorticotropic hormone (ACTH) 40 U IMI, b.d. for week 1, 40 U IMI, b.d. for week 2, 20 U IMI, daily for week 3

Interval therapy

- Beta-interferon has been found to reduce the number of relapses but is not yet generally available

Symptomatic treatment

- Spasticity: baclofen or diazepam, as above
- Fatigue: amantadine (Symmetrel), 100 mg capsules. Dosage one capsule two or three times daily has been recommended but is of doubtful benefit

- Urgency of micturition: propantheline bromide (Pro-Banthine) 15 mg, four times daily; penthienate bromide (Monodral), 5 mg tablets. Usual dose 5 mg three times daily; amitriptyline 25–100 g daily
- Tremor: Clonazepam and other agents as listed under tremor

Cerebral vascular disease

See Chapter 13.

Transient ischaemic attacks

- Aspirin, 50 mg, 100 mg or 300 mg tablets. Enteric-coated tablets containing 650 mg. The dose of 300 mg is of proven efficacy. 100 mg daily may be sufficient
- Ticlopidine 250 mg twice daily has also proved to be of benefit

Cerebral embolism of cardiac origin

- Anticoagulant agents, heparin initially and warfarin for a period of up to six months, are used in conventional doses.

Vertigo

See Chapter 4. Note that the following agents (except urea) may cause acute dystonic reactions requiring intravenous injection of 2 mg benztropine. Long-term use may cause tardive dyskinesia.

- Urea, 30 g orally is the most effective treatment for acute vertigo in Ménière's disease and should be taken at the onset of the attack
- Frusemide (Lasix) 40 mg daily with potassium supplements and low-salt diet is the treatment of choice for interval therapy
- Prochlorperazine (Stemetil), 5 mg tablets or suppositories of 5 mg and 25 mg. Injections of 12.5 mg, i.m. or suppositories given as required for nausea and vomiting associated with acute vertigo. Usual oral dose 5 mg three times daily
- Thiethylperazine (Torecan), 6.5 mg base tablets or suppositories. Injection 6.5 mg base in 1 mL. Injections or suppositories are given as required for nausea and vomiting associated with acute vertigo. Usual oral dose 6.5 mg base three times daily.

Myasthenia gravis

See Chapter 10.

Anticholinesterase agents

- Edrophonium (Tensilon). Injection of 10 mg in 1 mL, diluted to 10 mL in normal saline and injected intravenously, slowly over 2 minutes, as a diagnostic test

- Prostigmine, 15 mg tablets or injections of 1 mg. Usual oral dose 1–2 tablets, 3-hourly
- Pyridostigmine (Mestinon), tablets of 10 mg, 60 mg and 180 mg (sustained release). Usual dose 60 mg, 1–2 tablets, every 4–8 hours

Plasmapheresis or gamma globulin infusions
These may be indicated in severe cases.

Corticosteroids
Corticosteroids are prescribed in some cases after thymectomy or in some patients resistant to other forms of therapy.

Immunosuppressants
Azathioprine, for example, are used in resistant cases.

Guanidine
5–10 mg/kg, three times daily is used for Eaton-Lambert syndrome (myasthenia associated with malignant disease).

Myotonia
See Chapter 10.
- Quinine sulphate, 300 mg tablets. Usual dose one tablet once or twice daily
- Phenytoin (Dilantin), capsules of 100 mg. Usual dose 100 mg three times daily
- Procainamide (Pronestyl) is used for some severe cases but can produce a lupus-like syndrome

Pseudomyotonia, muscle cramps
- Carbamazepine (Tegretol), 100 mg and 200 mg tablets. Usual dose 100–200 mg three times daily
- Quinine sulphate, as above

Index